D0880809

The Scientific Basis
for the Treatment of
Parkinson's Disease

The Scientific Basis for the Treatment of Parkinson's Disease

Edited by C. W. Olanow and A.N. Lieberman

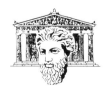

The Parthenon Publishing Group
International Publishers in Medicine, Science & Technology

Casterton Hall, Carnforth,
Lancs, LA6 2LA, UK

120 Mill Road, Park Ridge,
New Jersey 07656, USA

Published in the UK by
The Parthenon Publishing Group Limited
Casterton Hall, Carnforth,
Lancs, LA6 2LA, England

Published in the USA by
The Parthenon Publishing Group Inc.
120 Mill Road,
Park Ridge,
New Jersey 07656, USA

British Library Cataloguing in Publication Data
Scientific Basis for the Treatment of
Parkinson's Disease
I. Olanow, C. W. II. Lieberman, A.
616.8

ISBN 1-85070-355-8

Library of Congress Cataloging-in-Publication Data
The Scientific basis for the treatment of Parkinson's disease / edited
by C.W. Olanow and A. Lieberman.
    p.   cm.
Includes bibliographical references and index.
ISBN 1-85070-355-8 : $68.00
1. Parkinsonism.   I. Olanow, C. W. (Charles Warren), 1941–
II. Lieberman, A. (Abraham). 1938–
[DNLM: 1. Parkinson Disease--therapy.   WL 359 S416]
RC382.S383 1992
616.8'3306--dc20
DNLM/DLC
for Library of Congress   92-11897
                                                                    CIP

First published 1992

Typeset by Lasertext Ltd, Stretford, Manchester
Printed and bound in Great Britain by
Butler and Tanner Ltd., Frome and London

Contents

List of principal contributors

D. B. Calne
Division of Neurology
University Hospital
University of British Columbia
2211 Wesbrook Mall
Vancouver
British Columbia V6T 1W5
Canada

J. M. Cedarbaum
Department of Neurology and
  Neuroscience
Cornell University Medical
  College
New York
USA

S. Fahn
Neurological Institute
710 West 168th Street
New York
NY 10032-3784
USA

C. G. Goetz
Department of Neurological
  Sciences
Rush Presbyterian St Luke's
  Medical Center
1725 West Harrison Street
Chicago
Illinois 60612
USA

R. A. Hauser
Department of Neurology
University of South Florida
4 Columbia Drive 410
Tampa
Florida 33606
USA

J. H. Kordower
Department of Anatomy and
  Cell Biology
University of Illinois School of
  Medicine
808 S. Wood Street
Chicago
Illinois 60612
USA

J.W. Langston
The California Parkinson's
  Foundation
2444 Moorpark Avenue
Suite 316
San Jose
California 95128
USA

A.N. Lieberman
Division of Movement Disorders
Barrow Neurological Institute
Phoenix
Arizona 35013
USA

C.D. Marsden
University Department of
  Clinical Neurology
Institute of Neurology and
  National Hospital for
  Neurology and Neurosurgery
Queen Square
London WC1N 3BG
UK

C.W. Olanow
Movement Disorder Center
University of South Florida
4 Columbia Drive 410
Tampa
Florida 33606
USA

C.W. Shults
Department of Neurosciences
University of California,
  San Diego
Veterans Affairs Medical Center
3350 La Jolla Village Drive
San Diego
California 92161
USA

R.L. Watts
Department of Neurology
Emory University School of
  Medicine
PO Drawer V
Atlanta
Georgia 30322
USA

G.F. Wooten
Department of Neurology
Box 394
University of Virginia Medical
  Center
Charlottesville
Virginia 22908
USA

Foreword

C.W. Olanow

The initiation of levodopa therapy in the late 1960s revolutionized the treatment of Parkinson's disease. Levodopa provided patients with a reduction in morbidity and mortality. Symptomatic therapy with levodopa still remains the mainstay of therapy for Parkinson's disease but it has become clear that chronic treatment is associated with a high incidence of adverse effects and that levodopa does not prevent the chronic progressive neuronal degeneration which continues to occur. Research during the past quarter century has focused on attempts to enhance the symptomatic effects of levodopa and to limit the development of adverse side-effects. Recent advances in neuroscience now permit us to begin to address the critical issues of etiology and pathogenesis, and to formulate a scientific rationale for therapies designed to protect against neuronal progression and to restore functions lost as a consequence of cell degeneration.

The *Scientific Basis for the Treatment of Parkinson's Disease* provides state-of-the-art reviews on these areas with particular emphasis on current thinking regarding molecular biology, oxidative stress, neural transplantation and trophic factors. Reviews are provided regarding the current role of levodopa and dopamine agonists as well as on current information regarding the basis of adverse effects which complicates current therapy. There are, in addition, reviews regarding study design, attempts to develop quantitative scoring systems for evaluating new treatments and our current status with respect to the development of a marker of preclinical parkinsonism which is of particular importance in this era of 'neuroprotection', in which it would obviously be desirable to initiate a protective therapy as early as possible in the disease process.

We have reached a new stage in our approach to Parkinson's disease in which investigators are cautiously optimistic that the coming years will provide exciting therapies that may influence the natural progression of Parkinson's disease and lead to more effective treatment for our patients.

I

Early markers of idiopathic parkinsonism

D.B. Calne and B.J. Snow

INTRODUCTION

Opinions vary on the rate of progression of nigrostriatal decay in idiopathic parkinsonism[1-3] but there is general agreement that compensatory mechanisms prevent clinical expression of the disorder for some time. Substantial reductions of nigral dopaminergic neurons and striatal dopamine concentrations (up to 80%) have been argued to occur before symptoms appear, and the rate of advance of clinical deficits is usually slow. When idiopathic parkinsonism is diagnosed below the age of 40 years, it may run a course of over 30 years[4]. The earliest clinical features of idiopathic parkinsonism are usually subtle and difficult to identify with certainty; many patients cannot provide an exact time of onset of their illness.

Early detection of idiopathic parkinsonism is useful from the viewpoint of advising patients about their future, but the recent claims that deprenyl slows the progression of the underlying pathology[5,6] provide a new justification for attempting to make a diagnosis as soon as possible, perhaps even while the patient is still clinically normal. The combination of early detection and neuroprotective therapy could provide an invaluable addition to conventional treatment.

While the neurological history and examination provide the diagnostic criteria for idiopathic parkinsonism, recent developments in brain imaging and biochemical studies on blood samples are beginning to

3

raise the possibility of establishing the presence of idiopathic parkinsonism before symptoms become manifest. Physiological and pathological tests may extend the potential for screening for early idiopathic parkinsonism.

Tests are still being developed but, ultimately, they will be divisible into three groups:

(1) Those that identify the pathologic processes leading to the neuronal damage;
(2) Those that measure the degree of neuronal damage; and
(3) Those that pinpoint changes secondary to either of the above.

We have techniques that will be useful to classify tests into one of the above categories. Positron emission tomography (PET) is capable of demonstrating dopaminergic lesions in asymptomatic subjects. If a predictive test is negative in such subjects, this would suggest that the test is either insensitive or does not identify the pathological process leading to the dopaminergic lesion but relates, instead, to secondary phenomena that develop after the onset of neuronal damage. Similarly, if a test becomes more abnormal as parkinsonism progresses, then we would suspect that the test might also be measuring secondary phenomena. Finally, a test relating to the causal mechanism of idiopathic parkinsonism should not be positive in other diseases with a dopaminergic deficit such as progressive supranuclear palsy; although such a finding would be in accord with a shared pathogenetic pathway triggered by different etiologic factors.

BRAIN IMAGING

PET scanning

Two models of idiopathic parkinsonism have been studied in an attempt to identify impairment of the nigrostriatal pathway before parkinsonian deficits appear, namely, parkinsonism induced by 1,2,3,6-methylphenyl-tetrahydropyridine (MPTP), and that exhibited in Lytico–Bodig.

MPTP-induced parkinsonism

Intoxication with MPTP is known to produce a permanent parkinsonian syndrome in animals and humans[7,8]. PET with fluorodopa reveals a reduction in striatal uptake in idiopathic parkinsonism and in both humans and cynomolgus monkeys with the clinical features of parkinsonism induced by MPTP. More relevant to the current issue, PET with fluorodopa also displays a decrease in uptake, albeit less severe, in cynomolgus monkeys and humans exposed to MPTP in doses insufficient to result in any parkinsonian deficits[9,10]. These findings may be construed as evidence indicating that PET can detect subclinical impairment of nigrostriatal integrity of a type expected to occur early in the natural history of idiopathic parkinsonism, prior to the expression of clinical features.

Guamanian Lytico–Bodig parkinsonism

The ALS complex of Guam, called Lytico–Bodig by Guamanians, presents with a syndrome resembling idiopathic parkinsonism, ALS or Alzheimer's disease. While Lytico–Bodig may be manifest as either one of these syndromes, it can also exist in any combination. The parkinsonian signs of Lytico–Bodig are clinically indistinguishable from idiopathic parkinsonism, and PET with fluorodopa yields images that are also identical[11]. In the context of the present discussion, it is notable that patients with Lytico–Bodig expressed clinically as a pure ALS syndrome have been shown by PET to have impaired striatal uptake of fluorodopa[11]. This finding buttresses the argument, deriving from subclinical intoxication with MPTP, that nigrostriatal damage can be detected with PET at a stage that is clinically latent.

Magnetic resonance imaging (MRI)

MRI with high field strength allows localization of certain regions of the brain that possess a high concentration of iron. In particular, the substantia nigra, red nucleus and lentiform nuclei are readily discernible[12]. Initial reports indicate that in idiopathic parkinsonism the image of the substantia nigra is blurred, reflecting an increased accumulation of iron. Although this technique has not yet been applied to the specific task of detecting preclinical disturbance of the nigra, MRI is certainly a suitable technology to explore.

ANALYSIS OF BLOOD

Complex I in platelets

Recently, Parker and colleagues[13] have reported a reduction of mito-chondrial Complex I (NADH ubiquinone oxidoreductase) in the blood platelets of patients with idiopathic parkinsonism. This decrease was also noted in Huntington's disease and Leber's disease. Thus while the fall in Complex I was not specific, it may still be a useful marker of idiopathic parkinsonism. The assay of platelet Complex I may even have application as a test for subclinical evaluation. It is relevant to mention that Schapira and colleagues[14], and Mizuno and colleagues[15] have also reported a disorder of Complex I in idiopathic parkinsonism; their observation was based upon postmortem analysis of the substantia nigra. Brain abnormalities of other components of the electron transfer chain have also been recently detected by Riederer and colleagues[16].

The plasma ratio of cysteine/sulfate in plasma

In a recent survey of the plasma biochemistry in Parkinson's disease, Steventon and colleagues reported reduced S-oxidation capacity in patients with idiopathic parkinsonism[17]. The same group have sub-sequently reported an increase in the ratio of cysteine to sulfate in idiopathic parkinsonism, ALS and motoneuron disease[18]. An abnormality in this pathway may impair the body's ability to metabolize environmental toxins. If this finding is confirmed, it offers a further approach to early detection, and it may cast light on the etiology of and interrelationship between these neurodegenerative diseases.

Monoamine oxidase B in platelets

Monoamine oxidase B deaminates endogenous dopamine. This enzyme may contribute to substantia nigra degeneration in two ways. First, the enzyme may activate environmental protoxins, and, second, the oxidation of dopamine may produce increased free radicals which in turn may damage dopamine neurons. There are conflicting reports on monoamine oxidase B activity in idiopathic parkinsonism. When assayed with phenylethylamine, the activity is increased[19,20], but when assayed with dopamine, decreased activity is found[20]. This latter result suggests that the enzyme is not simply overactive and there may be some structural difference in the enzyme in idiopathic parkinsonism. If so, this finding may have relevance to elucidating etiopathogenesis, in addition to early detection.

Free radicals in leukocytes

Polymorphonuclear leukocytes produce free radicals. Recently Kalra and co-workers[21] have studied luminol-dependent chemiluminescence as an index of oxygen free radical production in polymorphonuclear leukocytes from parkinsonian patients and controls. They found a highly significant increase in the generation of oxygen free radicals in idiopathic parkinsonism.

Oxidative indices in serum

Malondialdehyde is a product of tissue injury by lipid peroxidation of membrane phospholipids. In a recent study[22] elevated concentrations of malondialdehyde were detected in the serum of patients with idiopathic parkinsonism. This finding has been claimed to suggest the involvement of oxygen free radicals in the pathogenesis of idiopathic parkinsonism; it also offers another possible approach to early detection.

PHYSIOLOGICAL TESTS

Long latency stretch reflexes

Tatton and Lee first described the large amplitude long latency stretch reflexes found in idiopathic parkinsonism[23]. Their observations were extended by Marsden and colleagues[24] and Evarts and colleagues[25]. Long latency motor responses were initially measured with a torque motor, but they can also be investigated by electrophysiological techniques[26]. Either type of investigation may be applied to the early detection of idiopathic parkinsonism.

Visual dysfunction

Several aspects of visual function appear to be distorted in idiopathic parkinsonism[27]. The latency of the visual evoked potentials is increased. The spatial frequency of stimulation seems to be an important determinant for detecting this disturbance. There is no definite evidence to distinguish between involvement of the dopaminergic retinal components, or abnormality of central processing. If the former is abnormal, visual assessment may provide a non-invasive measure of dopaminergic activity. Whether this correlates with nigrostriatal dopaminergic deficits remains to be seen.

Olfactory dysfunction

In 1975, Ansari and Johnson[28] showed that the threshold for detecting amylacetate was impaired in idiopathic parkinsonism, and subsequently Ward and colleagues demonstrated a deficit in olfactory discrimination[29]. These findings have been extended by others[30]. While such changes are not specific, being seen in other neurodegenerative conditions, they may still prove to be of some value in screening for early idiopathic parkinsonism.

PATHOLOGICAL TESTS

Lewy bodies are not limited to the substantia nigra in idiopathic parkinsonism. Importantly, they are also not confined to the central nervous system. They can be found in sympathetic ganglia, and in the mesenteric plexi of the whole gastrointestinal tract, particularly the lower esophagus[31]. The notion of a biopsy diagnosis for idiopathic parkinsonism stems from a unique observation of Stadlan and colleagues[32], who reported the presence of a Lewy body in the neuronal components of a sympathectomy performed 3 years prior to the development of clinically overt idiopathic parkinsonism. Lees has failed to detect Lewy bodies in a pilot study of rectal biopsies in idiopathic parkinsonism (personal communication), but further experience is desirable before this technique for early detection can be evaluated adequately.

SUMMARY

Possible approaches to early identification of subjects at risk for Parkinson's disease have been discussed. While PET provides an *in vivo* index of integrity of the nigrostriatal pathway, many other potential markers may also contribute to early detection. In addition, certain markers may provide some clue in the search for etiology. These tantalizing possibilities will undoubtedly be the subject of further exploration.

REFERENCES

1. Riederer, P. and Wuketich, S. (1976). Time course of nigrostriatal degeneration in Parkinson's disease. A detailed study of influential factors in human brain amine analysis. *J. Neural Trans.*, **38**, 277–301
2. McGeer, P.L., Itagaki, S., Akiyama, H. and McGeer, E.G. (1988). Rate of cell death in parkinsonism indicates active neuropathological process. *Ann. Neurol.*, **24**, 574–6
3. Wolters, E.C. and Calne, D.B. (1989). Is Parkinson's disease related to aging? In Calne, D.B., Donatella, C., Comi, G., Horowski, R. and Trabucchi, M. (eds.) *Parkinsonism and Aging*, pp. 125–33. (New York: Raven Press)
4. Hoehn, M.M. and Yahr, M.D. (1967). Parkinsonism: onset, progression and mortality. *Neurology, 17*, 427–42
5. Tetrud, J.W. and Langston, J.W. (1989). The effect of deprenyl (selegiline) on the natural history of Parkinson's disease. *Science, 245*, 519–22
6. The Parkinson Study Group (1989). Effect of deprenyl on the progression of disability in early Parkinson's disease. *N. Engl. J. Med.*, **321**, 1364–71
7. Burns, R.S., Markey, S.P., Phillips, J.M. and Chuang, C.C. (1984). The neurotoxicity of 1-methyl-4-phenyl-1,2,3,6-tetrahydropyridine in the monkey and man. *Can. J. Neurol. Sci.*, **11**, 166–8
8. Langston, J.W. and Ballard, P. (1984). Parkinsonism induced by 1-methyl-4-phenyl-1,2,3,6-tetrahydropyridine (MPTP): implications for treatment and the pathogenesis of Parkinson's disease. *Can. J. Neurol. Sci.,* **11**, 160–5
9. Guttman, M., Young, V.W., Kim, S.U., Calne, D.B., Martin, W.R.W., Adam, M.J. and Ruth, T.J. (1988). Asymptomatic striatal dopamine depletion: PET scans in unilateral MPTP monkeys. *Synapse, 2*, 469–73
10. Calne, D.B., Langston, J.W., Martin, W.R.W., Stoessl, A.J., Ruth, T.J., Adam, M.J., Pate, B.D. and Schulzer, M. (1985). Positron emission

tomography after MPTP: observations relating to the cause of Parkinson's disease. *Nature (London),* **317**, 246–8

11. Snow, B.J., Peppard, R.F., Guttman, M., Okada, J., Martin, W.R.W., Steele, J., Eisen, A., Schoenberg, B. and Calne, D.B. (1990). PET scanning demonstrates a presynaptic dopaminergic lesion in Lytico–Bodig (the ALS–PD Complex of Guam). *Arch. Neurol.,* **47**, 870–4

12. Olanow, C.W., Holgate, R.C., Murtaugh, R. and Martinez, C. (1989). MR imaging in Parkinson's disease and aging. In Calne, D.B., Donatella, C., Comi, G., Horowski, R. and Trabucchi, M. (eds.) *Parkinsonism and Aging,* pp. 155–64. (New York: Raven Press)

13. Parker Jn., W.D., Boyson, S.J. and Parks, J.K. (1989). Abnormalities of the electron transport chain in idiopathic Parkinson's disease. *Ann. Neurol.,* **26**, 719–23

14. Schapira, A.H.V., Cooper, J.M., Dexter, D., Clark, J.B., Jenner, P. and Marsden, C.D. (1990). Mitochondrial Complex I deficiency in Parkinson's disease. *J. Neurochem.,* **54**, 823–7

15. Mizuno, Y., Ohta, S., Tanaka, M., Takamiya, S., Suzuki, K., Sato, T., Oya, H., Ozawa, T. and Kagawa, Y. (1989). Deficiencies in complex I subunits of the respiratory chain in Parkinson's disease. *Biochem. Biophys. Res. Commun.,* **163**, 1450–5

16. Reichmann, H., Riederer, P., Seufert, S. and Jellinger, K. (1990). Disturbances of the respiratory chain in brain from patients with Parkinson's disease. *Movement Disorders,* **5** Suppl. 1, 28

17. Steventon, G.B., Heafield, M.T., Waring, R.H. and Williams, A.C. (1980). Xenobiotic metabolism in Parkinson's disease. *Neurology,* **39**, 883–7

18. Heafield, M.T., Fearn, S., Steventon, G.B., Waring, R.H., Williams, A.C. and Sturman, S.G. (1990). Plasma cysteine and sulphate levels in patients with motor neurone, Parkinson's and Alzheimer's disease. *Neurosci. Lett.,* **110**, 216–20

19. Danielcyzk, W., Streifler, M., Konradi, C., Riederer, P. and Moll, G. (1988). Platelet MAO-B activity and the psychopathology of Parkinson's disease, senile dementia and multi-infarct dementia. *Acta Psychiatr. Scand.,* **78**, 730–6

20. Steventon, G., Humfrey, C., Sturman, S., Waring, R.H. and Williams, A.C. (1990). Monoamine oxidase B and Parkinson's disease. *Lancet,* **1**, 180

21. Kalra, J., Rajput, A., Massey, K.L. and Prasad, K. (1990). Increased production of oxygen free radicals in Parkinson's disease. *Neurology,* **40** Suppl. 1, 169

22. Kalra, J., Rajput, A., Massey, K.L. and Prasad, K. (1990). Role of oxygen free radicals in Parkinson's disease – an increased level of malondialdehyde, a lipid peroxidation product. *Movement Disorders,* **5** Suppl. 1, 28

23. Tatton, W.G. and Lee, R.G. (1975). Evidence for abnormal long-loop reflexes in parkinsonian patients. *Brain Res.*, **100**, 671–6
24. Marsden, C.D. (1982). The mysterious motor function of the basal ganglia: the Robert Wertenberg Lecture. *Neurology*, **32**, 514–39
25. Evarts, E.V., Teravainen, H.T., Beuchert, D.E. and Calne, D.B. (1979). Pathophysiology of motor performance in Parkinson's disease. In Fuxe, K. and Calne, D.B. (eds.) *Dopamine Ergot Derivatives and Motor Function*, pp. 45–59. (New York: Pergamon Press)
26. Upton, A.R.M., McComas, A.J. and Sica, R.E.P. (1971). Potentiation of the 'late' responses evoked in muscles during effort. *J. Neurol. Neurosurg. Psychiatr.*, **34**, 699–711
27. Bodis-Wollner, I. and Onofrj, M. (1986). The visual system in Parkinson's disease. In Yahr, M.D. and Bergman, K.J. (eds.) *Adv. Neurol.*, Vol 45, pp. 323–7. (New York: Raven Press)
28. Ansari, K.A. and Johnson, A. (1975). Olfactory function in patients with Parkinson's disease. *J. Chron. Dis.*, **23**, 493–7
29. Ward, C.D., Hess, W.A. and Calne, D.B. (1983). Olfactory impairment in Parkinson's disease. *Neurology*, **33**, 943–6
30. Doty, R.L., Deems, D.A. and Stellar, S. (1988). Olfactory dysfunction in parkinsonism. *Neurology*, **38**, 1237–44
31. Wakabayashi, K., Takahashi, S., Ohama, E. and Ikuta, F. (1988). Parkinson's disease: the presence of Lewy bodies in Auerbac's and Meissner's plexuses. *Acta Neuropathol.*, **76**, 217–21
32. Stadlan, E.M., Duvoisin, R. and Yahr, M. (1966). The pathology of parkinsonism. In Luthy, F. and Bischoff, A. (eds.) *Proceedings of the 5th International Congress of Neuropathology*, pp. 569–71. (Amsterdam: Excerpta Medica)

2

Quantitative methods of evaluating Parkinson's disease

R.L. Watts and A.S. Mandir

INTRODUCTION

Technological advances have made it possible to quantify precisely motor disability related to Parkinson's disease. Clinicians generally use a scale of 1 + (mild) to 4 + (very severe), or a descriptive rating of mild, moderate, or severe to characterize parkinsonian motor signs and symptoms. These scales are somewhat variable from examiner to examiner, may not be as reproducible as one would like, and are relatively insensitive, particularly near the lower end of the range. Quantitative techniques have the advantage of providing precise numerical measures of parkinsonian disability that are reproducible and allow rigorous statistical analysis. Hence, new therapeutic approaches and disease progression can be assessed more objectively than with traditional clinical assessment alone. Furthermore, with the aid of a detailed database of normal and abnormal values, diagnostic accuracy can be improved using quantitative measures coupled with careful clinical assessment.

To optimize the usefulness of quantitative measures, the clinical state of a Parkinson's disease patient and experimental/measurement conditions must be controlled as carefully as possible. This is best exemplified in Parkinson's disease patients who exhibit motor response fluctuations related to levodopa administration ('off' and 'on' states). Controlling for timing after the last dosage of medication, time of day, degree of fatigue and/or anxiety, amount of practice when necessary, and familiarity with the testing procedure will help to improve the accuracy and reproducibility of the results. Correlation with a clinical rating of global parkinsonian disability at or near the time of testing and, when available, measurement of plasma levodopa levels provide an even better means of interpreting data obtained at different times.

We describe in this report some of the currently available techniques for the measurement of movement time (the physiological correlate of bradykinesia), reaction time (an index of premovement neural processing related to response initiation in motor tasks), rigidity and tremor. This discussion of techniques is related to our personal experience and is intended to be representative rather than exhaustive. As these objective measures of motor performance become more widely available, they will provide improved standards by which the efficacy of new therapeutic approaches can be assessed.

TIMED MOTOR PERFORMANCE MEASURES

As the simplest way of quantifying motor deficits, timed tests of motor function should complement standard clinical evaluation. It is important to perform these tests (adapted from the Core Assessment Program for Intracerebral Transplantation[1]) under different clinical circumstances. Suggested testing conditions are:

(1)   During a standard 'off' period (following 12 h of withdrawal of antiparkinsonian medications overnight);

(2)   During the 'best on' – defined as the condition in which the patient and physician both agree that functional improvement secondary to medications is maximal;

(3)   At the beginning of a 'single-dose L-dopa response test' and at 1-h intervals thereafter until 'off' again, or 3 h have passed.

Pronation–supination test

This test of motor performance is administered by measuring the time in seconds required for the patient to perform 20 successive cycles of alternating tapping movements of the palm and dorsum of the hand against the knee, while seated with both feet flat on the floor. One cycle consists of tapping both the palm and dorsum of the hand against the knee. Each hand should be tested with the ipsilateral knee, and the test should not be performed with both hands simultaneously. Two data sets consisting of 20 cycles each should be recorded with each hand, and the best set recorded as the result for each hand. The patient should be instructed to perform the movements as rapidly as possible, but they must make complete contact of the palmar and dorsal surfaces of the hand with the knee.

Hand/arm movement between two points

This motor performance test consists of measuring the time in seconds required for the patient to tap the index finger of the right or left hand between two points placed 30 cm (12 inches) apart horizontally, for 20 successive taps (10 cycles if tapping of both right and left targets are considered one cycle). The test should be performed independently for each hand. For consistency, each test should begin on the left target. Two data sets of 20 successive taps should be performed with each hand, and the best set for each hand saved as the final result.

Finger dexterity

The time required for tapping the thumb with the forefinger and then with each finger in rapid succession, for 10 cycles, should be measured in seconds with each hand independently. Two data sets should be recorded with each hand, and the best set for each hand saved as the final result[2].

Stand–walk–sit test

This timed performance test of postural and gait control should be administered as follows: the patient should be seated in a firm chair which has four legs (i.e. non-rocking or tilting) and no arms, with the seat located 45 cm (18 inches) off the floor. The time required to stand, walk 7 meters (23 feet), turn and walk back to the chair and sit down should be measured in seconds. If freezing episodes occur, they should be counted and this noted with the test result. This test should be performed twice, and the best time should be recorded as the final result.

ELECTROPHYSIOLOGICAL METHODS

Bradykinesia: movement time and reaction time measurements

Defective initiation and execution of movement are principal abnormalities of Parkinson's disease. Akinesia (paucity of spontaneous movement) and bradykinesia (slowness of movement execution) are the cardinal Parkinson's disease symptoms that relate to these fundamental movement deficits. Voluntary motor tasks are used to study movement initiation and execution in Parkinson's disease patients. Such motor tasks can be fractionated into a 'preparation phase' and an 'execution phase', and parkinsonian subjects demonstrate abnormalities of both phases[3-13].

The physiological measures related to movement initiation and movement execution are reaction time (RT) and movement time (MT), respectively. Motor tasks that measure RT and MT involve a 'preparatory period', a 'reaction time period', and a 'movement time period' (Figure 1). The preparatory period is the time elapsed between a 'prepare to move' or 'get set' signal and the 'go' signal. This preparatory period is pseudo-randomly varied (e.g. between 0.8 and 2.5 s) to prevent anticipation and false starts. The RT period has two components: the time elapsed between the 'go' signal and the onset of agonist muscle electromyographic (EMG) activity (RT_{EMG}, the 'true' reaction time); and the time elapsed between the onset of agonist EMG activity and movement onset (electromechanical delay, EMD). Some investigators measure RT from the 'go' signal to movement onset (MO) ($RT_{MO} = RT_{EMG} + EMD$), but RT_{EMG} is a more accurate measure of the time elapsed between the 'go' signal and when the neural activity first excites the muscle. Hence, RT_{EMG} more precisely reflects the abnormal premovement neural activity in Parkinson's disease, but if the transducer that detects movement onset is very sensitive, RT_{MO} provides essentially the same information[13]. The 'MT period' is the time elapsed between movement onset and achievement of the final target (i.e. time required to execute the movement).

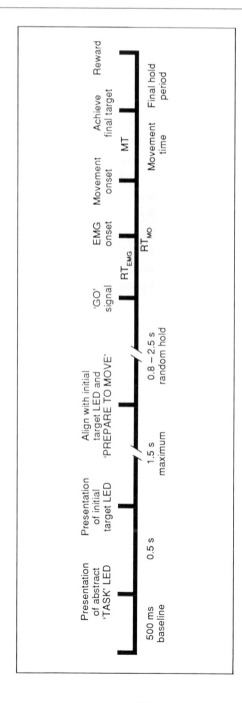

Figure 1 Schematic timing diagram of one cycle of a stimulus-initiated motor task used to obtain reaction time and movement time measurements

Wrist movement task

To assess RT and MT, a motor task requiring wrist flexion or extension in response to visual signals can be employed (Figure 2). Subjects sit in front of a computer-controlled visual display which presents instruction signals such as 'get set' and 'go', initial and final target locations, and handle position. The subject's hand is placed into a plexiglass handle which allows movement about the wrist only. On the visual display a light–emitting-diode (LED) presents the 'get set' signal, and 500 ms later

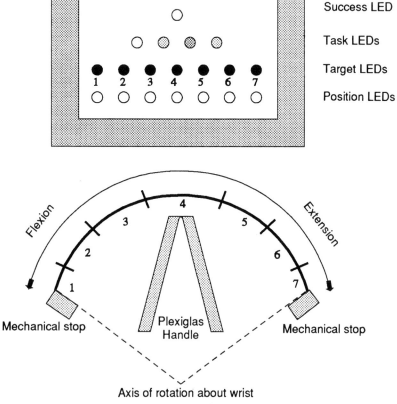

Figure 2 Schematic diagram of the apparatus used in the right wrist movement task for measuring movement time and reaction time

the initial target LED ('start' position) is illuminated. The subject moves the handle to align with the initial target location. After a random hold period (0.8–2.5 s) designed to prevent anticipatory movements, a 'go' signal in the form of illumination of a final target LED appears at a predetermined position (requiring either a 60° flexion or extension movement, depending upon the location of the initial target). The goal of the subject is to move the handle into the final target LED position (12° window) as rapidly and accurately as possible. Upon reaching the final target position, the subject is required to hold that position for 500 ms and an auditory signal is presented indicating a successful trial. A procedural error during the trial will blank the screen and prompt the subject to restart. A potentiometer records wrist angular displacement (position signal), and surface electromyographic electrodes are used to record EMG activity from the wrist flexor and extensor (agonist and antagonist) muscles (see Figure 3).

Three behavioral measures are calculated. RT_{MO} represents the time from the presentation of the 'go' signal to the onset of movement, and RT_{EMG} represents the time from presentation of the 'go' signal to the onset of agonist EMG activity. MT is the time elapsed from movement onset to achievement of the final target (see Figure 4). Following a practice session of 100 trials for each hand, two data sets consisting of 35 trials each are recorded for every subject.

Whole arm movement task

Simple and directional choice RT and MT measurements can also be made using a touchpad device connected to a computer. The configuration of the touchpads consists of one 'start' and two 'target' locations forming an equilateral triangle of 12 in (30 cm) sides (see Figure 5). The 'start' location is closest to the subject, and the two 'target' locations are equal distances away. For the simple RT task, the subject places his finger on a 1 in square that is sensitive to touch ('start' pad). Then, a 'get set' red LED is displayed at the designated 'target' pad. After a random hold period (0.8–2.5 s), a 'go' signal appears at the 'target' pad in the form of a green LED. The goal is to move the arm and touch the finger to the 'target' pad as rapidly and accurately as possible. An auditory signal ('beep') indicates the completion of a successful trial.

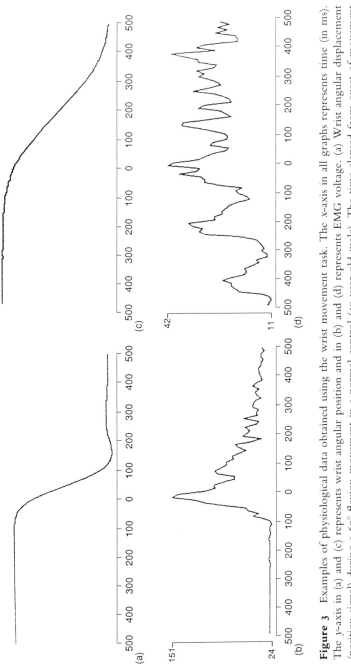

Figure 3 Examples of physiological data obtained using the wrist movement task. The x-axis in all graphs represents time (in ms). The y-axis in (a) and (c) represents wrist angular position and in (b) and (d) represents EMG voltage. (a) Wrist angular displacement (position signal) during a 60° flexion movement in a normal control (59-year-old male). The time elapsed from onset of movement to achievement of final target is the movement time (MT). (b) Rectified and integrated signal of agonist EMG activity during a rapid wrist flexion in the same subject. (c) Wrist position signal during a 60° flexion movement in a 57-year-old male Parkinson's disease patient. Note the prolongation of MT (bradykinesia). (d) Rectified and integrated agonist EMG signal from the same Parkinson's disease patient, demonstrating disorganized muscle activity (and superimposed tremor bursting at 5–6 Hz)

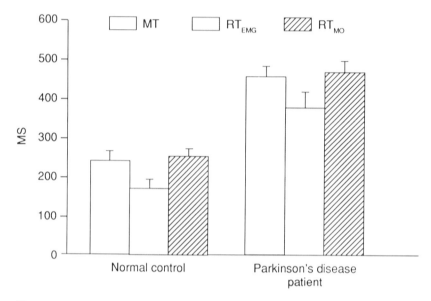

Figure 4 Histogram representation of prolongation of movement time (MT), reaction time to onset of agonist EMG (RT_{EMG}), and reaction time to movement onset (RT_{MO}) in a 57-year-old male with advanced Parkinson's disease compared with a 59-year-old normal male control. The bar graphs represent the mean of 30 consecutive trials of wrist flexion movement and the error bars represent the standard error from the mean (SEM). The y-axis represents time in ms

In the simple RT task the final target location is specified from the onset of the trial. In the choice RT task, either of the two locations are possible final targets. The direction of movement and the final target location are not specified until presentation of the 'go' signal. The 'go' signal appears randomly at either target pad forcing the subject to choose before making the movement towards the designated target, a cognitively more complex task than the simple RT task (Figure 6).

Rigidity measurements

Rigidity is defined in simple terms as an increased resistance to passive stretch of a muscle or group of muscles that is steady throughout the movement. Even though it is at times interrupted periodically in a

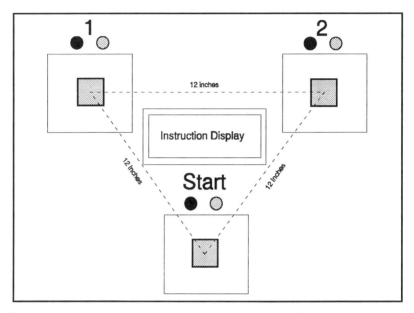

Figure 5 Schematic diagram of a touchpad device which requires whole-arm movements to obtain measurements of simple RT, directional choice RT, and MT with each hand (see text for explanation)

'cogwheel' manner, it is still described as plastic or steady to contrast it with spasticity, which builds in a crescendo manner as the muscle is stretched until it suddenly 'gives away' (clasp-knife phenomenon).

Muscular 'tone' is assessed clinically by passively stretching and shortening a muscle or group of muscles (e.g. those spanning a particular joint such as the wrist or elbow) with the patient as relaxed as possible. It is typically tested with a patient in a standard position, such as sitting with the arms at rest in the lap. If abnormally increased tone is present, an attempt is made to grade it on a scale of 1+ (mild) to 4+ (very severe). This method of evaluating tone, while being useful clinically, suffers from the limitations described in the first paragraph of this chapter. As Schwab noted, 'it is exceedingly difficult to obtain by routine clinical examination a specific value for rigidity at a given time for comparison with rigidity in the same joint at another time – a requisite for evaluating precisely the effect of an anti-rigidity medication or of physiotherapy directed against the rigidity'[14].

To measure rigidity objectively we have developed a technique using a torque motor to move the upper arm passively about the elbow[15,16]. Subjects are seated in a chair with the upper arm supported on a table at shoulder height. The forearm, wrist and hand are secured to a lever arm which is connected to the torque motor with elbow rotation centered over the axis of rotation of the torque motor. Subjects are instructed to relax, close their eyes, and neither help nor hinder their arm movements. Torque pulses are applied to the relaxed arm which starts out in the neutral position (the position to which the arm returns when manually deflected and allowed to move freely until it comes to rest). Surface electrodes are used to monitor EMG activity from the triceps and biceps muscles. A computer provides a torque pattern to the motor so that the elbow is first slowly extended and then slowly flexed during a single trial. This torque pattern consists of a series of four positive (extending) and four negative (flexing) torque levels which generate arm velocities far below those required to excite muscle stretch reflexes[15,16]. Angular position is measured by a goniometer on the motor

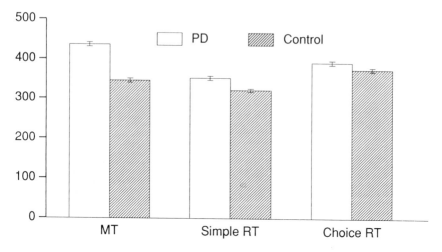

Figure 6 Histogram representation of summary right-hand movement times, simple reaction times, and directional choice reaction times, comparing ten unmedicated patients with recent onset Parkinson's disease (Parkinson's disease duration of less than 3 years) (grey bars) to ten age- and gender-matched normal controls (hatched bars). The bar graphs represent the mean, and the error bars the SEM. The y-axis represents time in ms. Note that in early Parkinson's disease patients, movement time is prolonged to a greater degree than simple and choice reaction times

shaft, and strain gauges on the lever arm measure torque. The slope of an angular position versus measured torque plot yields a measure of limb compliance, since limb compliance is linear over the range of limb movement tested (see Figure 7)[15,16]. Stiffness is proportional to the inverse of compliance. To correct for the effects of muscle mass, upper arm volume is estimated assuming a cylindrical model. The circumference of the arm is measured at three equidistant points between the acromion and the lateral epicondyle. The length of the arm is measured across the same two anatomical points. Using this correction, a normalized value of stiffness is obtained which can be compared across all subjects (see Figure 8).

Tremor measurements

Tremor is defined as an involuntary rhythmic oscillation of a body part. Electrophysiological tremor studies can be performed using two electronic accelerometers attached in perpendicular planes to the index finger (or any body part) of either the most affected side in the Parkinson's disease subjects or the dominant side in normal subjects

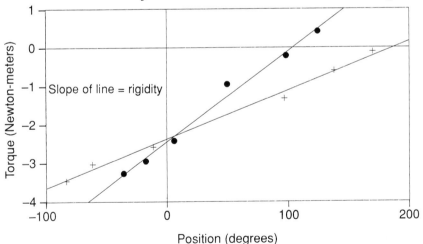

Figure 7 Rigidity profiles as demonstrated by linear regression fit of measured torque values at given elbow angular positions for a Parkinson's disease patient (●) and a normal control (+). The slope of each line provides a numerical measurement of muscular stiffness at the elbow (rigidity). The Parkinson's disease patient has a greater muscle stiffness value than the control (see text)

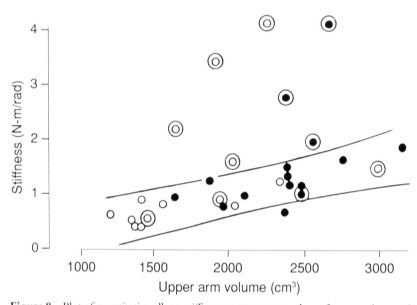

Figure 8 Plot of quantitative elbow stiffness vs. upper arm volume for normal controls (○, female, ●, male, not enclosed in circle) and Parkinson's disease subjects (○ or ●, enclosed in circle). The two lines represent 95% confidence limits for normal subjects. The majority of Parkinson's disease subjects' values fall well outside the normal range[15,16]

(Figure 9)[17]. Bipolar surface electrodes are placed over the deltoid, wrist extensor, and wrist flexor muscle groups on the most affected or dominant side. Additional surface EMG electrodes are placed on the contralateral wrist extensor muscles (or other muscles of interest). Subjects are studied while at rest and while performing standard motor tasks (holding a cup of water, writing or holding a pen, performing finger-to-nose coordination tests, holding the upper limbs outstretched, etc.). In addition, subjects may perform the motor tasks under two testing conditions since mental activity may accentuate tremor[18]: an 'activated' condition (during performance of a mental task consisting of serial counting backwards from 100) and a 'non-activated' condition (no counting, only performance of the motor task).

ELECTROPHYSIOLOGICAL DATA: DISCUSSION

Movement time/reaction time measurements

The most uniformly abnormal measure of movement performance in Parkinson's disease is prolongation of movement time (MT), that is,

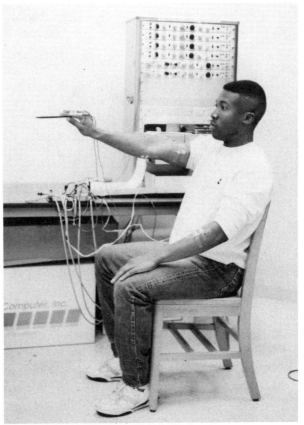

Figure 9 A patient undergoing an accelerometric and electromyographic tremor recording. The patient is holding the upper limb outstretched to assess for the presence of postural tremor. Accelerometers are attached to the right index finger in a perpendicular plane and surface EMG electrodes are applied to muscles of interest (see text)

bradykinesia. Figure 3c provides a graphical representation of bradykinesia during the performance of the rapid wrist flexion motor task (contrast this with the normal movement profile in Figure 3a). Underlying the slowed movement is abnormal agonist muscle activity, as shown graphically in Figure 3d. The prolongation of movement time is more pronounced in Parkinson's disease patients with more severe disability. In a recent study of ten Parkinson's disease patients, with mild symptoms and mean duration of disease just under 3 years, we found that prolongation of MT was the most uniformly encountered movement deficit. Figure 4 demonstrates the typical prolongation of MT during performance of the wrist movement task in a 57-year-old male Parkinson's disease patient with longstanding disease, compared with a 59-year-old normal male subject. Figure 6 demonstrates prolongation of MT during performance of the whole arm movement task in a group of ten early Parkinson's disease patients compared with ten age- and gender-matched controls.

While movement time relates directly to movement execution, reaction time relates more to premovement neural processing which helps facilitate rapid movement initiation. Simple reaction time is a measure of 'motor set', or the ability to take advantage of a 'prepare to move' or 'get set' cue prior to a 'go' signal. In a simple RT task, the position of the final target and trajectory of movement are known from the outset. In a normal subject, 'getting set' shortens simple reaction time (i.e. results in more rapid movement initiation). In contrast to simple RT tasks, choice RT tasks require the subject to make a decision about what type of movement is required when the 'go' signal is presented. In a directional choice RT task, the subject knows that he will have to make a movement in one of two different directions upon presentation of the 'go' signal, but he cannot 'set' to one specific location. Hence, at the time of the 'go' signal he must make a choice about the direction in which to move depending on from which target the 'go' signal arises. In normal subjects, choice RT is greater than simple RT because less specific information is conveyed in the 'prepare to move' cue and the subject must make a decision at the time of the 'go' signal; hence, it requires greater neural processing time.

In Parkinson's disease subjects, reaction time measurements are less consistently abnormal than MT measurements, especially in recent onset patients (see Figure 6). As the Parkinson's disease progresses, RT abnormalities are more readily observed. In general, simple RT is more consistently abnormal than choice RT[13]. In a study of Parkinson's disease patients who exhibited a stable 'wearing-off' effect with L-dopa, simple RT was significantly prolonged in the 'on' and 'off' conditions (331 ± 36 'on', and 371 ± 20 'off', vs. 251 ± 7 normal; mean $\pm$ SEM, ms), but directional choice RT was significantly prolonged only in the 'off' condition (373 ± 26 'on', and 464 ± 21 'off', vs. 360 ± 15 normal; mean $\pm$ SEM, ms)[13]. In other words, directional choice RT was sensitive to L-dopa replacement therapy whereas simple RT was not. The importance of when a given test is performed in relation to medication therapy is readily evident.

Rigidity measurements

Using the computerized torque motor system described above, we have found that reliable and reproducible measurements can be obtained of muscle stiffness (rigidity) at the right elbow. In a previous study of 11 patients with Parkinson's disease[16] we observed that Parkinson's disease patients had a mean stiffness value of 2.1 newton-meters/radian (range 0.52–4.1) compared to 1.0 Nm/rad (range 0.4–1.8) for controls. We also observed that the neutral elbow angle is more flexed in Parkinson's disease subjects (92 ± 15°, mean ± SD) compared to normal control subjects (107 ± 10°), an observation consistent with clinical observations that Parkinson's disease patients exhibit a flexion postural bias.

Since this technique utilizes a linear spring model of the muscles spanning the elbow joint, it is necessary to correct for upper arm volume (i.e. size of the spring) when comparing Parkinson's disease subjects with normal controls. When this is done, 5–95% confidence limits for normal stiffness values can be obtained, against which the stiffness value of a given Parkinson's disease patient can be compared to determine whether it falls outside the normal range (see Figure 8)[15,16].

Tremor measurements

With accelerometric and electromyographic recording techniques, specific characteristics of tremor can be identified, and tremor which may not be readily evident clinically can be detected. Most typical of Parkinson's disease is a 4–5 Hz 'rest' tremor which is best recorded when the patient is sitting with the hands resting in the lap or standing with the arms resting at the side. Typically, an alternating EMG bursting tremor pattern is seen in the agonist and antagonist muscles[17]. This type of tremor may be exacerbated during performance of mental tasks ('activated' condition)[18]. Also, a 5–6 Hz postural tremor is commonly observed in Parkinson's disease patients with rest tremor when they outstretch their upper limbs (Figure 10). This may take one to several

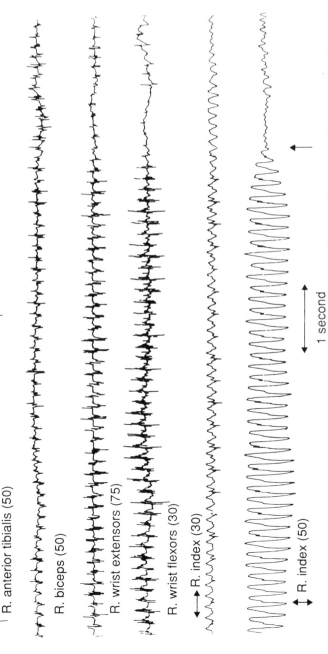

R. anterior tibialis (50)

R. biceps (50)

R. wrist extensors (75)

R. wrist flexors (30)

→ R. index (30)

R. index (50)

↕ R. index (50)

1 second

Figure 10 An example of an accelerometric and electromyographic tremor recording in a Parkinson's disease patient with postural tremor with some action component. This patient is 'off' Sinemet®, the last dose being given 2 h 15 min previously. Surface EMG electrodes are placed over the right wrist flexors, right wrist extensors, right biceps, and right anterior tibialis muscles. The accelerometers are placed in perpendicular planes on the right index finger. When the upper limbs are outstretched there is a 6 Hz postural tremor of moderate amplitude. The large arrow denotes when the patient places the upper limbs in a resting position in the lap (tremor significantly attenuated in the upper limbs)

seconds to emerge after the upper limbs are extended, and like rest tremor, it is accentuated during an activated condition (e.g. counting backwards from 100). When the upper limbs are used during performance of a particular action, this type of postural tremor is usually attenuated (as is rest tremor). This is in contrast to essential-familial tremor (usual frequency 6–8 Hz), which is most evident during performance of precision movements and maintenance of various postures. Essential-familial action/postural tremor may occur in Parkinson's disease patients[19], but it is much less common and less specific than rest tremor and 5–6 Hz postural tremor.

FUTURE DIRECTIONS AND APPLICATIONS

The techniques outlined in this chapter provide precise numerical measurements of three cardinal features of Parkinson's disease (bradykinesia, rigidity and tremor) at a particular time. While a single set of measurements in a given patient is useful (cross-sectional data), multiple measurements over time are likely to be much more valuable. This type of longitudinal analysis of motor deficits provides long-term objective data which can aid in the assessment of new therapeutic agents and provide a more accurate reflection of disease progression.

The electrophysiological techniques that have been described herein are laboratory based and provide a sample of data which is relatively brief (e.g. 1–2 h of a day). Movement monitoring devices which could be worn for extended periods during more natural daily activities (e.g. providing ambulatory recordings) may provide more useful and characteristic data about movement deficits related to Parkinson's disease. These types of data may relate more closely to the proportion of 'on' time in a given day, an important clinical measure employed in the assessment of Parkinson's disease with motor fluctuations in response to therapy. Some preliminary studies using long-term, ambulatory recording techniques to measure tremor[20] and hypokinesia[21] have been performed, and further development of this approach holds promise.

REFERENCES

1. Langston, J.W., Widner, H., Brooks, D., Fahn, S., Freeman, T., Goetz, C. and Watts, R.L. (1991). Core assessment program for intracerebral

transplantations. In Lindvall, O., Bjorklund, A. and Widner, H. (eds.) *Intracerebral Transplantation in Movement Disorders: Experimental Basis and Clinical Experiences*, pp. 221–30. (Amsterdam: Elsevier)

2. Lindvall, O., Rehncrona, S., Brundin, P., Gustavii, B., Astedt, B., Widner, H., Lindholm, T., Bjorklund, A., Leenders, K.L., Rothwell, J.C., Frackowiak, R., Hoffer, B., Seiger, A., Bygdeman, M., Stromberg, I. and Olson, L. (1989). Human fetal dopamine neurons grafted into the striatum in two patients with severe Parkinson's disease. *Arch. Neurol.*, **46**, 615–31

3. Heilman, K.M., Bowers, D., Watson, R.T. and Greer, M. (1976). Reaction times in Parkinson's disease. *Arch. Neurol.*, **33**, 139–40

4. Hallett, M. and Khoshbin, S. (1980). A physiological mechanism of bradykinesia. *Brain*, **103**, 301–14

5. Evarts, E.V., Teravainen, H. and Calne, D.B. (1981). Reaction time in Parkinson's disease. *Brain*, **104**, 167–86

6. Bloxham, C.A., Mindel, T.A. and Frith, C.D. (1984). Initiation and execution of predictable and unpredictable movements in Parkinson's disease. *Brain*, **107**, 371–84

7. Rafal, R.D., Posner, M.I., Walker, J.A. and Friedrich, F.J. (1984). Cognition and the basal ganglia. *Brain*, **107**, 1083–94

8. Stern, Y., Mayeux, R. and Cote, L. (1984). Reaction time and vigilance in Parkinson's disease. Possible altered norepinephrine metabolism. *Arch. Neurol.*, **41**, 1086–9

9. Yokochi, F., Nakamura, R. and Narabayashi, H. (1985). Reaction time of patients with Parkinson's disease, with reference to asymmetry of neurological signs. *J. Neurol. Neurosurg. Psychiatr.*, **48**, 702–5

10. Benecke, R., Rothwell, J.C., Dick, J.P., Day, B.L. and Marsden, C.D. (1986). Performance of simultaneous movements in patients with Parkinson's disease. *Brain*, **109**, 739–57

11. Benecke, R., Rothwell, J.C., Dick, J.P., Day, B.L. and Marsden, C.D. (1987). Simple and complex movements off and on treatment in patients with Parkinson's disease. *J. Neurol. Neurosurg. Psychiatr.*, **50**, 296–303

12. Sheridan, M.R., Flowers, K.A. and Hurrell, J. (1987). Programming and execution of movement in Parkinson's disease. *Brain*, **110**, 1247–71

13. Pullman, S.L., Watts, R.L., Juncos, J.L., Chase, T.N. and Sanes, J.N. (1988). Dopaminergic effects on simple and choice reaction time performance in Parkinson's disease. *Neurology*, **38**, 249–54

14. Schwab, R.S. (1964). Problems in the clinical estimation of rigidity (hypertonia). *Clin. Pharmacol. Ther.*, **5**, 942–6

15. Wiegner, A.W. and Watts, R.L. (1986). Elastic properties of muscles measured at the elbow in man. I. Normal controls. *J. Neurol. Neurosurg.*

Psychiatr., **49**, 1171–6

16. Watts, R.L., Wiegner, A.W. and Young, R.R. (1986). Elastic properties of muscles measured at the elbow in man. II. Patients with parkinsonian rigidity. *J. Neurol. Neurosurg. Psychiatr.*, **49**, 1177–81

17. Shahani, B.T. and Young, R.R. (1976). Physiological and pharmacological aids in the differential diagnosis of tremor. *J. Neurol. Neurosurg. Psychiatr.*, **39**, 772–83

18. Cleeves, L., Findley, L.J. and Gresty, M. (1986). Assessment of rest tremor in Parkinson's disease. *Adv. Neurol.*, **45**, 349–52

19. Young, R.R. (1984). Pathophysiology and pharmacology of tremors. In Shahani, B.T. (ed.) *Electromyography in CNS Disorders: Central EMG*, pp. 143–59. (Boston, London: Butterworth)

20. Scholz, E., Bacher, M., Bellenberg, A., Hart, S., Diener, H.C. and Dichgans, J. (1989). Long-term measurement of tremor: early diagnostic possibilities. In Przuntek, H. and Riederer, P. (eds.) *Early Diagnosis and Preventive Therapy in Parkinson's Disease*, pp. 93–102. (Vienna, New York: Springer-Verlag)

21. Laux, G., Kuhn, W. and Classen, W. (1989). Psychomotor investigations in depressed patients by comparison with Parkinson patients. In Przuntek, H. and Riederer, P. (eds.) *Early Diagnosis and Preventive Therapy in Parkinson's Disease*, pp. 55–63. (Vienna, New York: Springer-Verlag)

3

Etiology of Parkinson's disease

J.W. Langston, W.C. Koller and L.T. Giron

INTRODUCTION

What causes Parkinson's disease? While this fundamental question remains unanswered, during the last few years plausible mechanisms about neuronal cell death and therapeutically important theories of etiology have been put forth in ever increasing numbers[1-5]. In this chapter, we will critically evaluate current concepts on the etiology of idiopathic parkinsonism or Parkinson's disease, indicating, where appropriate, the constraints that pathological, biochemical and cell biology data currently impose. The main focus will be on recent genetic and epidemiological studies, especially those that bear on possible environmental causes. In addition, we will try to predict the most promising avenues for future research.

When dealing with the central nervous system (CNS), it is necessary to take into account at least three major considerations. First, the nervous system may be constrained in its response to different types of insult, toxic or otherwise, including a loss of endogenous maintenance factors. The implication is that vastly different agents could have the same final effects on the central nervous system, resulting in the clinicopathological complex that we call Parkinson's disease. It may also be true that critical interactions between causative factors are necessary for clinical expression of disease. Second, the agent or agents held responsible for the disease must be capable of accounting for its major features. From a cell biology perspective, these features include such things as the selective vulnerability of dopaminergic (and other monoaminergic) neurons and the rate of cell death. From a clinical perspective, these features are reflected in the characteristic signs and symptoms of the disease, including its predilection for the aging nervous system and the rate of progression of the disorder. A third and crucial issue from an epidemiological perspective is the necessity of explaining not only why some individuals get the disease, but why others do not.

IS PARKINSON'S DISEASE A SINGLE ENTITY?

The presumption in this discussion is that Parkinson's disease is distinct etiologically from the multisystem atrophies (MSAs). This group of atypical parkinsonian disorders includes such diseases as striatonigral degeneration and olivopontocerebellar atrophy. Certainly, differences in clinical symptomatology favor a separation of these other disorders from Parkinson's disease; notable among these are:

(1) The presence of both tremor at rest as well as rigidity in Parkinson's disease as opposed to the high prevalence of rigidity alone in the MSAs;

(2) The tendency for more rapid progression in the MSAs;

(3) A clearer tendency for familial transmittance in some of the MSAs; and

(4) The poor response to levodopa, which is typically but not always seen in the MSAs.[6].

Since there may be some degree of overlap between these conditions and Parkinson's disease, it could be argued that the etiology of these disorders may be shared. However, from an analytic as well as from an investigational point of view, we will presume that etiologies differ, and will exclude MSAs from consideration. Given the differences in their neuropathological substrate, this seems a reasonable assumption.

On a practical note, however, it should be pointed out that various forms of atypical parkinsonism, including striatonigral degeneration and progressive supranuclear palsy (PSP), are likely to continue to confound epidemiological studies. For example, many earlier accounts of the clinical and pathological features as well as the natural history of Parkinson's disease are likely to have included these atypical disorders.

Even experienced clinicians may not be able to make the distinction early in the course of these disorders. Therefore, erroneous conclusions about Parkinson's disease may have been drawn from populations not homogeneous for the disease. Assuming different etiologies for each of these conditions, this 'diluting factor' is likely to make identifying the etiological agent or agents even more difficult from an epidemiological perspective.

Since we will consider primarily idiopathic parkinsonism or Parkinson's disease in this chapter, it is appropriate to provide a brief description of the disease. By 'Parkinson's disease' we are referring to a distinct clinicopathological disorder as defined by typical clinical features (e.g. rest tremor, rigidity, bradykinesia and postural instability), neuropathological evidence of cell loss in the substantia nigra and the presence of Lewy bodies[3]. In this chapter, we will not discuss other forms of parkinsonism, such as the amyotrophic–lateral–sclerosis/parkinsonism–dementia –complex (ALS/PDC) of the Western Pacific, PSP and MSAs in any detail. Rather, they will be considered only as they are relevant to a discussion of the pathogenesis of Parkinson's disease.

CELLULAR AND NEUROCHEMICAL PROCESSES IN PARKINSON'S DISEASE

Parkinson's disease is characterized by loss of neurons in the substantia nigra and other pigmented nuclei[7,8]. While these neurons are known selectively to degenerate in Parkinson's disease, several fundamental aspects of this process are unknown, i.e. the mechanism of cell death, the exact anatomic localization of vulnerable cells within the nigra, and the rate of cell death. Striatal dopamine deficiency is the primary neurochemical lesion of Parkinson's disease[9]. This deficiency results from the disruption of the nigrostriatal pathway caused by the degenerative process in the substantia nigra. Other monoaminergic transmitters may likewise be reduced in concentration, but to a lesser degree and with less clear clinical consequences.

The relation between diminished striatal dopamine concentration and its cellular substratum has implications for the etiology and treatment of Parkinson's disease. It is estimated that a loss of 70% or greater of substantia nigra neurons and a loss of 80% or more of striatal dopamine are necessary for the production of clinical symptoms in Parkinson's disease[10,11]. Therefore, a substantial functional reserve capacity must be present in the substantia nigra, since a considerable degree of cell loss and dopamine decline is apparently required before clinical expression of the disease. This suggests a long presymptomatic phase, during which the fundamental disease process, selective neuronal cell death, progresses[1,12].

A long presymptomatic phase is consistent with continuous or intermittent dosing with an agent possessing minimal one-time effects on neuronal death; in this setting, disease progression would be the result of cumulative effects after multiple exposures. This contrasts with the short presymptomatic period that would be expected after a one-time exposure to a very potent agent. At the present time, investigation of this issue is planned with sequential dopamine uptake studies by positron emission tomography (PET) scans of subjects with exposure to MPTP who are likely to be vulnerable to the development of parkinsonism[13]. Many investigations are currently proceeding with the presumption that a long presymptomatic phase is the rule; hence, the early detection of presymptomatic individuals becomes a realistic goal[14].

UNEXPLAINED FEATURES IN THE PATHOLOGY OF PARKINSON'S DISEASE

In addition to cell loss in the substantia nigra, another neuropathological hallmark of Parkinson's disease is the Lewy body. Although other types of intracellular inclusions may be seen in the disease, such as neurofibrillary tangles[7] and colloid (hyaline) inclusion bodies[15], only the Lewy body is considered to be highly characteristic, though not specific for Parkinson's disease. These intraneuronal eosinophilic inclusions are invariably found in the substantia nigra and the locus ceruleus. They distribute, with lesser frequency, to other regions of the central nervous system, including raphe nuclei, hypothalamus and substantia innominata. They have also been observed in the autonomic nervous system, the adrenal medulla[16], and the myenteric plexus in the gastrointestinal tract[16]. The distribution of these structures is characteristic, and suggests a specificity of neuronal susceptibility (or reactivity) to degenerative stimuli.

At present, the exact chemical composition of these structures is unknown, but histochemical staining[17,18] suggests a high sphingomyelin content, while immunocytochemical stains indicate tyrosine hydroxylase protein in the Lewy bodies of catecholaminergic neurons but not of other transmitter-specific neurons[19]. Neurofilament antigens have been identified in Lewy bodies[20]. Although its cytosolic origins are uncertain, the ultrastructural features of the Lewy body implicate filamentous cytoskeletal components as constituents; the contribution of specific organelles is unknown.

How and why these inclusions develop is yet to be determined. Similarly, their relation to the etiology and the pathophysiology of Parkinson's disease is unknown but intriguing. Curiously enough, these inclusions are present in the central nervous system in about 2–10% of asymptomatic individuals over the age of 50 at the time of death[21–23]. Although they have been identified in other disorders[7], these 'incidental' Lewy bodies have been suggested to represent the histological picture of preclinical Parkinson's disease[23,24]. One provocative report supports this thesis[25]; in this case, a Lewy body was identified in the stellate ganglion of an asymptomatic patient who later developed parkinsonism. However, the relationship of these 'incidental' Lewy bodies to Lewy body dementia[26], to psychiatric disease[22], or even to Parkinson's disease itself[27] is still unclear at the present time.

Any etiological hypothesis must explain the role of the Lewy bodies in Parkinson's disease, including their:

(1) Distribution,
(2) Apparent labeling of the selectively vulnerable neuronal populations,
(3) Mechanism of formation,
(4) Cytosolic derivation,
(5) Chemical composition, and
(6) Relation to Lewy body dementia.

Finally, it will be necessary to explain the lack of specificity of Lewy bodies since, as noted above, they have been observed occasionally in other diseases that are clinically dissimilar to Parkinson's disease.

Many, but certainly not all, investigators would limit the definition of Parkinson's disease only to patients who have typical clinical features as well as the pathological confirmation of regional cell loss and of the presence of Lewy bodies. However, a question has recently been raised about the exact identity of similar-appearing inclusions that have been referred to as hyaline (colloid) inclusions. Pappolla and colleagues[15] have asserted that these bodies are histochemically distinct from Lewy bodies, but are nearly pathognomonic, representing the preferred marker for the disease when they appear in the substantia nigra. Further evaluation of this observation will be of interest.

During the last few years, Forno and colleagues[28,29] have been using the parkinsonogenic neurotoxin MPTP to produce an animal model of the Lewy body. When aged primates are given this neurotoxin repeatedly, they develop eosinophilic intraneuronal inclusions that bear a certain resemblance to Lewy bodies. Although classic Lewy bodies have yet to be replicated in this model, these MPTP-induced inclusions have a distribution that is very similar to that of human Lewy bodies, and they react weakly to antibodies raised against phosphorylated neurofilaments. In fact they are quite reminiscent of so-called pale bodies seen in Parkinson's disease, which some consider 'pre-Lewy bodies'. At the very least, this promising animal model for Lewy bodies deserves further investigation, and could prove quite fruitful in unraveling the secrets of these mysterious inclusions. Since the MPTP-induced inclusions are induced by an exogenous neurotoxin, they may also provide a bridge between Lewy bodies and the environmental hypothesis of Parkinson's disease, as discussed later in this chapter.

Other monoaminergic systems besides the dopaminergic system can be affected in Parkinson's disease. In cases studied biochemically by Hornykiewicz[30], norepinephrine as well as dopamine concentrations were markedly dininished in the substantia nigra. Since these observations, the findings of reduced striatal dopamine, serotonin and norepinephrine in Parkinson's disease have been replicated many times. Further, cortical concentrations of these neurotransmitters have been found to be reduced[31]. Conventional and histochemical studies confirm degeneration of both the noradrenergic locus ceruleus system[32,33] and the serotonergic raphe nuclear groups[33,34]. Therefore, any explanation for the selective vulnerability of dopaminergic systems must also account for the vulnerability of these other aminergic systems.

The cholinergic system is also affected in Parkinson's disease[35,36], most notably in the nucleus basalis of Meynert[37], a structure of particular importance in Alzheimer's disease. Besides the monoaminergic and cholinergic systems, other neuropeptide systems, such as substance-P[38], opioid[39] and cholecystokinin-like[40] systems, are affected in Parkinson's disease. It is interesting to note that MPTP has been reported to affect many of these systems as well, further highlighting the possibility that an exogenous neurotoxin might orchestrate some, if not all, of the neuropathological and neurochemical alterations that are seen in the idiopathic disease.

THE ROLE OF AGING

The relationship between normal aging and the clinical expression of Parkinson's disease is likely to be complex[41]. Part of the problem is that what passes for 'normal' aging may be the cumulative result of a number of otherwise subclinical pathological processes. For example, cross-sectional studies may include asymptomatic subjects who may have subclinical disease, confounding the problem of analysis considerably.

As might be expected, the evidence on the exact role of aging is mixed. A decline in dopaminergic function has been postulated to explain certain 'parkinsonian' features of aging. However, most evidence indicates that Parkinson's disease is not simply an exaggeration of 'normal' aging. Dopamine concentrations in the putamen show a probable plateau, then a sharp drop between 60 and 90 years[42]. Nigrostriatal attrition has been quantitated, showing a decline of 7% between ages 15 and 65, and another fall of 21% between 65 and 84[43,44]. Martin and colleagues[45] but not Sawle and colleagues[46] documented an age-related decline in [18F]dopa uptake in the striatum. In a quantitative PET study of a normal living population, Wagner[47] has documented a 'striking' decline in dopaminergic receptors with age, more marked for men than for women. In aging, a rostrocaudal gradient for aromatic acid decarboxylase in the human striatum becomes more marked, but is less steep than that for Parkinson's disease[48]. Using the binding of tritiated α-dihydrotetrabenazine as a measure of vesicular monoamine transport, Sherman and co-workers[49] demonstrated a decline in binding in the caudate with age; however, an exponential decline was observed in samples from Parkinson's disease independent of age at onset.

If the postulated decline in dopaminergic function during 'normal' aging does contribute to neurologic dysfunction, then pharmacological

39

enhancement of dopaminergic function should partially restore it. In fact, dopaminergic stimulation restores the posture and vigor of swimming aged rats to that of younger animals[50]. However, in humans, levodopa does not affect the mild extrapyramidal impairment of normal elderly subjects[51].

From a pathological point of view, the problem of defining a normal population of aging subjects notwithstanding, the dilemma is that neuronal aging is not uniform[52]. Also, to compound the dilemma, the same subcortical structures seem to be affected by aging as well as by Alzheimer's disease and Parkinson's disease[52,53].

Gibb and Lees[54] argue that Parkinson's disease and normal aging are separable processes. They studied four groups pathologically: controls, postencephalitic parkinsonian syndrome (PEPS), young patients with idiopathic parkinsonism (mean age of onset 40 years), and older patients with idiopathic parkinsonism (mean age at onset 59). Patients with idiopathic parkinsonism all had classic Lewy body Parkinson's disease (LB-Parkinson's disease). They documented that PEPS patients had 70% fewer cells in the substantia nigra than in LB-Parkinson's disease and 90% fewer than in controls; further nigral cell breakdown was not documented in PEPS but was present (gliosis, cell breakdown, extra-neuronal melanin) in LB-Parkinson's disease (interestingly, the number of remaining nigral cells was the same for the old LB-Parkinson's disease group as for the young). Thus, in contrast to PEPS, in LB-Parkinson's disease, the cell counts and pathological reactivity were consistent with 'continuous or self-perpetuating injury to the substantia nigra' that was not evident in postencephalitic parkinsonism after years of subsequent 'normal aging'.

This review suggests that, exclusive of the recognized decline in dopamine with age, the pathological alterations in catecholaminergic neurons in Parkinson's disease cannot be explained by the aging process alone. This conclusion is also supported by the data of McGeer and colleagues[55], who found a striking difference in the degree of microglial proliferation and number of neuronophagias when parkinsonians brains were compared to those of age-matched controls.

AUTOIMMUNITY AND PARKINSON'S DISEASE

The brisk microglia proliferation observed by McGeer and colleagues[55] (see previous section) raises the possibility of an autoimmune component in Parkinson's disease and indeed, there is some evidence of altered immune function in the disease. Autoantibodies have been shown to react to caudate[56], sympathetic ganglion cells[57], locus ceruleus and substantia nigra[58]. Sera from patients with Parkinson's disease revealed no autoantibodies against pituitary gland while ten other assays revealed low frequency or low titers[59]. Increased antibodies have been observed against herpes simplex virus (HSV) antigen in parkinsonians[60], without evidence of increased HSV antigen production in the brain[61]. Furthermore, in the later stages of Parkinson's disease, the number of peripheral blood lymphocytes is decreased and lymphocytes respond subnormally to T cell mitogens[62]. Among peripheral blood mononuclear cells of patients with Parkinson's disease, reduced numbers spontaneously secrete immunoglobulins; after stimulation, these cells also had reduced capacity to elaborate immunoglobulin *in vitro*[63].

These early studies have been interpreted to reflect an exaggerated effect of Parkinson's disease on the immune processes superimposed on those changes accompanying normal aging. The mechanisms are speculative but might include:

(1) Altered autonomic function in Parkinson's disease which subsequently perturbs lymph node reactivity; or

(2) Altered neurotransmitter function interfering with lymphocytic responses.

Barbeau[2] speculated that, in Parkinson's disease, damaged neurofilaments, after intracellular release, would be recognized as non-self and attacked by an autoimmune mechanism, and then converted into Lewy bodies; however, no evidence has substantiated this mechanism for the formation of Lewy bodies. Interestingly, however, an antibody directed against dopamine neurons has been detected in the cerebrospinal fluid of 78% of patients with Parkinson's disease, but in only 3% of controls[64]. Cerebrospinal fluid from the same Parkinson's disease patients also enhanced mesencephalic growth compared to controls[64]. However, in other studies[65,66], both the cerebrospinal fluid and serum of patients with Parkinson's disease has been cytotoxic to neurons in mesencephalic culture.

A formulation that accounts for the latter results is that, irrespective of the initial cytotoxic stimulus, autoimmmune mechanisms continue to propagate the destruction of nigral neurons. In this setting, the net result and the rate of destruction might be dependent on the competition between the cytotoxic stimulus and autoimmune destructive mechanism on the one hand, and neurotrophic maintenance on the other.

While all of this evidence is provocative, few would currently accept the proposition that Parkinson's disease is primarily autoimmune in nature. This is mainly because of the lack of pathological hallmarks of an immune process in the central nervous system of patients who have died with the disease. Nonetheless, the evidence cited above suggests that we should keep an open mind to the possibility that an autoimmune process might play at least a contributing role in the disease.

On the other hand, an autoimmune mediation may explain the unusual case reported by Golbe and co-workers[67]; in this case, parkinsonism was presumed to result from paraneoplastic degeneration of the substantia nigra; an autoimmune mechanism was sought but not confirmed by immunohistochemistry. Clearly, the case was atypical in many instances, including its association with ductal carcinoma of the breast, its resistance to levodopa, the prominent dystonia, and the absence of Lewy bodies.

THE GENETIC HYPOTHESIS OF PARKINSON'S DISEASE

The role of genetics in Parkinson's disease has been debated for many years and that controversy continues[68,69]. Unfortunately, family studies have been of variable quality and the value of early studies has been repeatedly questioned because of a host of methodological flaws. The issue of precise diagnosis has been touched on earlier; in many of these studies, the problem is compounded by reliance on chart-recorded diagnoses and on secondary evidence, as well as the contamination of the cohort by patients with essential tremor.

Two recent family studies, in which careful attention was paid to methodologic issues, are noteworthy. First, Golbe and co-workers[70] have described a large kindred of four generations, with early age of onset, an aggressive course, and a low incidence of tremor. Nonetheless, the subjects were levodopa-responsive and postmortem examinations have shown typical Lewy bodies. In this kindred, inheritance is ascribed to an autosomal dominant transmittance with incomplete penetrance. The second is a report by Maraganore and colleagues[71], who studied families of 20 probands with clinically typical Parkinson's disease who had at least one similarly affected relative; the latter were clinically indistinguishable from sporadic cases of idiopathic Parkinson's disease. The findings were interpreted as most compatible with an autosomal dominant transmittance, although the possibilities of other kinds of inheritance could not be excluded.

Studies of monozygotic (MZ) and dizygotic (DZ) twins with an index case of Parkinson's disease have been variably interpreted. The study of Ward and colleagues[72] yielded 43 index cases with definite Parkinson's disease and a single case of a co-twin with definite Parkinson's disease. Of 19 DZ pairs, all index cases had definite Parkinson's disease but no co-twin had definite Parkinson's disease. The authors concluded that genetics do not bear on the cause of Parkinson's disease. But this interpretation did not take into account:

(1)   That even Parkinson's disease-concordant MZ twins may differ in age of onset by 6.5–10 years[72,73], and

(2)   The possibility of subclinical Parkinson's disease in the non-affected twin.

Duvoisin and his co-workers[74] have recently reassessed the original interpretation of their own twin studies, and conclude the following:

(1)   Low MZ concordance can be compatible with a substantial genetic contribution, and

(2)   The broad confidence limits of the twin studies for the coefficient of genetic determination make it impossible for these studies to prove or disprove a substantial genetic component.

These issues, considered in combination with their own views regarding changing ideas about the definition of Parkinson's disease, led them to question conclusions of the twin studies.

They discuss three possible modes of genetic transmittance which have been postulated for Parkinson's disease:

(1)   Multifactorial threshold inheritance, by which environmental risk factors as well as genetic influences contribute to the risk for Parkinson's disease (e.g. a low caudate nucleus dopamine concentration);

(2)   Autosomal dominance with reduced penetrance; and

(3)   Mitochondrial inheritance.

They also predict the usefulness of additional family investigations, and studies of gene linkage, as well as positron emission tomography (PET) examinations and/or pathological studies of more unaffected twins to search for preclinical Parkinson's disease. In fact, Brooks[75] has reported that three out of six MZ and two of three DZ clinically unaffected co-twins have been shown to have reduced labelled fluorodopa uptake in the putamen. While all of these observations have re-opened the issue of inheritance, which originally appeared to be settled by the twin study of Ward and colleagues[72], additional PET scans in both MZ and DZ twin pairs are indicating that there may be an equal prevalence of preclinical disease in the non-concordant MZ and DZ co-twins[76]. If this observation holds, it would constitute additional evidence against a classic mode of inheritance for Parkinson's disease.

THE MITOCHONDRIAL CONNECTION

Recently, the activity of complex I of mitochondria from both substantia nigra and platelets of patients with Parkinson's disease has been reported to be less than that of controls[77–80]. Complex I is also the site of action of 1-methyl-4-phenylpyridinium ion (MPP+), the toxic metabolite of MPTP. With the examples of mitochondrial DNA deletions causing Kearns-Sayre syndrome[81] and other neurologic disorders[82], these findings suggest that complex I could be the site of confluence for both a genetic defect and a toxin.

The evidence for a mitochondrial genetic defect is provocative. Seven of the genes that code for mitochondrial complex are localized to the mitochondrial genome; therefore, mitochondrial DNA (mtDNA) deletions should be readily detectable[83]. Lestienne and co-workers[84] described normal mtDNA in brain of patients with Parkinson's disease. Subsequently, Ikebe and colleagues[85], using more sensitive techniques of polymerase chain reaction, detected small amounts of deleted mtDNA in the striatum of patients with Parkinson's disease. Utilizing the latter techniques, Ozawa and co-workers[86] have described nine-point and seven-point mutations in two patients with Parkinson's disease, and

44

compared them with those of patients with metabolic encephalomyopathies; they conclude that, although these patients are members of the same gene family diverged from a common ancestor, the type and number of overall mutations may be important factors for disease. In a later communication, Lestienne and co-workers[87] found that the deleted genome could also be present in small amounts in aged controls; they conclude that the deleted genome is not a specific property of Parkinson's disease but rather the result of aging. Our own data suggest that this same large deletion probably occurs even in young individuals, indicating that its presence may be quite non-specific (M. Sandy, D. DiMonte, J.W. Langston, unpublished observations).

Some unresolved experimental issues remain, including:

(1) The role of aging in regard to the number, location, and kind of mtDNA deletions;

(2) Whether the degenerative process itself causes or is caused by the mtDNA abnormalities; and

(3) If the mtDNA abnormalities must be amplified by a toxin to result in clinical Parkinson's disease.

A separate issue is whether the patients studied by Ikebe and colleagues[85] and Ozawa and associates[86] were typical clinically and pathologically for Parkinson's disease.

Another reason why the possibility that mitochondrial inheritance has attracted such interest is that it might explain the apparently low MZ concordance for Parkinson's disease and the delay in the clinical expression of the co-twin with Parkinson's disease, in that mitochondrial genetic material may be asymmetrically distributed between daughter cells at the time of mitosis. Thus, the twin with more normal mitochondrial DNA would have dopaminergic cells that would be more resistive to the degenerative process, in parallel to studies with inbred strains of mice who differ genetically in the numbers of dopaminergic neurons[88].

This experimental data must be considered in relation to the clinical information. Primary among these considerations is that only maternal transmittance can confer mitochondrial disorders that are dependent on mitochondrial DNA. Thus, a mitochondrial defect alone cannot explain why maternal transmittance has not been confirmed in any published family study of Parkinson's disease to date.

The mitochondrial genetic hypothesis does provide the promise of a biochemical test that can identify preclinical Parkinson's disease at an early age. Furthermore, the earlier the detection of such a defect, the more likely that the defect is the cause rather than the result of the disease or age, and importantly, the more likely that therapeutic intervention will be beneficial. At the very least, one can say that these observations on mitochondrial dysfunction have opened up an entirely new avenue of investigation into Parkinson's disease, and one which bears close scrutiny during the decade to come.

THE ENVIRONMENTAL HYPOTHESIS

During the last few years, interest has increasingly focused on the possibility that Parkinson's disease may be due, at least in part, to environmental causes. This was precipitated in large part by the discovery of MPTP[89] (a compound that selectively damages the substantia nigra after systemic exposure, and induces virtually all of the motor features of the disease in humans and experimental animals), combined with the near simultaneous publication of the twin study by Ward and colleagues[72], indicating a low concordance of Parkinson's disease in MZ twins (see above discussion). In the following sections we will discuss at least three possible environmental causes of the disease: infection, trauma, and toxic agents.

Infection and Parkinson's disease

The striking temporal relation between encephalitis lethargica (von Economo's encephalitis) and parkinsonism suggested that viral infections may cause idiopathic parkinsonism. However, a definite causal relation to a specific virus has never been established[90]. After the pandemic of encephalitis lethargica (1919–26), many cases of parkinsonism were observed[91,92]. Currently, most of this cohort of patients with postencephalitic parkinsonism have died[93].

The differences in clinical expression between postencephalitic parkinsonism and Parkinson's disease[94] suggest differences in etiology. In general, patients with postencephalitic parkinsonism were younger

46

(often in their twenties and thirties) at the onset of illness, more often experienced oculogyric crises, had many more hyperkinesias (e.g. chorea, dystonia, tics), had non-progressive courses, and more commonly had behavioral disturbances. Based on an analysis of the age of onset, Poskanzer and Schwab[95] had predicted, incorrectly, that all cases of Parkinson's disease were due to encephalitis lethargica, and that the disease would vanish. Transient parkinsonian features may occur during the acute or convalescent phases of a variety of viral encephalitides, including measles[96], Japanese B[97] and Western equine[98]. Rarely, parkinsonism may remain as a permanent sequela.

More recent investigations have not supported a viral etiology for Parkinson's disease. Case-controlled serological surveys have not found a higher incidence of viral exposure[99,100] and pathological studies do not support a viral etiology. Attempts to transmit Parkinson's disease by inoculation have been unsuccessful, suggesting that a 'slow virus' is not the cause[101]. A speculative hypothesis is that intrauterine influenza infection may lead to Parkinson's disease[102].

Trauma and Parkinson's disease

Early workers speculated that trauma causes Parkinson's disease[103–105]. However, many if not all of these studies were probably influenced by the problem of recall bias (i.e. individuals affected with the disease are more likely to recall such episodes). In support of this, recent epidemiological data from Olmstead county[106,107] indicate that individuals who have sustained severe head trauma are no more likely to acquire Parkinson's disease than those who have not.

Trauma may cause a parkinsonian syndrome, but the presentation is almost invariably atypical for the idiopathic disease, including such features as corticospinal findings and focal cortical signs, and diffuse encephalopathy (dementia pugilistica). Only rarely will trauma cause lesions sufficiently localized to be expressed as parkinsonism without other signs. In these instances, the computed tomography radiological features show low-density lesions, not consistent with the conventional pathology for Parkinson's disease.

On the other hand, trauma might have a minor role in triggering Parkinson's disease in susceptible individuals. For example, in the presence of existing Parkinson's disease, head trauma may result in transient worsening of symptoms[108]. Further, a trend has been suggested in a recent study relating severity of head trauma to later development of Parkinson's disease[109].

Toxins and Parkinson's disease

Recent epidemiological evidence suggests that an environmental factor may well play a role in the pathogenesis of Parkinson's disease. As we will see, the major culprits are suspected to be industrial chemicals and, in rural communities, herbicides/pesticides in well water. However, theories about etiology must conform to the known epidemiology of Parkinson's disease. If a man-made toxin causes the disease, a natural first question is when did the disease first begin? The earliest clinical description of the disorder was by James Parkinson in his *Essay on the Shaking Palsy*, published in 1817[110]. Although he quoted other scientists who wrote about tremor, it is unclear whether they described the same entity.

Did Parkinson's disease exist before 1817? This question is probably unanswerable because of the lack of clinical distinction between essential tremor and Parkinson's disease before that time. With this qualification, the manuscripts of Leonardo da Vinci[111,112] and of Ayurvedic medical text of 1000 BC[113] suggest that Parkinson's disease much predates James Parkinson. However, if the disease arose for the first time during Parkinson's lifetime, then an etiological relation of 18th and 19th century industrialization to Parkinson's disease is emphasized.

The current potential epidemiological constraints are:

(1) The higher prevalence of Parkinson's disease in different rural areas in Canada[114];

(2) Within rural areas, an association with drinking-well water in Canada[115];

(3) A higher prevalence in regions associated with market gardening and with wood-pulp mills[116]; and

(4) In China, an association with occupational or residential exposure to industrial chemicals, printing plants, or quarries[117].

Another consideration is the difference in prevalence between developed and undeveloped countries: the prevalences of Parkinson's disease in Nigeria[118] and China[119] are lower than that of the United States. Superficially, the evidence suggests a water-borne metal, pesticide or herbicide, such as paraquat[120,121]. The chemical similarity between paraquat and MPTP has been noted[116]. However, to date no specific environmental agent has been confirmed or even tentatively identified as an etiological agent[120].

The fact that no single chemical has been identified unequivocally suggests either that:

(1)   The chemical is present in extraordinarily low concentrations, requires prolonged exposure, is structurally dissimilar to MPTP, and has not been characterized chemically; or

(2)   A number of chemicals, perhaps in combination, can be toxic and etiologic in Parkinson's disease.

Recently, there has been increasing interest in the possibility that the failure to identify an agent in the environment may be because both exposure to such an agent and an inherited susceptibility may be prerequisites to develop the disease.

THE COMBINED ENVIRONMENTAL AND GENETIC HYPOTHESIS

Barbeau and colleagues[122] posited that inherited defects in the detox-ification of certain chemicals would enhance susceptibility to an environ-mental toxin, thus increasing the risk for developing Parkinson's disease. The first such risk factor to be suggested was a deficiency in the enzyme responsible for debrisoquine metabolism, which these investigators found more frequently in patients with Parkinson's disease compared to controls. Although this observation has not been fully replicated, this combined 'genetic–environmental' mechanism certainly warrants further exploration; indeed, a number of investigators are looking at other potential enzymatic deficits that could represent risk factors for the disease. For example, Williams and co-workers[123] have reported increased monoamine oxidase type B (MAO B) activity in platelets from parkinsonian patients when phenylethylamine was used as a substrate, but decreased activity when dopamine was the substrate. These findings are suggestive of a pharmacogenetic lesion that could predispose to parkinsonism by at least two mechanisms:

(1) The inefficient conversion of an MPTP-like substance systemically might allow entrance of similar molecules to the brain; and/or

(2) The inefficient enzymatic oxidation of dopamine could give rise to toxicity due to the build-up of dopamine autoxidation products.

This same group[124] has also suggested that defects in hepatic cytochrome oxidase P_{450} detected in Parkinson's disease could be inherited as a recessive trait, cause defects in S-oxidation, and be responsible for defective cysteine deoxygenase. This defect is also present in Haller-vorden–Spatz disease, in which nigral degeneration and abnormal basal ganglia iron deposition occur.

Thus, a more complete explanation of the events that lead to Parkinson's disease may entail two processes: first, a genetically inherited susceptibility factor (whether it be in the nuclear or mitochondrial genome), and second, an additional but necessary environmental trigger, with the prime candidate still remaining a toxin in the environment. It may be that a more sophisticated approach to the question of etiology that allows for an interaction between both of these factors will be the key to solving this mystifying neurodegenerative disease.

REFERENCES

1. Calne, D.B. and Langston, J.W. (1983). Aetiology of Parkinson's disease. *Lancet*, **2**, 1457–9
2. Barbeau, A. (1984). Etiology of Parkinson's disease: a research strategy. *Can. J. Neurol. Sci.*, **11**, 24–8
3. Langston, J.W. (1987). Etiology. In Koller, W.C. (ed.) *Handbook of Parkinson's Disease*, pp. 297–308. (New York: Marcel-Dekker)
4. Langston, J.W. (1989). Mechanisms underlying neuronal degeneration in Parkinson's disease: an experimental and theoretical treatise. *Mov. Disord.*, **4** (Suppl.1), S15–25
5. Burton, K. and Calne, D.B. (1990). Aetiology of Parkinson's disease. In Stern, G. (ed.) *Parkinson's Disease*, pp. 269–94. (Baltimore: Johns Hopkins Press)
6. Quinn, N.P. (1989). Multiple system atrophy – the nature of the beast. *J.*

Neurol. Neurosurg. Psychiatr., Special Suppl., 78–89

7. Alvord, E.C. and Forno, L.S. (1987). Pathology. In Koller, W.C. (ed.) *Handbook of Parkinson's Disease*, pp. 209–36. (New York: Marcel-Dekker)

8. Forno, L.S. (1990). Pathology of Parkinson's disease; the importance of the substantia nigra and Lewy bodies. In Stern, G. (ed.) *Parkinson's Disease*, pp. 185–238. (Baltimore: Johns Hopkins Press)

9. Forno, L.S. and Alvord, E.C. (1971). The pathology of Parkinson's disease. 1. Some new observations and correlations. *Contemp. Neurol.,* **8**, 120–30

10. Jellinger, K. (1987). The pathology of parkinsonism. In Marsden, C.D. and Fahn, S. (eds.) *Movement Disorders*, Vol. 2, pp. 124–65. (London: Butterworth)

11. Riederer, P. and St. Wuketich, S. (1976). Time course of nigrostriatal degeneration in Parkinson's disease. *J. Neural. Transm.,* **38**, 277–301

12. Koller, W.C., Langston, J.W., Hubble, J.P. *et al.* (1991). Does a long preclinical period occur in Parkinson's disease? *Neurology,* **41** (Suppl. 2), 8–13

13. Calne, D.B., Langston, J.W., Martin, W.R.W. *et al.* (1985). Positron emission tomography after MPTP: observations relating to the cause of Parkinson's disease. *Nature* (London), **45**, 19–34

14. Langston, J.W. and Koller, W.C. (1991). The next frontier in Parkinson's disease: presymptomatic detection. *Neurology,* **41** (Suppl. 2), 5–7

15. Pappolla, M.A., Shank, D.L., Alzofon, J. and Dudley, A.W. (1988). Colloid (hyaline) inclusion bodies in the central nervous system: their presence in the substantia nigra is diagnostic of Parkinson's disease. *Hum. Pathol.,* **19**, 27–31

16. Wakabayahi, K., Takahashi, H., Takeda, S., Ohama, E. and Ikuta, F. (1989). Lewy bodies in the enteric nervous system in Parkinson's disease. *Arch. Histol. Cytol.,* **52** (Suppl. 1), 191–4

17. Den Hartog Jager, W.A. (1970). Histochemistry of adrenal bodies in Parkinson's disease. *Arch. Neurol.,* **23**, 528–33

18. Den Hartog Jager, W.A. (1969). Sphingomyelin in Lewy inclusion bodies in Parkinson's disease. *Arch. Neurol.,* **21**, 615–19

19. Nakashima, S. and Ikuta, F. (1984). Tyrosine hydroxylase protein in Lewy bodies of parkinsonian and senile brains. *J. Neurosci.,* **66**, 91–6

20. Cork, L.C., Kitt, C.A., Struble, R.G.H., Griffin, J.W. and Price, D.L. (1987). Animal models of degenerative neurological disease. *Prog. Clin. Biol. Res.,* **229**, 241–69

21. Gibb, W.R.G. (1986). Idiopathic Parkinson's disease and the Lewy body disorders. *Neuropathol. Appl. Neurobiol.,* **12**, 223–34

22. Perry, R.H., Irving, D. and Tomlinson, B.E. (1990). Lewy body

prevalence in the aging brain: relationship to neuropsychiatric disorders, Alzheimer-type pathology and catecholaminergic nuclei. *J. Neurol. Sci.,* **100**, 223–33

23. Forno, L.S. (1969). Concentric hyalin intraneuronal inclusions of Lewy type in the brains of elderly persons (50 incidental cases): relationship to parkinsonism. *J. Am. Ger. Soc.,* **17**, 557–75

24. Gibb, W.R.G. and Lees, A.J. (1988). The relevance of the Lewy body to the pathogenesis of idiopathic Parkinson's disease. *J. Neurol. Neurosurg. Psychiatr.,* **51**, 745–52

25. Standlan, E.M., Duvoisin, R. and Yahr, M.D. (1965). The pathology of parkinsonism. In Luthy, F. and Bischoff, A. (eds.) *Proceedings of the 5th International Congress of Neuropathology,* Vol. 100, pp. 569–71. (Amsterdam: Excepta Medica International Congress Series)

26. Gibb, W.R.G., Esiri, M.M. and Lees, A.J. (1985). Clinical and pathological features of diffuse Lewy body disease (Lewy body dementia). *Brain,* **110**, 1131–53

27. Sage, J.I., Miller, D.C., Golbe, L.I. *et al.* (1990). Clinically atypical expression of pathologically typical Lewy-body parkinsonism. *Clin. Neuropharmacol.,* **13**, 37–47

28. Forno, L.S., Langston, J.W., DeLanney, L.E., Irwin, I. and Ricaurte, G.A. (1986). Locus ceruleus lesions and eosinophilic inclusions in MPTP-treated monkeys. *Ann. Neurol.,* **20**, 449–55

29. Forno, L.S., Langston, J.W., DeLanney, L.E. and Irwin, I. (1988). An electron microscopic study of MPTP-induced inclusion bodies in an old monkey. *Brain Res.,* **448**, 150–7

30. Hornykiewicz, O. (1963). Die topische Lokalisation und das verhalten von Noradrenalin und Dopamine (3-hydroxytyramin) in der Substantia Nigra des normalen und parkinsinkranken Menschen. *Wien Klin. Wschr.,* **75**, 309–12

31. Scatton, B., Javoy-Agid, F., Rouguier, L., Dubois, B. and Agid, Y. (1983). Reduction of cortical dopamine, noradrenaline, serotonin and their metabolites in Parkinson's disease. *Brain Res.,* **275**, 321–8

32. Mann, D.M., Yates, P.O. and Hawkes, J. (1983). The pathology of the human locus ceruleus. *Clin. Neuropathol.,* **2**, 1–7

33. Halliday, G.M., Ki, Y.W., Blumbergs, P.C. *et al.* (1990). Neuropathology of immunohistochemically identified brainstem neurons in Parkinson's disease. *Ann. Neurol.,* **27**, 373–85

34. Scatton, B., Dennis, T., L'Heureux, R., Monfort, J.C., Duyckaerts, C. and Javoy-Agid, F. (1986). Degeneration of noradrenergic and serotonergic but not dopaminergic neurones in the lumbar spinal cord of parkinsonian patients. *Brain Res.,* **380**, 181–5

35. Dubois, B., Ruberg, M., Javoy-Agid, F., Plasica, A. and Agid, Y. (1983). A subcortico-cortical cholinergic systems is affected in Parkinson's disease. *Brain Res.*, **288**, 213–18

36. Ruberg, M., Ploska, A., Javoy-Agid, F. and Agid, Y. (1982). Muscarinic binding and choline acetyltransferase in parkinsonian patients with reference to dementia. *Brain Res.*, **232**, 129–39

37. Nakano, I. and Hirano, A. (1984). Parkinson's disease: neuron loss in the nucleus basalis without concomitant Alzheimer's disease. *Ann. Neurol.*, **15**, 415–18

38. Halliday, G.M., Blumbergs, P.C., Cotton, R.G., Blessing, W.W. and Geffen, L.B. (1990). Loss of brainstem serotonin- and substance P-containing neurons in Parkinson's disease. *Brain Res.*, **510**, 104–7

39. Sandyk, R. (1985). The endogenous opioid system in neurological disorders of the basal ganglia. *Life Sci.*, **37**, 1655–63

40. Studler, J.M., Javoy-Agid, F., Cesselin, F., Legrand, J.C. and Agid, Y. (1982). CCK-8-immunoreactivity distribution in human brain: selective decrease in the substantia nigra from parkinsonian patients. *Brain Res.*, **243**, 176–9

41. Koller, W.C., O'Hara, R., Weiner, W.J. *et al.* (1986). Relationship of aging to Parkinson's disease. *Adv. Neurol.*, **45**, 317–21

42. Carlsson, A., Nyberg, P. and Winblad, B. (1984). The influence of age and other factors on concentrations of monoamines in the human brain. In Nyberg, P. (ed.) *Brain Monoamines in Normal Aging and Dementia*, pp. 53–84. (Ummea: Ummea University Medical Dissertations)

43. Mann, D.M.A. (1984). Dopamine neurons of the vertebrate brain: some aspects of anatomy and pathology. In Winlow, W. and Markstein, R. (eds.) *The Neurobiology of Dopamine Systems*, pp. 87–103. (Manchester: Manchester University Press)

44. Mann, D.M.A. and Yates, P.O. (1983). Possible role of neuromelanin in the pathogenesis of Parkinson's disease. *Mech. Age Dev.*, **21**, 193–203

45. Martin, W.R.W., Palmer, M.R., Patlak, C.S. and Calne, D.B. (1989). Nigrostriatal function in humans studied with positron emission tomography. *Ann. Neurol.*, **26**, 535–42

46. Sawle, G.V., Colebratch, J.G., Shah, A., Brooks, D.J., Marsden, C.D. and Frackowiak, R.S.J. (1990). Striatal function in normal aging: implications for Parkinson's disease. *Ann. Neurol.*, **28**, 799–804

47. Wagner, H.N. Jr. (1986). Quantitative imaging of neuroreceptors in the living human brain. *Sem. Nucl. Med.*, **16**, 51–62

48. Garnett, E.S., Lang, A.E., Chirakal, R., Firnau, G. and Nahmias, C. (1987). A rostrocaudal gradient for aromatic acid decarboxylase in the human striatum. *Can. J. Neurol. Sci.*, **14** (Suppl. 3), 444–7

49. Sherman, D., Desnos, C., Darchen, F., Pollak, P., Javoy-Agid, F. and Agid, Y. (1989). Striatal dopamine deficiency in Parkinson's disease: role of aging. *Ann. Neurol.*, **26**, 551–7

50. Marshall, J. and Berrios, N. (1979). Movement disorders of aged rats: reversal by dopamine receptor stimulation. *Science,* **206**, 477–9

51. Newman, R.P., LeWitt, P.A., Jaffe, N., Calne, D.B. and Larsen, T.A. (1985). Motor function in the normal aging population: treatment with levodopa. *Neurology,* **35**, 571–3

52. McGeer, P.L. (1984). The 12th J.A.F. Stevenson memorial lecture. Aging, Alzheimer's disease, and the cholinergic system. *Can. J. Physiol. Pharmacol.,* **62**, 741–54

53. Jellinger, K. (1987). Quantitative changes in some subcortical nuclei in aging, Alzheimer's disease and Parkinson's disease. *Neurobiol. Aging,* **8**, 556–61

54. Gibb, W.R.G. and Lees, A.J. (1987). The progression of idiopathic Parkinson's disease is not explained by age-related changes. Clinical and pathological comparisons with post-encephalitic parkinsonian syndrome. *Acta Neuropathol.* (Berl.), **73**, 195–201

55. McGeer, P.L., Itagaki, S., Akiyama, H. and McGeer, E.G. (1988). Rate of cell death in parkinsonism indicates active neuropathological process. *Ann. Neurol.,* **24**, 574–6

56. Husby, G., Li, L., Davis, L., Wedge, E., Kokmen, E. and Williams, R.C. Jr. (1977). *J. Clin. Invest.,* **59**, 922–32

57. Pouplard, A., Emile, J., Pouplard, F. and Hurez, D. (1979). Parkinsonism and autoimmunity – antibody against human sympathetic ganglion cells in Parkinson's disease. *Adv. Neurol.,* **24**, 321–6

58. Pouplard, A. and Emile, J. (1984). Autoimmunity in Parkinson's disease. *Adv. Neurol.,* **40**, 307–13

59. Moller, A., Perrild, H., Pedersen, H. and Hoier-Madsen, M. (1989). Parkinson's disease and autoimmunity. *Acta Neurol. Scand.,* **79**, 175–6

60. Marttila, R.J., Arstila, P., Nikoskelainen, J., Halonen, P. and Rinne, U.K. (1977). Viral antibodies in the sera from patients with Parkinson's disease. *Eur. Neurol.,* **15**, 25–33

61. Schwartz, J. and Elizan, T.S. (1979). Search for virus particles and virus-specific products in idiopathic Parkinson's disease brain material. *Ann. Neurol.,* **6**, 261–3

62. Marttila, R.J., Eskola, J., Paivarinta, M. and Rinne, U.K. (1984). Immune functions in Parkinson's disease. *Adv. Neurol.,* **40**, 315–23

63. Martilla, R.J., Eskola, J., Soppi, E. and Rinne, U.K. (1985). Immune functions in Parkinson's disease lymphocyte subsets, concanavalin A-induced suppressor cell activity and *in vitro* immunoglobulin production.

J. Neurol. Sci., **69**, 121–31

64. Carvey, P.M., McRae, A., Lint, T.F. *et al.* (1991). The potential use of a dopamine neuron antibody and a striatal-derived neurotrophic factor as diagnostic markers in Parkinson's disease. *Neurology,* **41** (Suppl. 2), 53–8

65. Dahlstrom, A., Wigander, A., Lundmark, K. *et al.* (1990). Investigations on auto-antibodies in Alzheimer's and Parkinson's disease using defined neuronal cultures. *J. Neural. Transm.,* **29** (Suppl.), 195–206

66. Dal Tosa, R., DeFazio, G., Benvegnu, D. *et al.* (1990). Specific dopaminergic cytotoxicity in sera of idiopathic parkinsonian patients. *Soc. Neurosci. Abstr.,* **16**, 809

67. Golbe, L.I., Miller, D.C. and Duvoisin, R.C. (1989). Paraneoplastic degeneration of the substantia nigra with dystonia and parkinsonism. *Mov. Disord.,* **4**, 147–52

68. Lang, A.E. (1987). Genetics. In Koller, W.C. (ed.) *Handbook of Parkinson's Disease,* pp. 81–97. (New York: Marcel-Dekker)

69. Golbe, L.I. (1990). The genetics of Parkinson's disease: a reconsideration. *Neurology,* **40** (Suppl. 3), 7–14

70. Golbe, L.I., Di Ioria, G., Bonavita, V., Miller, D.C. and Duvoisin, R.C. (1990). A large kindred with autosomal dominant Parkinson's disease. *Ann. Neurol.,* **27**, 276–82

71. Maraganore, D.M., Harding, A.E. and Marsden, C.D. (1991). A clinical and genetic study of familial Parkinson's disease. *Mov. Disord.,* **6**, 205–11

72. Ward, C.D., Duvoisin, R.C., Ince, S.E., Nutt, J.D., Eldridge, R. and Calne, D. (1983). Parkinson's disease in 65 pairs of twins and in a set of quadruplets. *Neurology,* **33**, 815–24

73. Koller, W.C., O'Hara, R., Nutt, J. *et al.* (1990). Monozygotic twins with Parkinson's disease. *Ann. Neurol.,* **27**, 276–82

74. Johnson, W.G., Hodge, S.E. and Duvoisin, R. (1990). Twin studies and the genetics of Parkinson's disease – a reappraisal. *Mov. Disord.,* **5**, 187–94

75. Brooks, D.J. (1991). Detection of preclinical Parkinson's disease with PET. *Neurology,* **41** (Suppl. 2), 24–7

76. Golbe, L.I. and Langston, J.W. (1992). The etiology of Parkinson's disease: new directions for research. In Jankovic, J. and Tolosa, E. (eds.) *Parkinson's Disease and Movement Disorders.* (Baltimore: Williams & Wilkins) in press

77. Bindoff, L.A., Birch-Machlin, M., Carlidge, N.E.R, Parker, W.D. and Turnbull, D.M. (1989). Mitochondrial function in Parkinson's disease. *Lancet,* **2**, 49

78. Mizumo, Y., Ohta, S., Tanaka, M. *et al.* (1989). Deficiencies in complex I subunits of the respiratory chain in Parkinson's disease. *Biochem. Biophys. Res. Commun.,* **163**, 1450–5

79. Parker, W.D. Jr., Boyson, S.J. and Parks, J.K. (1989). Abnormalities of the electron transport chain in idiopathic Parkinson's disease. *Ann. Neurol.,* **26**, 719–23

80. Schapira, A.H.V., Cooper, J.M., Dexter, D., Jenner, P., Clark, J.B. and Marsden, C.D. (1989). Mitochondrial complex I deficiency in Parkinson's disease. *Lancet,* **1**, 269

81. Moraes, C.T., DiMauro, S., Zeviani, M. *et al.* (1989). Mitochondrial DNA deletions in progressive external ophthalmoplegia and Kearns-Sayre syndrome. *N. Engl. J. Med.,* **320**, 1293–9

82. Wallace, D.C., Zheng, Y., Lott, M.T. *et al.* (1988). Familial mitochondrial encephalomyopathy (MERRF): genetic, pathophysiological and biochemical characterization of a mitochondrial DNA disease. *Cell,* **55**, 601–10

83. DiMonte, D.A. (1991). Mitochondrial DNA and Parkinson's disease. *Neurology,* **41** (Suppl. 2), 38–42

84. Lestienne, P., Nelson, I., Riederer, P., Jellinger, K. and Reichmann, H. (1990). Normal mitochondrial genome in brain from patients with Parkinson's disease and complex I defect. *J. Neurochem.,* **55**, 1810–12

85. Ikebe, S., Tanaka, M., Ohno, K. *et al.* (1990). Increase of deleted mitochondrial DNA in the striatum in Parkinson's disease and senescence. *Biochem. Biophys. Res. Commun.,* **170**, 1044–8

86. Ozawa, T., Tanak, M., Ino, H. *et al.* (1991). Distinct clustering of point mutations in mitochondrial DNA among patients with mitochondrial encephalomyopathies and with Parkinson's disease. *Biochem. Biophys. Res. Commun.,* **176**, 938–46

87. Lestienne, P., Nelson, I., Riederer, P., Reichmann, H. and Jellinger, K. (1991). Mitochondrial DNA in postmortem brains from patients with Parkinson's disease. *J. Neurochem.,* **56**, 1819

88. Baker, H., Joh, T.H. and Reis, D.J. (1980). Genetic control of the number of midbrain dopaminergic neurons in inbred strains of mice – relationship to size and neuronal density of the striatum. *Proc. Natl. Acad. Sci. USA,* **77**, 4369–73

89. Langston, J.W., Ballard, P., Tetrud, J.W. and Irwin, I. (1983). Chronic parkinsonism in humans due to a product of meperidine-analog synthesis. *Science,* **219**, 979–80

90. Elizan, T.S. and Casals, J. (1983). The viral hypothesis in parkinsonism. *J. Neural. Transm.,* Suppl. **19**, 75–88

91. Dimsdale, H. (1946). Changes in the parkinsonian syndrome in the twentieth century. *Q.J. Med.,* **14**, 155–70

92. Harris, J.S. and Cooper, H.A. (1937). Late results of encephalitis lethargica. *Med. Press Circular*, **194**, 12–14

93. Sacks, O. (1973). *Awakenings*. (London: Duckworth)

94. Duvoisin, R.C. and Yahr, M. (1965). Encephalitis and parkinsonism. *Arch. Neurol.*, **12**, 227–39

95. Poskanzer, D.C. and Schwab, R.S. (1961). Studies in the epidemiology of Parkinson's disease predicting its disappearance as a major clinical entity by 1980. *Trans. Am. Neurol. Assoc.*, **86**, 234–5

96. Sasco, A.J. and Paffenberger, R.S. (1985). Measles infection and Parkinson's disease. *Am. J. Epidemiol.*, **122**, 1017

97. Goto, A. (1962). A followup study of Japanese B encephalitis. *Psychiatr. Neurol. Jap.*, **64**, 236–66

98. Mulder, D.W., Parrott, M. and Thaler, M. (1951). Sequelae of Western equine encephalitis. *Neurology*, **1**, 318–27

99. Eadie, M.J., Sutherland, J.M. and Doherty, R.L. (1965). Encephalitis in etiology of parkinsonism in Australia. *Arch. Neurol.*, **12**, 240–5

100. Elizan, T.S., Madden, D.L., Noble, G.R. *et al.* (1979). Viral antibodies in serum and CSF of parkinsonian patients and controls. *Arch. Neurol.*, **36**, 529–34

101. Gibbs, C.J. and Gajdusek, D.C. (1982). An update on long term *in vivo* and *in vitro* studies designed to identify a virus as the cause of amyotrophic lateral sclerosis and Parkinson's disease. *Adv. Neurol.*, **36**, 1–41

102. Mattock, C., Marmot, M. and Stern, G. (1988). Could Parkinson's disease follow intra-uterine influenza? A speculative hypothesis. *J. Neurol. Neurosurg. Psychiatr.*, **51**, 753–6

103. Crouzon, O. and Justin Besanco, L. (1929). Le parkinsonisme traumatique. *Presse Med.*, **37**, 1325–7

104. Factor, S.A., Sanchez-Ramos, J. and Weiner, W.J. (1988). Trauma as an etiology of parkinsonism: a historical review of the concept. *Mov. Disord.*, **3**, 30–6

105. Koller, W.C., Wong, G.F. and Lang, A.E. (1989). Posttraumatic movement disorders: a review. *Mov. Disord.*, **4**, 20–36

106. Williams, D.B., Annegers, J.F., Kokmen, E. and Kurland, L.T. (1990). Brain injury and its neurological sequelae: a prospective study of dementia, parkinsonism, and amyotrophic lateral sclerosis. *Neurology*, **40** (Suppl. 1), 419

107. Williams, D.B., Annegers, J.F., Kokmen, E., O'Brien, P.C. and Kurland, L.T. (1991). Brain injury and neurologic sequelae: a cohort study of dementia, parkinsonism, and amyotrophic lateral sclerosis. *Neurology*, **41**, 1554–7

108. Goetz, C.G. and Stebbins, G.T. (1991). Effects of head trauma from

motor vehicle accidents on Parkinson's disease. *Ann. Neurol.,* **29**, 191–3
109. Factor, S.A. and Weiner, W.J. (1991). Prior history of head trauma in Parkinson's disease. *Mov. Disord.,* **6**, 225–9
110. Parkinson, J. (1817). *Essay on the Shaking Palsy.* (London: Whittingham and Rowland)
111. Calne, D.B., Dubini, A. and Stern, G.M. (1989). Did Leonardo describe Parkinson's disease? *N. Engl. J. Med.,* **320**, 594
112. Stern, G. (1989). Did parkinsonism occur before 1817? *J. Neurol. Neurosurg. Psychiatr.,* Special Suppl., 11–12
113. Manyam, B.V. (1990). Paralysis agitans and levodopa in 'Ayurveda' ancient Indian medical treatise. *Mov. Disord.,* **5**, 47–8
114. Barbeau,, A., Roy, M., Bernier, G., Campanella, G. and Paris, S. (1987). Ecogenetics of Parkinson's disease: prevalence and environmental aspects in rural areas. *Can. J. Neurol. Sci.,* **14**, 36–41
115. Rajput, A.H., Uitti, R.J., Stern, W. and Laverty, W. (1986). Early onset Parkinson's disease and childhood environment. *Adv. Neurol.,* **45**, 295–306
116. Barbeau, A., Roy, M., Cloutier, T., Plasse, L. and Paris, S. (1986). Environmental and genetic factors in the etiology of Parkinson's disease. *Adv. Neurol.,* **45**, 299–306
117. Tanner, C.M., Chen, B., Wang, W. *et al.* (1989). Environmental factors and Parkinson's disease: a case-control study in China. *Neurology,* **39**, 660–4
118. Li, S.C., Schoenberg, B.S., Wang, C.C. *et al.* (1985). A prevalence survey of Parkinson's disease and other movement disorders in the People's Republic of China. *Arch. Neurol.,* **42**, 655–7
119. Schoenberg, B.S., Osuntokun, B.O., Adeuja, A.O.G. *et al.* (1988). Comparison of the prevalence of Parkinson's disease in black populations in the rural United States and in rural Nigeria: door-to-door community studies. *Neurology,* **38**, 645–6
120. Koller, W.C. (1986). Paraquat and Parkinson's disease. *Neurology,* **36**, 1147
121. Rajput, A.H., Uitti, R.J., Stern, W. *et al.* (1987). Geography, drinking water chemistry, pesticides and herbicides and the etiology of Parkinson's disease. *Can. J. Neurol. Sci.,* **14**, 414–18
122. Barbeau, A., Roy, M., Paris, S. *et al.* (1985). Ecogenetics of Parkinson's disease: 4-hydroxylation of debrisoquine. *Lancet,* **2**, 1213–16
123. Williams, A., Steventon, G., Sturman, S. and Waring, R. (1991). Xenobiotic enzyme profiles and Parkinson's disease. *Neurology,* 41 (Suppl. 2), 29–32
124. Steventon, G.B., Heafield, M.T.E., Waring, R.H. and Williams, A.C. (1989). Xenobiotic metabolism in Parkinson's disease. *Neurology,* **39**, 883–7

4

The pathogenesis of Parkinson's disease

C. W. Olanow and G. Cohen

Oxygen is essential for aerobic life. However, oxidative reactions can generate toxic species and lead to tissue damage. Normally, antioxidant mechanisms prevent tissue damage and an equilibrium exists between pro-oxidant and antioxidant forces. An imbalance favoring oxidative changes is termed oxidant stress and has been implicated in a wide variety of diseases including cancer, heart disease, stroke, cataracts and arthritis. An accumulating body of information now suggests that oxidative stress may also play a role in the pathogenesis of Parkinson's disease[1-4].

Oxidation and reduction (redox) reactions involve the transfer of electrons and can, at times, generate by-products known as free radicals. This is particularly true for reactions involving molecular oxygen (Equation i).

$$O_2 \xrightarrow[\text{electron}]{+1} O_2^- \xrightarrow[\substack{\text{electron}\\ +2H}]{+1} H_2O_2 \xrightarrow[\text{electron}]{+1} \cdot OH + OH^- \qquad (i)$$

| Molecular oxygen | Superoxide radical | Hydrogen peroxide | Hydroxyl radical | Hydroxide ion |

The reduction of molecular oxygen demonstrates how the continued addition of an electron leads to the formation of superoxide radical, hydrogen peroxide and hydroxyl free radical.

These reactions generate the superoxide and hydroxyl free radicals as well as hydrogen peroxide. Free radicals are atoms or molecules that contain an orbital with an unpaired electron. Most radicals are unstable and tend to react with neighboring biological molecules. Molecules which donate an electron to free radicals through these reactions are, by definition, 'oxidized' and may be damaged in this process. The hydroxyl radical is a particularly reactive oxidizing agent. Free radical interactions have the capacity to damage many critical biological molecules including DNA, membrane lipids, enzymes and structural proteins[5-7]. In the central nervous system, with its abundance of cellular processes, there is a risk that free radicals will interact with membrane lipids and initiate the chain reaction of lipid peroxidation (Equation ii).

$$.OH + RH \longrightarrow R^{\cdot} + H_2O$$

.OH
Hydroxyl
radical

RH
Lipid

R˙
Lipid
radical

$$R^{\cdot} + O_2 \longrightarrow ROO^{\cdot} \qquad (ii)$$

R˙
Lipid
radical

O$_2$

ROO˙
Peroxyl
radical

$$ROO^{\cdot} + RH \longrightarrow ROOH + R^{\cdot}$$

ROO˙
Peroxyl
radical

RH
Lipid

ROOH
Lipid
hydroperoxide

R˙
Lipid
radical

The sequence of reactions in which hydroxyl radical generated from oxidation reactions interacts with lipids to form hydroperoxides. Note that these reactions generate lipid radicals (R˙) which can react directly with molecular O$_2$ and subsequently regenerate R˙ to continue the chain reaction of lipid peroxidation.

Lipid peroxidation can lead to alterations in the structural integrity of neuronal membranes and ultimately the death of the cell. Hydrogen peroxide itself is not a free radical but it is an oxidizing species capable of inducing tissue damage. It's major threat, however, lies in its potential to accept an electron from transition metals such as iron or copper and generate the highly reactive and damaging hydroxyl radical (Equation iii).

A series of naturally occurring protective mechanisms prevent or limit oxygen toxicity under normal circumstances (Table 1). The preventative

Fenton reaction:

$$H_2O_2 + Fe^{2+} \longrightarrow OH^{\cdot} + OH^- + Fe^{3+}$$

Iron catalyzed Haber–Weiss reaction: (iii)

$$H_2O_2 + O_2^{\cdot -} \xrightarrow{\text{Fe}} O_2 + OH^{\cdot} + OH^-$$

Hydroxyl radical generated from the Fenton Reaction or the Haber–Weiss reaction is catalyzed by the transition of iron from its ferrous to ferric form.

system consists of enzymes which defend against the formation of the hydroxyl radical. The enzyme superoxide dismutase catalyzes the conversion of the superoxide free radical to hydrogen peroxide and oxygen (Equation iv).

$$2O_2^{\cdot -} + 2H^+ \xrightarrow{\text{superoxide dismustase}} H_2O_2 + O_2 \qquad \text{(iv)}$$

Hydrogen peroxide is normally detoxified by interaction with the enzymes glutathione peroxidase or catalase (Equation v).

$$2\,GSH + H_2O_2 \xrightarrow{\text{glutathione peroxidase}} GSSG + 2H_2O \qquad \text{(v)}$$

$$2\,H_2O_2 \xrightarrow{\text{catalase}} 2H_2O + O_2$$

Chain-breaking antioxidants or free radical scavengers such as α-tocopherol (vitamin E) or ascorbate (vitamin C) have the potential to prevent or limit the interaction of free radicals with critical biological molecules.

Molecular oxygen contains two orbitals with unpaired electrons and is, by definition therefore, a free radical (a di-radical). However, the electronic structure of molecular oxygen limits its oxidizing properties and serves as a protective mechanism which impedes the direct oxidation of most molecules and therefore consequent tissue damage. Normally, molecules have orbitals containing two electrons with opposite spin.

Table 1 Naturally occurring defense mechanisms to prevent free radical damage

(1) Preventative mechanisms: enzymes which remove species of reactive oxygen
    (a) superoxide dismutase (SOD),
    (b) glutathione peroxidase,
    (c) catalase.
(2) Chain-breaking mechanisms: agents that react with free radicals
    (a) α-tocopherol (vitamin E),
    (b) β-carotene,
    (c) ascorbate (vitamin C),
    (d) uric acid.
(3) Relatively unreactive nature of molecular oxygen.
(4) Storage of iron in unreactive forms such as ferritin and transferrin.

Molecular oxygen, in its unexcited ground state, has two electrons with identical spin which are housed in two separate orbitals. This creates a spin restriction and limits the ability of molecular oxygen to accept electrons to fill the vacancies in its orbitals. For molecular oxygen to accept both electrons at the same time, a spin inversion must take place so that both electrons in the reacting molecule exhibit parallel spin. Under this circumstance, molecular oxygen can then accept the two electrons and complete the oxidation reaction. A large amount of energy is required for this sequence of events to occur, so molecular oxygen tends to react sluggishly with other biological molecules.

Molecular oxygen can accept a single electron and promote auto-oxidation if it reacts with an easily oxidizable molecule such as dopamine (Equation vi). In this case two free radicals are generated: a superoxide radical and a semiquinone[8].

$$DA + O_2 \longrightarrow .SQ + O_2^- + H^+$$
$$DA + O_2^- + 2H^+ \longrightarrow .SQ + H_2O_2 \qquad \text{(vi)}$$
$$.SQ + O_2 \longrightarrow Q + O_2^- + H^+$$

Auto-oxidation of dopamine, where SQ is the semiquinone formed by one electron transfer and Q is the corresponding quinone formed by transfer of a second electron. Note that hydrogen peroxide is also generated when dopamine undergoes auto-oxidation.

Molecular oxygen is *most* likely to react by accepting a single electron from a *transition metal*. Transition metals are molecules, such as iron, copper, or manganese, which can exist in more than one valence state. They have the capacity to either accept or donate an electron to promote redox reactions (Equation vii).

$$O_2 + Fe^{2+} \longrightarrow O_2^- + Fe^{3+} \qquad \text{(vii)}$$

Ferrous iron donates an electron to molecular oxygen to promote the formation of superoxide radical and is converted to ferric iron.

Oxidation reactions in biological tissues can be influenced by the regional concentration of a transition metal. For example, an increased concentration of iron is associated with an increased likelihood that a redox reaction involving molecular oxygen will occur. In contrast, chelation of iron such that it is in an unreactive form can retard or prevent the occurrence of the oxidative process[9]. Recycling of transition metals, such as iron, from the oxidized to the reduced state by tissue ascorbate, glutathione, or dopamine can drive an oxidation reaction and the formation of a cascade of free radicals.

Alterations in the concentration of transition metals have been implicated in the pathogenesis of several basal ganglia disorders, such as Wilson's disease (copper), parkinsonism (manganese) and Hallervorden Spatz disease (iron). Recently, interest has focused on the possibility that iron may contribute to the pathogenesis of Parkinson's disease. Iron is known to promote lipid peroxidation and to play an important role in oxidative processes[10]. Iron is most likely to enhance oxidation when it exists in a low molecular weight form complexed with either citrate, ATP or amino acids. When iron is bound to proteins such as ferritin or transferrin, it is relatively inactive and has a markedly diminished capacity to promote oxidation reactions[11,12]. While iron is suspected of playing a role in neurodegeneration, surprisingly little is known about brain iron.

Initial traces of iron in the human or mammalian brain are first detected between the first and second year of life[13,14]. Thereafter, there is a gradual accumulation of iron in brain-specific regions including the substantia nigra pars reticularis (SNR), the red nucleus, the globus pallidus and the dentate nucleus. In some of these areas, iron is present at a higher concentration than in the liver. Adult levels are reached by approximately 20 years of age and remain relatively constant until the sixth or seventh decades when iron concentrations again appear to rise, particularly in the putamen. Iron is thought to enter the brain bound to transferrin, by way of transferrin receptors[15]. In normal adults, iron does not readily cross the blood–brain barrier and patients with hemochromotosis or iron deficiency do not have alterations in brain iron concentration. Transferrin receptors are present in greatest concentration in sites remote from areas of iron accumulation, suggesting that axonal transport may account for the regional distribution of iron[16]. Iron is primarily localized in oligodendrocytes and is stored bound to ferritin[17]. In older individuals some accumulation in astrocytes is also seen. It remains unknown why iron accumulates in a regional distribution, and its specific microscopic localization has yet to be defined. Furthermore, it is not clear why iron accumulates in concentrations which appear to be far higher than are necessary to fulfill its known physiological functions, and also in what form iron is present, bearing in mind that it is most likely to promote oxidation when present in a low molecular weight reactive form.

There is concern that the brain may be vulnerable to oxidant-mediated tissue damage, for the following reasons:

(1) The brain contains large concentrations of polyunsaturated lipids which are components of neuronal membranes and are substrates for lipid peroxidation;

(2) The brain utilizes a disproportionately large percentage of body oxygen;

(3) Iron is present in large concentrations in specific regions of the brain;

(4) The brain is relatively deficient in protective mechanisms (e.g. within the basal ganglia there is very little catalase and a reduced concentration of glutathione compared to the liver); and

(5) The brain has a limited capacity for self-repair once it has been damaged.

Oxidation reactions have been implicated as a cause of dopamine neuronal damage caused by the neurotoxin 1-methyl-4-phenyl-1,2,3,6-tetrahydropyridine (MPTP). This compound is a synthetic byproduct of the illegal synthesis of a meperidine derivative. Some addicts who were injected with illicit drugs contaminated with MPTP developed a severe form of parkinsonism[18]. MPTP was subsequently demonstrated to cause parkinsonism in experimental animal models[19]. It is now known that the toxicity of MPTP results from its oxidation to the methylphenyl pyridinium ion (MPP[+]) by the monoamine oxidase type B (MAO-B) enzyme[20]. Inhibition of MAO-B by drugs such as deprenyl or Pargyline prevents the oxidation of MPTP to MPP[+] and the development of MPTP-parkinsonism in experimental animals[21-23].

The metabolism of dopamine (DA) also has the potential to contribute to oxidative stress and may render *dopamine* neurons vulnerable to free radical damage. Dopamine is metabolized either enzymatically by monoamine oxidase (MAO) (Equation viii) or by auto-oxidation (Equation vi) to form hydrogen peroxide, which is a potential source of hydroxyl radical formation (Equation iii).

$$DA + O_2 + H_2O \xrightarrow{MAO} 3,4 \, Dihydroxyphenylacetaldehyde + NH_3 + H_2O_2 \quad \text{(viii)}$$

Under physiological conditions, hydrogen peroxide generated from these reactions is cleared by glutathione (GSH) in a reaction which is catalyzed by glutathione peroxidase and which results in the formation of oxidized glutathione (GSSG). Glutathione is restored by the reduction of GSSG in a reaction catalyzed by glutathione reductase (Equation ix).

$$2\,GSH + H_2O_2 \xrightarrow{\text{glutathione peroxidase}} GSSG + 2H_2O \quad \text{(ix)}$$

$$GSSG + NADPH + H + \xrightarrow{\text{glutathione reductase}} 2GSH + NADP^+$$

In this manner, a pool of glutathione is continually available to detoxify newly formed hydrogen peroxide and prevent tissue damage. However, an increase in dopamine turnover or a reduction in glutathione could result in a change in the steady state and an increased concentration of hydrogen peroxide. These circumstances could lead to cellular damage by hydrogen peroxide itself, or by the increased likelihood that hydrogen peroxide could interact with low molecular weight iron complexes and produce the toxic hydroxyl free radical (see equation iii). An increased concentration of low molecular weight iron could also lead to a state of oxidant stress by promoting the formation of peroxides and free radicals. A scenario could be envisioned in which peroxides and free radicals generated from the metabolism of dopamine could induce a state of oxidant stress resulting in degeneration of dopamine neurons. Over the past several years a growing body of information has accumulated which supports the hypothesis that an oxidative stress involving peroxides and free radicals may contribute to the pathogenesis of Parkinson's disease. Some of these observations are described below.

(1) *An increase in the concentration of iron in the substantia nigra of patients with Parkinson's disease* Earle initially reported that the concentration of iron in the brain of patients with Parkinson's disease was 2-3 times higher than normal[24]. He did not report on the localization of iron or its potential clinical implication. High field strength (1.5 Tesla) magnetic resonance imaging (MRI) permitted the *in vivo* detection of iron on heavily T2-weighted sequences by virtue of its effect on water molecules[25]. MRI studies in patients with Parkinson's disease suggested that iron was increased in the substantia nigra[26]. Subsequent measurements of iron with biochemical and X-ray micro-analysis techniques confirmed these observations and noted that iron is primarily increased in the pars compacta of the substantia nigra (SNC)[27-29]. While it is possible that iron accumulation may simply be a marker of a degenerative process, iron is not reported to be increased in the nigra of patients with progressive supranuclear palsy (PSP), despite extensive neuronal degeneration[29]. The propensity of iron to enhance oxidation reactions with the generation of peroxides and free radicals raises concern that increased levels of iron in the nigra of patients with Parkinson's disease may contribute to cell death. Youdim and colleagues have suggested that iron may accumulate within the SNC because it contains neuromelanin which has an affinity to bind iron[30]. In this regard, it is noteworthy that melanized neurons appear to be preferentially lost in aging and Parkinson's disease[31,32]. Studies using Perl's stain suggest that iron is localized to areas devoid of melanin[33]. However, recent studies using X-ray microanalysis indicate that iron *is* increased in the vicinity of neuromelanin but in a form which is not detected by Perl's stain (M.B.H. Youdim, personal communication). More refined techniques such as LAMMA are necessary to establish the cellular and subcellular distribution of iron and to confirm whether increased iron is present in association with neuromelanin granules.

There are also conflicting reports in the literature regarding the concentration of ferritin in the brain of patients with Parkinson's disease.

Ferritin is a protein which binds iron in a way that decreases its capacity to promote oxidation reactions. One study using a monoclonal antibody directed against spleen-derived ferritin reported a reduction in brain ferritin in multiple brain areas including the substantia nigra in patients with Parkinson's disease[34]. The findings of reduced ferritin and increased iron suggest that iron in the nigra of patients with Parkinson's disease may be present as low molecular weight complexes capable of promoting oxidation reactions. However, ferritin levels were reported to be increased in another study[35], although this used a different monoclonal antibody (directed against hepatic ferritin) and the patients may have had a multisystem atrophy rather than Parkinson's disease. This issue remains to be clarified.

Further evidence of the potential role of iron in the degeneration of dopamine neurons is provided by studies which show that iron chelation may diminish the toxicity of 6-hydroxydopamine[36], and iron infusion into the nigra induces neuronal degeneration and a model of parkinsonism[37]. There remains a need for more definitive studies to ascertain in what form iron accumulates in the nigra of patients with Parkinson's disease, precisely where it is localized, how it gains access to the SNC, and whether it is the primary cause of cell injury or a non-specific consequence of cell degeneration. In this regard it should be noted, however, that the accumulation of iron secondary to tissue injury of any cause, might lead to a state of oxidant stress which jeopardizes the integrity of residual neurons. For the present, there remains concern that increased iron in the SNC of patients with Parkinson's disease promotes the formation of peroxides and free radicals and contributes to neuronal damage.

(2)   *A reduction in the concentration of glutathione in the substantia nigra of patients with Parkinson's disease*   There are reports that glutathione, which represents the primary mechanism for the removal of hydrogen peroxide, may be reduced in the nigra of patients with Parkinson's disease[35,38]. Preliminary studies also suggest that glutathione, but not iron, may be altered in the nigra of Lewy body-positive non-parkinsonian patients who may have presymptomatic Parkinson's disease (P. Jenner, personal communication). Thus, it appears that in Parkinson's disease, iron which accelerates oxidation reactions is increased and glutathione which protects against the formation of peroxides is

diminished. These factors might be expected to create an environment in the substantia nigra which is conducive to the formation of free radicals and lipid peroxidation. Indeed, one report suggests that in the nigra of patients with Parkinson's disease, malondialdehyde, a break-down product of lipid peroxides, is increased and polyunsaturated lipids, substrates for lipid peroxidation, are reduced[39]. These observations, taken together, may indicate that increased lipid peroxidation occurs within the substantia nigra of patients with Parkinson's disease.

(3) *Increased dopamine turnover in residual dopamine neurons* This would be expected to enhance free radical formation and could result in an additional oxidant stress in an already compromised system. As a consequence of dopamine neuronal loss, compensatory mechanisms take place which include increased dopamine neuronal firing and increased dopamine synthesis[40]. Increased dopamine turnover is associated with an increase in the production of hydrogen peroxide (equation viii) and an increased demand on the capacity of the remaining pool of glutathione to defend against free radical formation (equation ix). It has been shown that the increased dopamine turnover induced by treatment of animals with haloperidol or reserpine, or by treatment of striatal slices with levodopa creates an oxidant stress as shown by an increased concentration of oxidized glutathione[41-43]. This rise in oxidized glutathione can be suppressed by coadministration of MAO inhibitors, indicating that it is due to the oxidative metabolism of dopamine. Furthermore, recent experiments with isolated mitochondria from liver and brain demon-strate that within mitochondria there is either a significant increase in levels of GSSG, or a decrease in levels of GSH following the addition of various monoamines which are substrates for either MAO-A or MAO-B including dopamine[43,44]. This indicates that turnover of monoamines such as dopamine causes an oxidative stress within mito-chondria.

Oxidative stress induced by dopamine metabolism may also contribute to basal ganglia damage secondary to ischemic lesions. Ischemia has been shown to release striatal dopamine[46,47], and depletion of dopamine to protect against ischemic damage[48]. A dramatic reduction in the age-related decline of dopamine neurons in the substantia nigra and dopamine terminals in the striatum has been demonstrated in rats fed a diet enriched with the dopamine agonist, pergolide[49]. This effect was thought to be related to the capacity of low doses of pergolide to stimulate presynaptic dopamine autoreceptors, and thus decrease dopamine turnover and consequently oxidative stress. Dopamine has also been demonstrated to damage dopamine neurons in tissue culture[50]. Taken together, this information suggests that increased dopamine turnover may have adverse effects on dopamine neurons by way of oxidative stress.

(4) *A reduction in complex I of the mitochondrial respiratory chain* This has been reported in the substantia nigra, platelets and muscle of patients with Parkinson's disease[51-54]. The respiratory chain in mitochondria is the site of electron transfer reactions leading to the formation of ATP. A deficiency in mitochondrial complex I can be associated with a reduction in the synthesis of ATP which is essential for cellular metabolic processes. Among these is the biosynthesis of glutathione. A failure to generate ATP as a consequence of mitochondrial complex I deficiency might result in a reduction in glutathione formation and an increase in the likelihood that free radicals will be derived from peroxides. It is noteworthy that MPTP, by way of its conversion to MPP^+ induces a marked reduction in mitochondrial complex I[55]. A decrease in nigral complex I is thus observed in both MPTP-parkinsonism and human Parkinson's disease. Mitochondrial complex I is comprised of 26 peptides of which seven are encoded by mitochondrial DNA[56]. It is noteworthy that mitochondrial DNA exhibits a tenfold increase in spontaneous mutation rate compared with nuclear DNA and is particularly vulnerable to damage by toxins or free radicals[57].

It is intriguing to speculate that an interplay of decreased complex I, decreased glutathione, increased peroxide and free radical formation could represent a common pathway leading to dopamine neuronal damage as a result of oxidative stress. MPTP administration has been reported to be associated with a reduction in glutathione which is thought to be the result of complex I inhibition[58]. Alternatively, it has been observed that glutathione inhibition induced by buthionine sulfoximine results in changes in dopamine neurons that mimic MPTP[59] and that a deficiency of glutathione leads to mitochondrial damage[60]. One can envision a cycle in which a deficiency of glutathione promotes increased levels of peroxide, free radical formation, damage to complex I and a further reduction in glutathione. Alternatively, a process causing damage to mitochondrial complex I could lead to decreased formation of glutathione, increased levels of peroxide with the generation of free radicals and further damage to complex I (Figure 1).

There is, therefore, a body of evidence suggesting that oxidative stress may play a role in the pathogenesis of Parkinson's disease:

(1) Dopamine is oxidized and can generate hydrogen peroxide and free radicals;

(2) Oxidation derived free radicals have the capacity to damage dopamine neurons; and

(3) In the nigra of patients with Parkinson's disease, there is evidence of increased iron, decreased glutathione, decreased mitochondrial complex I and increased dopamine turnover which can all promote the formation of free radicals with consequent neuronal damage.

Oxidative stress in a given patient might result from different etiologies acting alone or in combination. This concept would help to explain much of the difficulty encountered by those who have sought to uncover a singular etiology for Parkinson's disease. It further raises the possibility that therapeutic strategies designed to interfere with oxidation reactions might be effective in slowing or stopping the progression of Parkinson's disease despite the uncertainty as to its specific etiology. Should this be

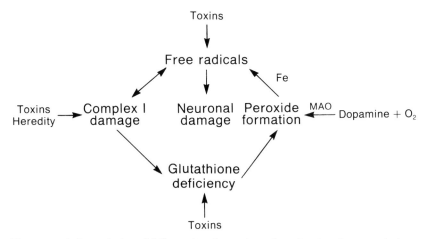

Figure 1 A theoretical model illustrating that an interplay of various factors including complex I, glutathione, peroxides and iron could lead to a cycle generating free radicals and neuronal damage

the case, it is possible that a biological marker of dopamine deficiency might permit the presymptomatic detection of patients who are at risk for the development of Parkinson's disease, and permit the introduction of antioxidant therapies prior to the development of symptoms or disability.

Attempts to confirm that oxidation reactions play a role in the pathogenesis of Parkinson's disease are currently being pursued in both clinical and laboratory studies. The DATATOP study, discussed elsewhere in this volume, demonstrates unequivocally that the MAO-B inhibitor deprenyl delays the emergence of disability in patients with early, otherwise untreated Parkinson's disease[61]. While it has not yet been established whether deprenyl acts by protective or symptomatic mechanisms[62], the findings are consistent with the notion that oxidative damage contributes to the pathogenesis of Parkinson's disease.

Other possible mechanisms of cell death in Parkinson's disease are also being explored. L-glutamate, and compounds which activate glutamate receptors can induce excitotoxic lesions[63], possibly by permitting an accumulation of intracellular calcium with activation of proteases and endonucleases. A specific brain-derived neurotropic factor has also been identified in the striatum and has been shown to stimulate growth of dopamine neurons in tissue culture and to protect them from the toxic effects of MPP^+[66]. It is possible that a deficiency of one or more neurotropic factors may play a role in the pathogenesis of cell death in Parkinson's disease.

It is conceivable that a combination of oxidation stress, excitatory neurotransmitters and tropic factors (or lack thereof) may play a role in the cell death that occurs in Parkinson's disease, and that therapeutic manipulation of these modalities will alter the natural progression of Parkinson's disease. It is certainly possible that multiple etiologies, acting through different mechanisms contribute to the pathogenesis of Parkinson's disease even in individual patients. At present, a single unifying etiologic or pathogenetic process to account for Parkinson's disease is far from established. Nevertheless, there are provocative clues for further research and it is hoped that enlightenment will be soon forthcoming.

REFERENCES

1. Olanow, C.W. (1990). Oxidation reactions in Parkinson's disease. *Neurology*, **40**, 32–7

2. Halliwell, B. (1989). Oxidants and the central nervous system: some fundamental questions. *Acta Neurol. Scand.*, **126**, 23–33

3. Halliwell, B. and Gutteridge, J.M.C. (1985). Oxygen radicals and the nervous system. *Trends Neurol. Sci.*, **8**, 22–9

4. Cohen, G. (1990). Monoamine oxidase and oxidative stress at dopaminergic synapses. *J. Neural. Trans.* (Suppl.), **32**, 229–38

5. Imlay, J.A. and Linn, S. (1988). DNA damage and oxygen radical toxicity. *Science*, **240**, 1302–9

6. Halliwell, B. and Gutteridge, J.M.C. (1985). *Free Radicals in Biology and Medicine*. (Oxford: Clarendon Press)

7. Cochrane, C.J., Schraufstatter, I., Hyslop, P. and Jackson, J. (1988). Cellular and biochemical events in oxidant injury. In Halliwell, B. (ed.) *Oxygen Radicals and Tissue Injury*, pp. 49–54. (FASEB)

8. Graham, D.G., Tiffany, S.M., Bell, W.R. Jr and Gutknecht, W.F. (1978). Auto-oxidation versus covalent binding of quinones as the mechanism of toxicity of dopamine, 6-hydroxy dopamine, and related compounds towards C1300 neuroblastoma cells in vitro. *Mol. Pharmacol.*, **14**, 644–53

9. Halliwell, B. and Gutteridge, J.M.C. (1988). Iron as a biological pro-oxidant. *ISI Atlas Sci. Biochem.*, **1**, 48–52

10. Halliwell, B. and Gutteridge, J.M.C. (1986). Oxygen free radicals and iron in relation to biology and medicine: some problems and concepts. *Arch. Biochem. Biophys.*, **246**, 501–14

11. Gutteridge, J.M.C., Halliwell, B., Treffry, A. *et al.* (1983). Effect of ferritin containing fractions with different iron loading on lipid peroxidation. *Biochem. J.*, **209**, 557–60

12. Puppo, A. and Halliwell, B. (1989). Oxidation of dimethylsulfoxide to formaldehyde by oxyhaemoglobin in the presence of hydrogen peroxide is not mediated by 'free' hydroxyl radicals. *Free Radical Res. Commun.*, **5**, 277–81

13. Hallgren, B. and Sourander, P. (1958). The effect of age on the non-haemin iron in the human brain. *J. Neurochem.*, **3**, 41–51

14. Olanow, C.W., Holgate, R.C., Murtagh, R. and Martinez, C. (1989). MR images in Parkinson's disease and aging. In Calne, D.B. *et al.* (eds.) *Parkinsonism and Aging*, pp. 155–64. (New York: Raven Press)

15. Fishman, J.B., Rubin, J.B., Handrahan, J.V. *et al.* (1987). Receptor-mediated transcytosis of transferrin across the blood–brain barrier. *J. Neurosci. Res.*, **18**, 299–304

16. Hill, J. and Switzer, R.C. III (1984). The regional distribution and cellular localization of iron in the rat brain. *Neuroscience*, **11**, 595–607

17. Connor, J.R., Menzies, S.L., St. Martin, S.M. and Musson, E.J. (1990). Cellular distribution of transferrin, ferritin and iron in normal and aged

human brains. *J. Neurosci. Res.*, **27**, 595–611

18. Langston, J.W., Ballard, J., Tetrud, J. and Erwin, I. (1983). Chronic parkinsonism in humans due to a product of meperidine-analog synthesis. *Science*, **219**, 979–80

19. Burns, R.S., Chieuh, C.C., Markey, S.P. *et al.* (1983). A primate model of parkinsonism: selective destruction of dopaminergic neurons in the pars compacta of the substantia nigra by N-methyl-4-phenyl-1,2,3,6-tetrahydropyridine. *Proc. Natl. Acad. Sci. USA*, **80**, 4546–50

20. Chiba, K., Trevor, A. and Castagnoli, N. Jr. (1984). Metabolism of the neurotoxic tertiary amine, MPTP, by brain monoamine oxidase. *Biochem. Biophys. Res. Commun.*, **120**, 547–78

21. Heikkila, R.E., Manzino, L., Cabbat, F.S. and Duvoisin, R.C. (1984). Protection against the dopaminergic neurotoxicity of 1-methyl-4-phenyl-1,2,5,6, tetrahydropyridine by monoamine oxidase inhibitors. *Nature (London)*, **311**, 467–9

22. Langston, J.W., Irwin, I., Langston, E.B. and Forno, L.S. (1984). Pargyline prevents MPTP-induced parkinsonism in primates. *Science*, **225**, 1480–2

23. Cohen, G., Pasik, P., Cohen, B. *et al.* (1984). Pargyline and deprenyl prevent the neurotoxicity of 1-methyl-4-phenyl-1,2,3,6-tetrahydropyridine (MPTP) in monkeys. *Eur. J. Pharmacol.*, **106**, 209–10

24. Earle, K.M. (1968). Studies in Parkinson's disease including X-ray fluorescent spectroscopy of formalin fixed brain tissue. *J. Neuropathol. Exp. Neurol.*, **27**, 1–14

25. Drayer, B., Burger, P., Darwin, R., Riederer, S. *et al.* (1986). Magnetic resonance imaging of brain iron. *AJNR*, **7**, 373–80

26. Olanow, C.W. and Drayer, B. (1987). Brain iron: MRI studies in Parkinson's syndrome. In Fahn, S., Marsden, C.D., Calne, D. and Goldstein, M. (eds.) *Recent Developments in Parkinson Disease*, Vol. II, pp. 135–43. (Florham Park, New Jersey: MacMillan Healthcare)

27. Dexter, D.T., Wells, F.R., Lees, A.J. *et al.* (1989). Increased nigral con content and alterations in other metal iron occurring in brain in Parkinson's disease. *J. Neurochem.*, **52**, 1830–6

28. Sofic, E., Riederer, P., Heinsen, H., Beckmann, H., Reynolds, G.P. *et al.* (1988). Increased iron (III) and total iron content in post mortem substantia nigra of parkinsonian brain. *J. Neural. Transm.*, **74**, 199–205

29. Hirsch, E.C., Brandel, J.P., Galle, P. *et al.* (1991). Iron and aluminium increase in the substantia nigra of patients with Parkinson's disease: an X-ray microanalysis. *J. Neurochem.*, **56**, 446–51

30. Youdim, M.B.H., Ben-Shachar, D. and Riederer, P. (1989). Is Parkinson's disease a progressive siderosis of substantia nigra resulting in iron and melanin-induced neurodegeneration? *Acta Neurol. Scand.*, **126**, 47–54

31. Mann, D.M.A. and Yates, P.O. (1974). Lipoprotein pigments – their relationship to aging in the human nervous system II. The melanin content of pigmented nerve cells. *Brain,* **97**, 489–98

32. Hirsch, E.C., Graybel, A.M. and Agid, Y.A. (1988). Melanized dopaminergic neurons are differentially susceptible to degeneration in Parkinson's disease. *Nature (London),* **334**, 345–8

33. Jellinger, K., Paulus, W., Grundke-Iqbal, I. *et al.* (1990). Brain iron and ferritin in Parkinson's and Alzheimer's disease. *J. Neural. Transm.,* **2**, 327–40

34. Dexter, D.T., Carayon, A., Vidaihet, M. *et al.* (1990). Decreased ferritin levels in brain in Parkinson's disease. *J. Neurochem.,* **55**, 16–20

35. Riederer, P., Sofic, E., Rausch, W. *et al.* (1989). Transition metals, ferritin, glutathione, and ascorbic acid in parkinsonian brains. *J. Neurochem.,* **52**, 515–20

36. Ben-Shachar, D., Eshel, G., Finberg, J.P.M. and Youdim, M. (1991). The iron chelator desferrioxamine (desferal) retards 6-hydroxy dopamine-induced degeneration of nigral striatal dopamine neurons. *J. Neurochem.,* **56**, 1441–4

37. Segstock, G.J., Olanow, C.W., Dunn, A.J. *et al.* (1991). Iron induces degeneration of substantia nigra neurons. *Mov. Disord.,* **6**, 272

38. Perry, T.L., Godin, D.V. and Hansen, S. (1982). Parkinson's disease: a disorder due to nigral glutathione deficiency? *Neurosci. Lett.,* **33**, 305–10

39. Dexter, D.T., Carter, C.J., Wells, F.R. *et al.* (1989). Basal lipid peroxidation in substantia nigra is increased in Parkinson's disease. *J. Neurochem.,* **52**, 381–9

40. Zigmond, M.J., Abercrombie, E.D., Berger, T.W. *et al.* (1990). Compensation after lesions of central dopaminergic neurons: some clinical and basic implications. *Trends Neurosci.,* **13**, 290–5

41. Spina, M.B. and Cohen, G. (1989). Dopamine turnover and glutathione oxidation: implications for Parkinson's disease. *Proc. Natl. Acad. Sci. USA,* **86**, 1398–400

42. Spina, M.B. and Cohen, G. (1988). Exposure of striatal synaptosomes to L-dopa elevates levels of oxidized glutathione. *J. Pharmacol. Exp. Ther.,* **247**, 502–7

43. Cohen, G. and Spina, M.B. (1989). Deprenyl suppresses the oxidant stress associated with increased dopamine turnover. *Ann. Neurol.,* **26**, 689–90

44. Werner, P. and Cohen, G. (1991). Intramitochondrial formation of oxidized glutathione during the oxidation of benzylamine by monoamine oxidase. *FEBS Lett.,* **280**, 44–6

45. Sandri, G., Panfili, E. and Ernster, L. (1990). Hydrogen peroxide production by monoamine oxidase in isolated rat brain mitochondria: its effect on

glutathione levels and Ca^{2+} efflux. *Biochem. Biophys. Acta GNL Subj.*, **1035**, 300–5

46. Phebus, L.A., Perry, K.W., Clemens, J.A. and Fuller, R.W. (1986). Brain anoxia release of strial dopamine in rats. *Life Sci.*, **38**, 2447–53

47. Slivka, A., Brannan, P.S., Weinberger, J. *et al.* (1988). Increase in extracellular dopamine in the striatum during cerebral ischemia. A study utilizing cerebral microdialysis. *J. Neuro. Chem.*, **50**, 1714–18

48. Clemens, J.A. and Phebus, L.A. (1988). Dopamine depletion protects striatal neurons from ischemia-induced cell death. *Life Sci.*, **42**, 707–13

49. Felten, D.L., Felten, S.Y., Fuller, R.W. *et al.* (1992). Chronic dietary pergolide preserves nigrostriatal neuronal integrity in aged Fischer 344 rats. *Neurobiol. Aging*, in press

50. Michel, P.P. and Hefti, F. (1990). Toxicity of 6-hydroxydopamine and dopamine for dopaminergic neurons in cultures. *J. Neurosci. Res.*, **26**, 428–35

51. Mizuno, Y., Ohta, S., Tanaka, M. *et al.* (1989). Deficiencies in complex I subunits of the respiratory chain in Parkinson's disease. *Biochem. Biophys. Res. Commun.*, **163**, 1450–5

52. Schapira, A.H.V., Cooper, J.M. *et al.* (1989). Mitochondrial complex I deficiency in Parkinson's disease. *Lancet*, **1**, 1269

53. Parker, W.D., Boyson, S.J. and Parks, J.K. (1989). Abnormalities of the electron transport chain in idiopathic Parkinson's disease. *Ann. Neurol.*, **26**, 719–23

54. Shoffner, J.M., Watts, R.L., Juncos, J.L., Torroni, A. and Wallace, D.C. (1991). Mitochondrial oxidative phosphorylation defects in Parkinson's disease. *Ann. Neurol.*, **30**, 332–9

55. Nicklas, W.J., Vyas, I. and Heikkila, R.E. (1985). Inhibition of NADH-linked oxidation in brain mitochondria by 1-methyl-4-phenyl-pyridinium, a metabolite of the neurotoxin 1-methyl-4-phenyl-1,2,5,6-tetrahydropyridine. *Life Sci.*, **36**, 2503–8

56. Chomyn, A., Mariotinni, P., Cleeter, M.J.W. *et al.* (1985). Functional assignment of the unidentified reading frames of human mitochondrial DNA. In Quagliariello, E., Slater, E.C., Palmierri, F., Saccone, C. and Kroon, E.M. (eds.) *Achievements and Prospectives in Mitochondrial Research*, Vol. 11, pp. 259–75. (Amsterdam: Elsevier)

57. Reichter, C., Park, J.W. and Ames, B.N. (1988). Normal oxidative damage to mitochondrial and nuclear DNA is extensive. *Proc. Natl. Acad. Sci. USA*, **85**, 6465–7

58. Yong, V.W., Perry, T.L. and Krisman, A.A. (1986). Depletion of glutathione in brain stem of mice caused by 1-methyl-4-phenyl-1,2,3,6-tetrahydropyridine is prevented by antioxidant pretreatment. *Neurosci. Lett.*, **63**, 56–60

59. McNeil, T.H., Koek, L.L., Haycock, J.W. and Gash, D.M. (1988). Glutathione reduction mimics MPTP neurotixicity and age correlated changes in dopamine neurons in substantia nigra of the C57BL/6NNIA mouse. *Soc. Neurosci.*, (Abstr. 1986), **12**, 1470

60. Jain, A., Martensson, J., Stole, E. *et al.* (1991). Glutathione deficiency leads to mitochondrial damage in brain. *Proc. Natl. Acad. Sci. USA.*, **88**, 1913–17

61. The Parkinson's Study Group. (1989). Effect of deprenyl on the progression of disability in early Parkinson's disease. *N. Engl. J. Med.*, **321**, 1364–71

62. Olanow, C.W. and Calne, D.B. (1991). Does deprenyl monotherapy in Parkinson's disease act by symptomatic or protective mechanisms? *Neurology*, in press

63. Olney, J.W. (1989). Excitatory and N-methyl-D-aspartate receptors. *Drug Dev. Res.*, **17**, 299–319

64. Hyman, C., Hofer, M., Barde, Y.A. *et al.* (1991). BDNF is a neurotrophic factor for dopaminergic neurons of the substantia nigra. *Nature (London)*, **350**, 230–2

5

Molecular biology of dopamine receptors: clinical implications

G.F. Wooten

INTRODUCTION

In the vertebrate central nervous system, dopamine initiates its physiological effects by binding to neuronal cell surface receptors. Such synaptic actions of dopamine are directly involved in the initiation and control of movement, the regulation of emotional states, and the inhibition of tonic prolactin release from the anterior pituitary. Based on several lines of evidence, Kebabian and Calne in 1979 proposed the existence of two types of dopamine receptors, now termed D_1 and D_2[1]. These two dopamine receptors are distinguished by their G-protein (guanine nucleotide-binding protein) coupling[1,2], selective binding to specific agonist and antagonist ligands[3], physiological and metabolic effects[4], and regional distribution in the brain[5] (Table 1).

CLONING OF THE D_2 DOPAMINE RECEPTOR

Occupation of the D_2 dopamine receptor activates second messenger systems via interactions with G-proteins. Previous studies of receptor families coupled to such G-proteins have revealed a significant similarity of amino acid sequences and a common topology consisting of seven lipophilic, hydrophobic, transmembrane domains[6]. Bunzow and colleagues, in the laboratory of Olivier Civelli, exploited the predicted

Table 1 Properties of D_1 and D_2 dopamine receptors

	D_1	D_2
G-protein coupling	G_s	G_i
Effect on adenylate cyclase activity	stimulates	inhibits or unlinked
Selective agonists	SKF 38393, A-68930	quinpyrole, PHNO
Selective antagonists	SCH 23390	raclopride, sulpiride
Effect on striatal acetylcholine release	little	inhibits
Effect on striatal GABA★ release	stimulates	no effect
Effect on nigral and medial pallidal glucose utilization	increases	no effect
Regional localization	striatum, substantia nigra, pars reticulata, medial globus pallidus	striatum, substantia nigra pars compacta

★ γ-aminobutyric acid

similarities in nucleotide sequence of the members of this gene family to isolate genes coding for related, but previously unisolated, receptors[7]. Using the hamster β_2-adrenergic receptor gene as a hybridization probe, they succeeded in isolating a cDNA encoding the rat brain D_2 receptor. This cDNA contained 2455 bases, the longest open reading frame coded for a 415 amino acid protein ($M_r = 47\,064$). A deglycosylated form of the D_2 dopamine receptor has been reported to have a similar relative molecular mass. Northern blot analysis of mRNA to this cDNA clone showed a regional distribution in rat brain similar to that of D_2 dopamine receptor binding sites. Furthermore, mouse fibroblast cells transfected with the cDNA expressed binding sites on their membranes, the binding properties of which were characteristic of the D_2 dopamine receptor (see Figure 1).

Using a different cloning strategy, Todd and colleagues have established a transfected mouse fibroblast cell line that expresses a binding site similar to the D_2 receptor which appears to be linked functionally to calcium channels[8]. In addition, this receptor appears to be distinct from the one reported by Bunzow and co-workers, but the new clone

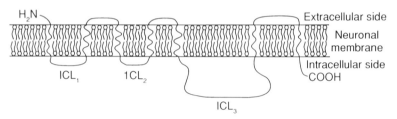

Figure 1 Proposed structure of D$_2$ dopamine receptor. Seven membrane-spanning segments of the polypeptide are postulated with three intracytoplasmic loops (ICL$_{1-3}$), an extracellular amino terminal and an intracellular carboxy terminal

of Todd and colleagues has not yet been sequenced for comparison purposes.

In 1989, at least two groups reported the successful cloning of the cDNA and gene for a human D$_2$ dopamine receptor. Grandy and colleagues isolated a clone from a human pituitary cDNA library with a deduced protein sequence 96% identical to that of the cloned rat receptor[9]. The one difference was that the human receptor contained an additional 29 amino acids in its third cytoplasmic loop. Similar findings were reported by Selbie and colleagues[10].

Molecular cloning and expression of a D$_2$ dopamine receptor from human retina have also been reported[11]. This clone encodes a protein that differs from the rat brain D$_2$ dopamine receptor by 18 amino acids.

MULTIPLE FORMS OF THE D$_2$ DOPAMINE RECEPTOR: ALTERNATIVE SPLICING

Since the initial report of the cloning and sequencing of the rat brain D$_2$ dopamine receptor in December 1988, many laboratories have reported the existence of at least two forms of the D$_2$ receptor in both brain and pituitary tissue from man and rat[12-16]. The gene for the D$_2$ receptor appears to produce two isoforms by alternative mRNA splicing. One isoform corresponds to the sequence reported by Bunzow and colleagues[7], but the second contains an additional sequence encoding a 29-amino acid fragment that is located within the third cytoplasmic loop that binds to G-proteins[12-16]. It seems that most genes coding for the superfamily of G-protein-coupled receptors do not have introns but rather encode a unique polypeptide product. Because the D$_2$ dopamine receptor gene appears to code for two isoforms, the potential exists for the two isoforms to interact with different G-proteins or even distinct second messenger systems.

Recent evidence suggests that the larger of the two forms predominates in both rat and human brain[14]. Whether these isoforms are regulated physiologically is not yet known.

HUMAN D₂ DOPAMINE RECEPTOR GENE ON CHROMOSOME ELEVEN

By probing a chromosome mapping panel with rat D_2 dopamine receptor cDNA, Grandy and colleagues succeeded in localizing the gene for the D_2 dopamine receptor on the long arm of chromosome eleven[17]. Further studies localized the gene to the q22–q23 junction of chromosome eleven, a gene locus containing a frequent TaqI RFLP. Recently, the gene for ataxia telangiectasia was assigned to the same region of chromosome 11.

The balance of current evidence suggests that there is a single gene encoding for brain and pituitary D_2 dopamine receptor protein and that this coding sequence is interrupted by introns, allowing different forms of the D_2 receptor to be synthesized by the mechanism of alternative splicing.

FUNCTIONAL CHARACTERIZATION OF THE D₂ DOPAMINE RECEPTOR PROTEIN

Knowledge of the amino acid sequence of the D_2 dopamine receptor and the ability to mass-produce cells that express the D_2 receptor provide a powerful new tool for pharmacologists. With knowledge of the primary structure and deduced tertiary conformation of the D_2 receptor, particularly of the ligand binding site, it will be possible to design drugs that optimally interact with the binding sites. Furthermore, screening of new drugs will be greatly facilitated, largely obviating the need for costly and time-consuming *in vivo* behavioral tests. Numerous studies of clonal cell lines expressing the D_2 receptor have already demonstrated their utility for binding studies.

Albert[18] and Neve[19] and their colleagues have functionally characterized the D_2 receptor expressed in pituitary-derived cell lines that do not normally express the receptor. Their work demonstrated several, critical, functional properties of the D_2 receptor: the D_2 dopamine receptor clearly interacted with one or more G-proteins because addition of guanosine triphosphate (GTP) and sodium chloride increased the IC_{50} value for dopamine competition for spiperone binding sites by two-fold; addition of dopamine decreased resting intra- and extracellular cAMP levels by 50-70% and completely blocked the capacity of vasoactive intestinal polypeptide (VIP) to increase cAMP levels; dopa-mine agonists inhibited forskolin-stimulated adenylate cyclase activity by almost 50%; and dopamine abolished the acute release of prolactin following treatment with either VIP or thyrotropin-releasing hormone.

Future studies in such transfected cell lines should provide more information as to the molecular interaction between the receptor protein, G-proteins, and adenylate cyclase. Insights into the mechanisms of how D_2 receptor occupation is transduced into effects on other second messenger systems should also evolve. New knowledge in these areas will provide the groundwork for novel drug strategies that would modify the effects of dopaminergic drugs.

REGULATION OF D_2 RECEPTOR EXPRESSION

Such diverse clinical phenomena as tardive dyskinesias and levodopa-induced psychosis have been hypothesized to occur as the result of the regulation or modification of dopamine receptor expression. The new molecular biological tools derived from cloning and sequencing the D_2 receptor will facilitate the study of the effects of dopamine denervation and chronic drug treatments on the expression of the D_2 dopamine receptor as manifested by changes in mRNA levels encoding the receptor. Studies of the rate of synthesis of new mRNA, of translation, of the insertion of receptor into membrane, and of receptor degradation are all now feasible. Hypotheses regarding the molecular mechanism(s) of change in sensitivity to dopamine can now be addressed with much less ambiguity than previous methods allowed.

A recent study by Autelitano and colleagues[20] elegantly demonstrated tissue-specific regulation of D_2 dopamine receptor mRNA in comparison to other receptor mRNAs in cells from anterior and intermediate lobes of the rat pituitary gland. Such studies represent the initial forays into an entirely new field addressing the question of how dopamine receptor occupation on cell surfaces is translated into regulation of the gene coding for the dopamine receptor.

REGIONAL AND CELLULAR LOCALIZATION OF THE D_2 DOPAMINE RECEPTOR

Since the sequence of the D_2 dopamine receptor has been reported, many groups have synthesized radiolabeled cDNA or oligonucleotide probes and performed *in situ* hybridization histochemical mapping studies of the regional distribution of mRNA encoding the D_2 receptor[21–25]. The results are similar to receptor autoradiographic studies of the regional binding of radiolabeled D_2 receptor-specific ligands, with the highest levels of D_2 mRNA reported in the substantia nigra, ventral tegmental area, caudate, putamen, nucleus accumbens, olfactory tubercle, and the neurointermediate lobe of the pituitary.

An important promise of *in situ* hybridization with radiolabeled probes for the D_2 receptor mRNA is to take mapping studies to the cellular level of resolution. No satisfactory irreversible binding ligands have been developed for the D_2 dopamine receptor; therefore, high resolution autoradiographic mapping studies are not technically feasible. All of the currently available ligands wash off the tissue when exposed to liquid emulsion. In contrast, cDNA and oligonucleotide probes hybridize to the receptor mRNA almost irreversibly under the conditions used.

Only a few reports of the cellular localization of D_2 dopamine receptor mRNA in the striatum have appeared as yet. Le Moine and colleagues[25] reported that all enkephalin-expressing neurons in the striatum also contained D_2 receptor mRNA, and that a separate population of large striatal neurons also expressed D_2 mRNA but not preproenkephalin mRNA. Also, Fink and colleagues[26] have reported that D_2 receptor mRNA was expressed in virtually all large neurons of the striatum, most of which are cholinergic, as well as in a subset of medium-sized striatal neurons. These findings are consistent and indicate that not all neurons in the striatum express the D_2 receptor. A full description of the co-localization of D_2 receptor expression and other transmitter-specific markers will surely provide a new layer of understanding regarding the functional anatomy of the basal ganglia.

CLONING OF THE D₁ DOPAMINE RECEPTOR

Several groups have reported the successful cloning of the D_1 dopamine receptor. Dearry and colleagues[27] have isolated a clone from a human genomic library, the open reading frame of which encodes a protein of 447 amino acids with the typical seven hydrophobic stretches presumed to be transmembrane domains. The homology of this clone was extensive with respect to the D_2 dopamine receptor and other catecholamine receptors, especially within the transmembrane domains. Expression of this DNA in COS-7 cells resulted in these cells expressing binding sites for [³H]SCH 23390 and [¹²⁵I]SCH 23982 with high affinity ($K_d = 100$ and $350\,pM$, respectively) and selective binding properties characteristic of the D_1 dopamine receptor. In cells expressing this clone, dopamine administration resulted in the elevation of cyclic AMP levels as would be predicted. Studies employing Northern analysis and *in situ* hybridization indicated that this clone is expressed primarily in the striatum.

Sibley and co-workers[28] utilized the polymerase chain reaction technique to amplify a putative D_1 dopamine receptor sequence using mRNA from NS20Y cells, which are known to express the D_1 receptor positively linked to adenylate cyclase. Using Northern blot analysis of brain tissue, transcripts were localized predominantly in striatal tissue. A high concentration of mRNA was also found in the striatum and the olfactory tubercle using *in situ* hybridization. Pharmacological studies of clones expressing this probe, in order to confirm its identity, have not yet been published.

Thus, it appears that the D_1 dopamine receptor has been sequenced and cloned but no information is yet available on the regulation, chromosomal localization, or cellular localization of the D_1 receptor using molecular biological techniques. Harrison and colleagues[29] have employed retrograde lesion techniques to obtain data suggesting that D_1 dopamine receptors are selectively, if not exclusively, expressed by striatonigral neurons. These data coupled with the studies of D_2 dopamine receptor mRNA expression cited above strongly suggest that striatonigral neurons selectively express D_1 receptors while intrinsic striatal neurons and striatal neurons projecting to the external segment of the globus pallidus selectively express D_2 receptors. Confirmation of this suggestion awaits double-label *in situ* hybridization studies, with probes for each dopamine receptor site.

CLINICAL IMPLICATIONS

Knowledge of the sequence and three-dimensional conformation of D_1 and D_2 dopamine receptor binding sites will permit structure–activity studies to define how agonists and antagonists bind to the receptor. This information should facilitate the rational design of new drugs. Such detailed information will also facilitate direct molecular studies of how binding site occupation is transduced into the generation of intracellular second messengers. This information could define new sites of drug action to modify the effects of dopamine agonists and antagonists.

Hypotheses regarding mechanisms of changes in sensitivity to agonists will be directly testable for the first time. Changes in receptor number may be recognized as due either to increased synthesis of receptor or decreased degradation.

With the knowledge of normal dopamine receptor structure, disease states due to abnormal D_1 and D_2 dopamine receptors may now be identified and characterized.

REFERENCES

1. Kebabian, J.W. and Calne, D.B. (1979). Multiple receptors for dopamine. *Nature (London)*, **277**, 93–6
2. Onali, P., Olianas, M.C. and Gessa, G.L. (1985). Characterization of dopamine receptors mediating inhibition of adenylate cyclase activity in rat striatum. *Mol. Pharmacol.*, **28**, 138–45
3. Stoof, J.C. and Kebabian, J.W. (1984). Two dopamine receptors: Biochemistry, physiology, and pharmacology. *Life Sci.*, **35**, 2281–96
4. Trugman, J.T. and Wooten, G.F. (1987). Selective D_1 and D_2 dopamine agonists differentially alter basal ganglia glucose utilization in rats with

unilateral 6-hydroxydopamine substantia nigra lesions. *J. Neurosci.*, **7**, 2927–35

5. Boyson, S.J., McGonigle, P. and Molinoff, P.B. (1986). Quantitative autoradiographic localization of the D_1 and D_2 subtypes of dopamine receptors in rat brain. *J. Neurosci.*, **6**, 3177–88

6. Lefkowitz, R.J. and Caron, M.G. (1988). Adrenergic receptors: Model for the study of receptors coupled to guanine nucleotide regulatory proteins. *J. Biol. Chem.*, **263**, 4993–6

7. Bunzow, J.R., Van Tol, H.H.M., Grandy, D.K., Albert, P., Salon, J., Christie, M., Machida, C.A., Neve, K.A. and Civelli, O. (1988). Cloning and expression of a rat D_2 dopamine receptor cDNA. *Nature (London)*, **336**, 783–7

8. Todd, R.D., Khurana, T.S., Sajovic, P., Stone, K.R. and O'Malley, K.L. (1989). Cloning of ligand-specific cell lines via gene transfer: Identification of a D_2 dopamine receptor subtype. *Proc. Natl. Acad. Sci. USA*, **86**, 10134–8

9. Grandy, D.K., Marchionni, M.A., Makam, H., Stofko, R.E., Alfano, M., Frothingham, L., Fischer, J.B., Burke-Howie, K.J., Bunzow, J.R., Server, A.C. and Civelli, O. (1989). Cloning of the cDNA and gene for a human D_2 dopamine receptor. *Proc. Natl. Acad. Sci. USA*, **86**, 9762–6

10. Selbie, L.A., Hayes, G. and Shine, J. (1989). The major dopamine D_2 receptor: Molecular analysis of the human D_{2A} subtype. *DNA*, **8**, 683–9

11. Stormann, T.M., Gdula, D.C., Weiner, D.M. and Brann, M.R. (1989). Molecular cloning and expression of a dopamine D_2 receptor from human retina. *Mol. Pharmacol.*, **37**, 1–6

12. Giros, B., Sokoloff, P., Martres, M.-P., Riou, J.-F., Emorine, L.J. and Schwartz, J.-C. (1989). Alternative splicing directs the expression of two D_2 dopamine receptor isoforms. *Nature (London)*, **342**, 923–6

13. Monsma Jr., F.J., McVittie, L.D., Gerfen, C.R., Mahan, L.C. and Sibley, D.R. (1989). Multiple D_2 dopamine receptors produced by alternative RNA splicing. *Nature (London)*, **342**, 926–9

14. Toso, R.D., Sommer, B., Ewert, M., Herb, A., Pritchett, D.B., Bach, A., Shivers, B.D. and Seeburg, P.H. (1989). The dopamine D_2 receptor: two molecular forms generated by alternative splicing. *EMBO J.*, **8**, 4025–34

15. Miller, J.C., Wang, Y. and Filer, D. (1990). Identification by sequence analysis of a second rat brain cDNA encoding the dopamine (D_2) receptor. *Biochem. Biophys. Res. Commun.*, **166**, 109–12

16. Chio, C.L., Hess, G.F., Graham, R.S. and Huff, R.M. (1990). A second molecular form of D_2 dopamine receptor in rat and bovine caudate nucleus.

Nature (London), **343**, 266–9

17. Grandy, D.K., Litt, M., Allen, L., Bunzow, J.R., Marchionni, M., Makam, H., Reed, L., Magenis, R.E. and Civelli, O. (1989). The human dopamine D_2 receptor gene is located on chromosome 11 at q22–q23 and identifies a TaqI RFLP. *Am. J. Hum. Genet.,* **45**, 778–85

18. Albert, P.R., Neve, K.A., Bunzow, J.R. and Civelli, O. (1990). Coupling of a cloned rat dopamine-D_2 receptor to inhibition of adenylyl cyclase and prolactin secretion. *J. Biol. Chem.,* **265**, 2098–104

19. Neve, K.A., Henningsen, R.A., Bunzow, J.R. and Civelli, O. (1989). Functional characterization of a rat dopamine D_2 receptor cDNA expressed in a mammalian cell line. *Mol. Pharmacol.,* **36**, 446–51

20. Autelitano, D.J., Snyder, L., Sealfon, S.C. and Roberts, J.L. (1989). Dopamine D_2-receptor messenger RNA is differentially regulated by dopaminergic agents in rat anterior and neurointermediate pituitary. *Mol. Cell. Endocrinol.,* **67**, 101–5

21. Weiner, D.M. and Brann, M.R. (1989). The distribution of a dopamine D_2 receptor mRNA in rat brain. *FEBS Lett.,* **253**, 207–13

22. Najlerahim, A., Barton, A.J.L., Harrison, P.J., Heffernan, J. and Pearson, R.C.A. (1989). Messenger RNA encoding the D_2 dopaminergic receptor detected by *in situ* hybridization histochemistry in rat brain. *FEBS Lett.,* **255**, 335–9

23. Meador-Woodruff, J.H., Mansour, A., Bunzow, J.R., Van Tol, H.H.M., Watson Jr., S.J. and Civelli, O. (1989). Distribution of D_2 dopamine receptor mRNA in rat brain. *Proc. Natl. Acad. Sci. USA,* **86**, 7625–8

24. Mengod, G., Martinez-Mir, M.I., Vilaró, M.T. and Palacios, J.M. (1989). Localization of the mRNA for the dopamine D_2 receptor in the rat brain by *in situ* hybridization histochemistry. *Proc. Natl. Acad. Sci. USA,* **86**, 8560–4

25. Le Moine, C., Normand, E., Guitteny, A.F., Fouque, B., Teoule, R. and Bloch, B. (1990). Dopamine receptor gene expression by enkephalin neurons in rat forebrain. *Proc. Natl. Acad. Sci. USA,* **87**, 230–4

26. Fink, J.S., DiFiglia, M. and Aronin, N. (1990). Two molecular forms of the D-2 receptor are expressed in subsets of neurons in the rat striatum. *Movement Disorders,* **5** (Suppl. 1), 88

27. Dearry, A., Gingrich, J.A., Falardeau, P., Fremeau, R., Bates, M.D. and Caron, M.A. (1990). Isolation and cloning of the D1 dopamine receptor. *Dopamine 90,* (Abstr.), p. 1. *Satellite Meeting of the XIth International Congress of Pharmacology,* Cono, Italy

28. Sibley, D.R., Monsma, F.J., McVittie, L.D., Gerfen, C.R. and Mahan,

L.C. (1990). Molecular biology of dopamine receptor subtypes. *Dopamine 90*, (Abstr.), p. 2. *Satellite Meeting of the XIth International Congress of Pharmacology*, Cono, Italy

29. Harrison, M.B., Wiley, R.G. and Wooten, G.F. (1990). Selective localization of striatal D_1 receptors to striatonigral neurons. *Brain Res.*, **528**, 317–22

6

Adverse effects of levodopa

S. Fahn

INTRODUCTION

It is generally believed that almost all symptoms in Parkinson's disease are due to progressive loss of monoaminergic neurons, with the consequent loss of monoamines in the nerve terminals normally found at the target structures. Theoretically then, all patients with Parkinson's disease or other causes of striatal dopamine deficiency, such as postencephalitic parkinsonism and reserpine-induced parkinsonism, should respond to dopamine replacement therapy provided that:

(1)   The postsynaptic dopamine receptors are intact,

(2)   The medication can reach the target (i.e. these dopamine receptors), and

(3)   The medication is not toxic and can be tolerated by the patient.

Indeed, there are rarely any failures with levodopa therapy in the early years of treatment with this drug. Unfortunately, such a good response is not commonly maintained. Most patients develop adverse effects after long-term usage of levodopa. In some, the benefit from levodopa seen in the early years of treatment wanes. Some patients who respond early in the course of their illness and then fail may actually have some other cause of parkinsonism, so-called parkinsonism-plus syndromes, such as striatonigral degeneration and supranuclear palsy. In this chapter, I will restrict my comments to Parkinson's disease and not discuss these other types of parkinsonism.

89

In this chapter, I review the adverse effects in 330 Parkinson's disease patients who had been receiving levodopa for more than 5 years. The data were obtained from the Parkinson's disease (PD) database of the Movement Disorder Group at the Neurological Institute, Columbia-Presbyterian Medical Center in New York City. The database listed 2161 patients with parkinsonism, of whom 1619 were diagnosed as having Parkinson's disease; the remainder had some other form of parkinsonism. Of the Parkinson's disease patients, there were sufficient data on 858 regarding their levodopa treatment history; 330 of them had been on levodopa for more than 5 years. This group of 330 patients consisted of 189 men and 141 women. The duration of levodopa therapy was 6–7 years: 35%; 8–9 years: 20%; 10–11 years: 16%; 12–15 years: 21%; > 15 years: 8%.

With long-term treatment with levodopa (defined as greater than 5 years), only approximately 25% of patients were continuing to have a good, smooth response at the time of this analysis. Most patients were having either troublesome fluctuations, troublesome dyskinesias, toxicity at therapeutic or sub-therapeutic dosages, or total or substantial loss of efficacy (Table 1). This review will cover only the major complications of levodopa. For a more detailed review of the complications, the reader is referred to the review article by Fahn[1]. A listing of the types of fluctuations and dyskinesias is presented in Table 2.

TROUBLESOME FLUCTUATIONS

The most common complication of long-term levodopa therapy is the development of fluctuations in clinical response (Table 1). By fluctuations, I refer to the presence of periods during the day when the patient is not responding as adequately as he/she normally does to levodopa; these periods of poor response are called 'off' periods. There are several types of fluctuations (Table 2), and I will review their highlights. Details of the clinical descriptions and pathophysiology of the fluctuations can be found in other reviews[2,3]. One should not mistake an 'off' phenomenon with transient 'freezing' or motor blocks that last only a few seconds, before the block is dissipated.

Table 1 Five major responses to more than 5 years of levodopa therapy (*n* = 330 patients). This table was derived from the Parkinson's disease database of the Movement Disorder Group at the Neurological Institute, Columbia-Presbyterian Medical Center in New York City. The database listed 2161 patients with parkinsonism, of whom 1619 were diagnosed as having Parkinson's disase, the remainder with some other form of parkinsonism. Of the Parkinson's disease patients, 858 were recorded as receiving levodopa, 330 of them being on levodopa for more than 5 years. This group of 330 patients consists of 189 men and 141 women. The duration of levodopa therapy was 6–7 years: 35%; 8–9 years: 20%; 10–11 years: 16%; 12–15 years: 21%; > 15 years: 8%. Thirty-six patients were considered to have both troublesome fluctuations and troublesome dyskinesias

	n	%
Smooth, good response	83	25
Troublesome fluctuations	142	43
Troublesome dyskinesias	67	19
Toxicity at therapeutic or subtherapeutic dosages	14	4
Total or substantial loss of efficacy	27	8

Table 2 Major fluctuations and dyskinesias as complications of levodopa

Fluctuations ('offs')	Dyskinesias
Slow 'wearing-off'	Peak-dose chorea and dystonia
Sudden 'off'	Diphasic chorea and dystonia
Random 'off'	'Off' dystonia
Yo-yo-ing	Myoclonus
Episodic failure to respond	Simultaneous dyskinesia and
Delayed 'on'	parkinsonism
Weak response at end of day	
Response varies in relationship to meals	
Sudden transient freezing	

'Wearing-off' phenomenon

The 'wearing-off' phenomenon, also known as the 'end-of-dose deterioration' is the most common type of fluctuation. Of 330 patients who had been treated with levodopa for more than 5 years, 172 of them had the wearing-off phenomenon (Table 3); in 117 of them the wearing-off

Table 3 Clinical fluctuations seen in patients who have been receiving levodopa therapy for more than 5 years ($n = 330$ patients). These recorded adverse effects were not necessarily considered to be troublesome, so they do not match with the data presented in Table 1

'Offs'	n	%	Comments
Wearing-off	172	52	117 had troublesome fluctuations
Sudden off	63	19	83% also had wearing-off phenomenon
			59% had random offs
Random off	74	22	80% also had wearing-off
Failure to respond to every dose	48	15	79% are troublesome fluctuators
Delayed 'on'	54	16	all except 12 had troublesome fluctuations
'Off' in morning	79	24	all except 18 had troublesome fluctuations
'Off' in afternoon	52	16	all except 12 had troublesome fluctuations
'Off' in evening	45	14	all except 10 had troublesome fluctuations
'Off' with high protein	32	10	75% are troublesome fluctuators

phenomenon represented a major problem (i.e. troublesome fluctuations). The wearing-off phenomenon is manifested as a gradual fading of benefit, occurring usually between 1 and 3 h after taking a dose of levodopa. The shorter the time period that a good response persists, the more severe the wearing-off problem is. Patients feel as if their medication is wearing off, hence its name. Although it can appear early in the course of therapy if the disease is severe, as in the patients with MPTP-induced parkinsonism[4], in Parkinson's disease the prevalence increases as a function of duration of therapy[5]. The major risk factors for this and other fluctuations appears to be duration[6,7] and dosage[8] of levodopa therapy.

In patients with the wearing-off problem, the clinical improvement from a dose of levodopa lasts only as long as the plasma level of levodopa is high[9]. As the plasma level gradually falls, there is a loss of clinical response. If the plasma level can be maintained, the clinical response can also be maintained[10,11]. Providing a continuous supply of dopamine or dopamine agonist to the striatum, such as by intravenous[12] or intestinal[13] infusion of levodopa, or by subcutaneous infusion of dopamine agonist[14] can overcome this type of fluctuation. Thus, benefit depends upon a steady supply of levodopa in the plasma to reach the brain in a constant influx. Patients with a smooth response to levodopa have the same pattern of plasma levels of levodopa. So, it seems likely that some central factors must differ between patients with the wearing-off problem and those who do not have this difficulty.

Loss of storage sites of dopamine in the striatum, where dopamine is usually present in the terminals of the dopaminergic nigrostriatal fibers, is probably one explanation, but not the sole cause, of this problem. Such a mechanism cannot explain why younger patients are more prone to develop fluctuations, compared to older patients[15]. Nor would it explain why using low doses of levodopa instead of high doses would delay the development of this problem[8].

Furthermore, treatment with direct-acting agonists does not eliminate the problem, although it does ameliorate it somewhat by making the depths of the 'off' state less severe. Rinne[16,17] showed that if dopamine agonists are used early in the course of treatment, the 'wearing-off' phenomenon is virtually avoided. This observation would imply that levodopa itself or the peaks and valleys of supplying the brain with levodopa may be responsible for contributing to this problem. How levodopa or dopamine could result in this phenomenon is unclear. The use of low doses of levodopa[8] or the delay of the introduction of levodopa delays the start of this problem[18]. It seems that central as well as peripheral pharmacokinetic and pharmacodynamic mechanisms are both involved in the pathophysiology of these problems[19-21].

Treatment of the wearing-off problem consists of utilizing selegiline, giving the doses of levodopa closer together, and utilizing direct-acting dopamine agonists, which have a longer biological half-life than levodopa. When Sinemet CR® becomes available, this drug should be tried[22].

'Sudden-off' phenomenon

Whereas the 'wearing-off' phenomenon is a gradual lack of benefit from levodopa that takes many minutes to develop its full depth, the 'sudden-off' phenomenon occurs within several seconds to reach full depth. Moreover, it tends to be more random and unpredictable, since it does not usually occur at a set time following a dose of levodopa. Of the 330 patients receiving levodopa for more than 5 years, 63 had sudden offs, and 74 had random offs (Table 3), with the majority in each group having the combination. In the 'sudden-off' disorder, the patient can improve just as suddenly, even without taking another dose of levodopa. Pharmacological studies have revealed that plasma levels of levodopa were in the declining phase when the 'offs' appear[23]. It has been speculated that the 'sudden-off' problem is due to a sudden and transient desensitization blockade of the dopamine receptors that would be compatible with the receptor switching from a high-affinity to a low-affinity state[23]. Response to an injection of apomorphine[24,25] is compatible with the stimulation of a desensitized receptor, and this result is not incompatible with the hypothesis. It is now clear that direct-acting dopamine agonists amantadine and selegiline are ineffective, and the 'sudden-off' phenomenon remains a difficult problem to overcome. The 'sudden-off' phenomenon is predominantly a pharmacodynamic problem, whereas the 'wearing-off' phenomenon is a pharmacokinetic one.

Episodic failure to respond

Another fairly common type of fluctuation is the episodic failure to respond to each dose. This problem is related to poor gastric empty-ing[26,27]. This problem can be overcome by dissolving levodopa in liquid prior to ingesting it. This type of fluctuation is probably more common than is usually recognized. In a survey of their patients Melamed and colleagues[28] found a number of patients with this difficulty. It is not clear if the delayed gastric emptying is due to levodopa therapy itself or if the disorder develops because frequent dosing will statistically result in some tablets not passing through the stomach quickly enough to reach the small intestine where absorption takes place. This problem was present in 48 of the 330 patients taking levodopa for more than 5 years (Table 3).

Delayed 'on'

Melamed and Bitton[29] reported that patients with fluctuations often also have a problem in getting an 'on' with the first dose in the morning. These patients tend to have a longer delay with this dose than the non-fluctuator. Fifty-four of the 330 patients receiving levodopa for more than 5 years had this problem (Table 3). The mechanism is not clear, but it may have to do with obtaining adequate plasma levels. I have noticed that many patients need a larger dosage of levodopa as their first dose of the day in order to 'kick-in' a response to the medication. Since the first dose is often accompanied by a higher plasma level of levodopa than later doses[2,10], the problem may not be entirely pharmacokinetic. Rather, it is possible that the dopamine receptors are in a low-affinity state and require more dopamine agonism to activate them. To treat the delayed 'on' by obtaining a higher plasma level of levodopa sooner, the patient should dissolve Sinemet before swallowing.

We noted whether patients tended to have more parkinsonism in the beginning, middle or end of the day. Of the 330 patients receiving levodopa for more than 5 years, 79 tended to be 'off' in the morning, 52 tended to be 'off' in the afternoon, and 45 'off' in the evening (Table 3).

Table 4 examines only those fluctuations that were considered severe enough to be 'troublesome' and not all recorded fluctuations. Patients can have more than one type of troublesome fluctuations, but 82% of the troublesome fluctuations were of the wearing-off type (Table 4).

TROUBLESOME DYSKINESIAS

Choreic movements can occur early in the treatment with levodopa, but the incidence of these involuntary movements increases with continuing treatment[30]. However, the major risk factor for peak-dose dyskinesia has been considered to be severity of the disease[31]. In the early stages of levodopa therapy, chorea is more common than dystonia, but with continuing treatment individual patients can develop more dystonic dyskinesias and less chorea. Many probably have a combination

Table 4 Troublesome fluctuations ($n = 142$)

	n	%
Wearing-off phenomenon	117	82
Delayed 'on'	48	34
Sudden on/off	52	37
Failure to respond to each dose	38	27
Less response after a protein meal	24	17

of chorea and dystonia. Dystonia is a more serious problem than chorea because it is more disabling.

There are several types of dyskinesia, and each appears to have a different pathophysiological mechanism.

Peak-dose dyskinesias

The most common type of dyskinesia is the chorea and dystonia that appears when the plasma levels of levodopa are high, so-called peak-dose dyskinesia. This problem occurred in 128 of the 330 patients on levodopa for more than 5 years (Table 5).

Peak-dose dyskinesias are due to too high a dose of levodopa and are representative of a toxic state. When the plasma levels of levodopa are high[32], there is presumably increased striatal dopamine. Reducing the individual dose can resolve this problem. The patient may need to take more frequent doses at this lower amount because reducing the amount of an individual dose also reduces the duration of benefit[33]. It was once believed that chorea only appeared in the presence of supersensitive dopamine receptors, but if the dosage of levodopa is high enough, chorea can occur in normal individuals.

Another method to reduce peak-dose dyskinesia is to substitute higher doses of a dopamine agonist while lowering the dose of Sinemet.

Table 5 Dyskinesias seen in patients who have been receiving levodopa therapy for more than 5 years ($n = 330$). These recorded adverse effects were not necessarily considered to be troublesome, so they do not match with the data presented in Table 1

Dyskinesias	*n*	*%*	*Comments*
Peak-dose dyskinesia	128	39	41% had troublesome dyskinesias
			16% were considered mild
			63% also had troublesome fluctuations
D-I-D	36	11	89% had troublesome fluctuations
Early morning dystonia	57	17	16% had other types of 'off' dystonia
Other 'off' dystonia	25	8	
Yo-yo phenomenon	16	5	
Excess response on empty stomach	15	5	80% had troublesome fluctuations

Dopamine agonists are less likely to cause dyskinesias, and therefore can usually be used in this situation quite safely. If lowering the dose of Sinemet results in more severe 'off' states, then the agonists become more important.

In the early stages of levodopa therapy, peak-dose chorea is more common than peak-dose dystonia, but with continuing treatment individual patients may develop more dystonic dyskinesias and less chorea. Many probably have a combination of chorea and dystonia. Peak-dose dystonia, like peak-dose chorea, also develops when plasma levels of levodopa are high, and subside when the dosage is lower. Dystonia is a more serious problem than chorea because it is more disabling. In many patients dystonia occurs at subtherapeutic doses, and lowering the dosage will render a patient with inadequate response from levodopa even more parkinsonian. There is little choice but to use smaller and more frequent doses, often coupled with dopamine agonists and other antiparkinsonian drugs, such as amantadine.

Diphasic dyskinesia

Diphasic dyskinesias were first described by Muenter and his colleagues[32] who labeled them as the 'D-I-D' phenomenon, for 'dystonia-impro-vement-dystonia'. The D-I-D phenomenon occurred in 39 of the 330 patients taking levodopa for more than 5 years (Table 5). Although most of the affected individuals have dystonia as their pattern of dyskinesia, some have choreic movements, and others have a mixture of the two types. Diphasic dyskinesia is a situation where the dyskinesia develops as the plasma levels of levodopa are rising or falling, but not during the peak plasma level[32,34].

The mechanism of this phenomenon is difficult to explain. It is possible that there is a differential sensitivity of at least two dopamine receptors. The more sensitive one would respond to lower levels of levodopa to induce the dyskinetic state. The other receptor would be activated at higher levels and will inhibit the dyskinesia. Treatment of the problem is difficult. Although Lhermitte and colleagues[34] proposed treating this condition with higher doses of levodopa, my own experience is that higher dosages merely induce peak-dose dyskinesia and possibly other forms of central adverse effects. On the other hand, lowering the dosage is equally unsatisfactory because increasing parkinsonism ensues. My own personal experience has led me to use pergolide, a direct-acting dopamine agonist with a long duration of action. When used as the major pharmacological agent with supplementary levodopa, it is usually effective in reducing the severity of this problem. Perhaps sustained release levodopa will also prove beneficial.

'Off' dystonia and 'off' painful cramps

Dystonic spasms are not always a sign of levodopa overdosage. This is particularly true in many instances of painful sustained contractions. Painful dystonic cramps occur most often when the plasma level of levodopa is low, particularly in the early morning. Originally called early-morning dystonia[35] because of its timing, this problem is now recognized as appearing at other times of the day in susceptible patients. Its characteristic feature is dystonic spasms when the patient is 'off' and therefore can be seen with accompanying features of parkinsonism. But this type of dystonia can occur at any time the patient goes 'off'[36]. In this sense, 'off' dystonia has some relationship to pharmacokinetics. But why painful dystonic spasms should occur in addition to parkinsonism during low plasma levels of levodopa is not clear. This phenomenon may relate to some peculiarity of the dopamine receptors as well as the low plasma levels of levodopa in these patients. de Yebenes and colleagues[37] have proposed that dystonia may occur when the ratio of norepinephrine to dopamine is high. However, there are only speculations about the pathophysiology of the dystonia in general, and it is difficult to be certain of the explanation of either peak-dose dystonia or of 'off' dystonia and early-morning dystonia. Preventing 'offs' is the best way to control 'off' dystonia. The use of pergolide is often effective when it is the major dopaminergic agent. Perhaps sustained release levodopa will also prove beneficial. Early-morning dystonia occurred in 53 patients and other types of 'off' dystonia in 25 patients of the 330 who had been taking levodopa for more than 5 years (Table 5).

One should not forget that dystonia can also occur as a feature of Parkinson's disease. However, 'off' dystonia does not appear to be merely a reflection of the dystonia of parkinsonism. If patients with 'off' dystonia are given a drug holiday from levodopa, after a few days the painful dystonia will disappear, and the patient will be left with the baseline parkinsonian state and without painful dystonia (unpublished observations).

Yo-yo-ing

Yo-yo-ing is a combination of dyskinesia and fluctuation, and refers to the bouncing up and down of a yo-yo. Phenomenologically, the patient responds rapidly to a dose of levodopa with a peak-dose dyskinesia, followed by a predictable wearing-off[2]. The dopamine receptors are obviously intact, and they would seemingly be extremely supersensitive to lead to such dyskinesias. Hence there appears to be a pharmacodynamic factor to account for the dyskinesias. At the same time, the short plasma half-life and the need for constant bioavailability of levodopa in the plasma accounts for the 'off' states. Thus, the 'offs' are the result of a pharmacokinetic factor. This condition should be considered as a combined pharmacokinetic and pharmacodynamic problem. Treatment is virtually impossible with standard Sinemet. Perhaps Sinemet CR will prove to be useful, but it is unlikely. We have had success with direct acting agonists when used as the sole or dominant form of pharmacotherapy, and with plain levodopa (without carbidopa) used as a supplement.

Simultaneous dyskinesias with parkinsonism

Many patients have different responses to levodopa therapy in different parts of the body. For example, the head and neck regions may be more sensitive to levodopa than are the legs. When the upper part of the body responds in this situation, the legs may remain parkinsonian and the patient may not be able to walk well. In this example, on higher dosages of levodopa, the legs improve, but now the head and neck regions are dyskinetic. This problem may be due to different sensitivities of the striatal dopamine receptors on a somatotopic basis. That is, in the case described, the head and neck areas of the striatum would have more sensitive receptors than the leg area. This problem is difficult to treat, and one can only titrate the dosage to the optimum response between the two extremes for each individual patient.

Table 6 examines only those dyskinesias that were considered severe enough to be 'troublesome' and not all recorded dyskinesias. Patients can have more than one type of troublesome dyskinesia, but 78% of the troublesome dyskinesias were of the peak-dose chorea or dystonia type.

TOXICITY AT A SUBTHERAPEUTIC DOSE

Toxicity from levodopa can be divided into the cases due to central nervous system dysfunction (referred to as central side-effects) and those of a peripheral mechanism (known as peripheral side-effects). The former are much more common since the introduction of a peripheral decarboxylase inhibitor used in combination with levodopa. Table 7 lists the types of toxicity states encountered in 330 patients who had been taking levodopa for ore than 5 years.

Mental adverse effects

The most common types of central toxic side-effects are mental changes. These consist of confusion, agitation, hallucinosis, hallucinations, delusions, depression, mania and excessive sleeping. These symptoms are probably related to activation of dopamine receptors in non-striatal regions, particularly the cortical and limbic structures. Elderly patients and patients with cortical Lewy body disease or concomitant Alzheimer's disease are extremely sensitive to small doses of levodopa. But all patients with Parkinson's disease, regardless of age, can develop psychosis if they take excess amounts of levodopa as a means to overcome 'off' periods. This is difficult to remedy, except by reducing the dosage of levodopa,

Table 6 Troublesome dyskinesias ($n = 67$)

	n	%
Peak dose dyskinesia/dystonia	52	78
Diphasic dyskinesia (D-I-D)	32	48
Early morning dystonia	22	33
Other 'off' dystonia	13	19
Yo-yo	9	13

Table 7 Toxic states seen in patients who have been receiving levodopa therapy for more than 5 years (*n* = 330)

Toxicities	*n*	%
Gastrointestinal effects	44	13
Psychosis	26	8
Confusion, dementia	54	16
Hallucinosis	51	15
Sleep disturbances	83	25
Postural hypotension	24	7
Episodic sweating	6	2
Fatigue after dose	12	4
Myoclonus	5	2
Freezing when 'on'	40	12
Hypersexuality	9	3

thereby possibly lessening the beneficial response to levodopa as well. Clearly, a dopamine agonist that would be specific for striatal receptors would be welcome. Alternatively, a dopamine antagonist that would be specific for non-striatal receptors would theoretically be effective.

A promising approach to treat psychosis associated with levodopa is the use of clozapine, an antipsychotic agent that does not cause parkinsonism or antagonize the antiparkinson effect of levodopa[38,39], but not all investigators report satisfactory results[40]. Unfortunately, clozapine induces agranulocytosis in approximately 1–2% of patients. If it is not tolerated, one can try molindone, pimozide or other relatively weak antipsychotics. If the antipsychotics produce an increase of parkinsonism, it is preferable to lower the dosage of Sinemet to avoid the psychosis, rather than maintain the antipsychotic at that high dosage. An intact mental function is more important than an intact motor function.

It should be mentioned that it is not safe to discontinue levodopa suddenly, for such action can induce the neuroleptic malignant syndrome[41,42].

Altered sleep–wake cycle

The adverse effects of drowsiness during the daytime, particularly after a dose of levodopa, and insomnia at night are fairly common. Of the

330 patients receiving levodopa for more than 5 years, 83 had sleep disturbances. This problem often accompanies the central adverse effects of confusion. Like mental adverse effects, changes in the sleep–wake cycle most likely represent activation of non-striatal dopamine receptors. Perhaps those located in the hypothalamus are responsible for this set of symptoms. If a patient becomes drowsy after each dose of medication, this is a sign of overdosage. Reducing the dosage is the only means of correcting this problem. If the patient is generally drowsy during the daytime and remains awake at night, this alteration of the sleep–wake cycle makes it difficult for those caring for the patient to look after him effectively. It is important to get the patient onto a sleep–wake schedule that fits with the rest of the household. To correct the problem, it may be necessary to use a combination of approaches. Efforts must be made to stimulate the patient physically and mentally during the daytime and force him to remain awake, otherwise he would not be able to sleep at night. At night he should then be drowsy enough so that he will be able to sleep.

It may be necessary to use stimulants in the morning and sedatives at night in order to reverse the altered state of affairs. This should be done in addition to prodding the patient to remain awake during the day. Drugs such as methylphenidate and amphetamine are usually well tolerated by patients with Parkinson's disease. A 10 mg dose of either of these two drugs, repeated once if necessary, may be helpful. To encourage sleep at night, a hypnotic may be necessary in addition to using daytime stimulants. It should be noted that strong sedatives, such as barbiturates, are poorly tolerated by patients with Parkinson's disease. Milder hypnotics, such as benzodiazepines, are usually taken without difficulty. Short-acting benzodiazepines would be preferable, but if the patient awakens too early, a longer acting one may need to be used.

LOSS OF EFFICACY

A debated point in the treatment of parkinsonism is the cause of declining efficacy from continuing treatment with levodopa in many patients[43]. If the postsynaptic dopamine receptors in the striatum are not lost in this disease, why should a patient receive less response from medication over time? Progression of the illness with further loss of dopamine storage sites in the presynaptic terminals is the most invoked explanation. However, loss of these structures does not automatically produce a loss of response to levodopa. For example, postencephalitic parkinsonism with its much greater loss of dopamine in the striatum[44,45] has more, not less, sensitivity to levodopa[46,47]. This observation is sufficient to argue against the concept that reduced storage sites for dopamine is responsible for the declining efficacy of levodopa. Perhaps Parkinson's disease is associated with loss of striatal dopamine receptors as well as the presynaptic dopaminergic neuron.

Even so, there may be additional factors contributing in part to the loss of efficacy seen with continuous treatment with levodopa. Some decline may arise in part from gradual down-regulation of striatal dopamine receptors[48]. Not all patients develop this problem, but it appears to be due to the receptors being constantly exposed to high levels of dopamine. Evidence to support this concept comes from the studies of drug holidays from levodopa. After levodopa is eliminated for a short period, restoration of levodopa therapy usually provides enhanced temporary benefit[49,50]. Unfortunately, this enhanced sensitivity is short-lived, and the potential risks of aspiration during the drug holiday render this approach undesirable for the short-term benefit that can be obtained.

OTHER COMPLICATIONS

Increased tachyphemia and increased running gait

A number of patients overdosed with levodopa will speak faster, running syllables together, so that it is difficult for the listener to understand what the patient is saying. At the same time as the speech is rapid (tachyphemia), the amplitude is lower so that the voice is softer, aggravating the situation. If the patient purposely tries to enunciate each syllable distinctly, he is able to do so for a few words, but then the tachyphemia takes over again. With speech therapy, sometimes using a metronome for pacing, a patient can improve the pattern of speaking, but only during the treatment session. There seems to be little carry-over. Associated with tachyphemia are rapid voluntary movements in other parts of the body, displayed as such when the patient is asked to perform rapid successive movements. These are usually very fast and of small amplitude, i.e. tachykinetic and hypokinetic.

This type of tachykinetic problem can also involve walking. Usually the patient moves more rapidly but with smaller steps. Gait in this instance can be mistaken for festination, which it resembles. If postural instability is impaired, such a running gait can lead to falling. Often, lowering the dosage of levodopa will allow the patient to slow down, with a resulting clarity of speech and gait. However, parkinsonian bradykinesia can become more of a problem.

Freezing (motor blocks)

Freezing takes many forms (Table 8), and these have different names, such as start hesitation, target hesitation, turning hesitation, startle (fearfulness) hesitation, and sudden transient freezing. However, it is not clear if any of these types has a different pathophysiological mechanism. It is of major therapeutic importance to distinguish between 'off freezing' and 'on freezing'. 'Off freezing' is best explained as a feature of Parkinson's disease and treatment involves keeping the patient from becoming 'off'. 'On freezing' remains an enigma, and this problem tends to be aggravated by increasing the dosage of levodopa. It is not benefited by adding direct-acting dopamine agonists. Rather, it is lessened by reducing the dosage of levodopa. Although Narabayashi and colleagues[51] reported benefit with L-threo-dops, supposedly a precursor of brain norepinephrine, I have not seen any benefit with this drug in the treatment of 'on freezing'. Furthermore, we have found no evidence that this drug increases norepinephrine in rat brain or human cerebrospinal fluid. Interestingly, in the intravenous infusions of levodopa

Table 8 Motor blocks occurring in patients treated with levodopa for more than 5 years ($n = 330$)

Freezing of gait	n	%
Start-hesitation	131	40
When turning	70	21
In doorways	39	12
In open walkway	38	12
At destination	30	9

performed by Shoulson and colleagues[10], a sudden stimulus, such as tilting the patient upright on a tilt table, resulted in sudden transient worsening of parkinsonism. This can be interpreted as indicating the induction of sudden transient freezing. It may be a useful model for future studies.

Falling due to intractable loss of postural reflexes

Falling is a common feature of Parkinson's disease as the illness progresses and there is increasing loss of postural reflexes. Since this particular cardinal sign of Parkinson's disease is little benefited by levodopa therapy[52], this problem persists and worsens despite pharmacotherapy. Because levodopa may allow the patient to be more mobile, such as allowing him to arise more easily from a chair and walk independently, the persistence of postural instability becomes a particular problem because it raises the hazard of increased likelihood of falling. Thus, this complication of levodopa therapy in this particular subpopulation of patients with Parkinson's disease is technically not a true adverse effect of the medication, but a complication of the improvement in mobility in a patient at risk for falling, thereby increasing that risk. In this situation the patient should use physical assistance, such as a walker. An alternative approach is to keep the patient sufficiently parkinsonian so that he/she cannot arise without assistance.

Postural hypotension

Postural hypotension as a complication of levodopa can be either a peripheral or central adverse effect. Since this problem persists in the presence of carbidopa, a central mechanism is clearly responsible, but a peripheral action could also play a role in addition. Postural hypotension from levodopa is aggravated by other drugs taken by the patient, such as tricyclic antidepressants. The central site for producing this complication by levodopa is uncertain, but the hypothalamus should be considered since it gives rise to autonomic fibers that descend to the spinal cord. The treatment of postural hypotension can sometimes be managed by using support stockings, sodium chloride, and fludrocortisone[53], but often the dosage of levodopa needs to be reduced.

Excessive sweating

The problem of episodic sweating remains an enigma, both in its mechanism and its treatment. These episodes, seemingly unrelated to timing of medication, cause the patient to be drenched in sweat, and could potentially cause an electrolyte imbalance. At the minimum it is an unpleasant, uncomfortable problem, and requires frequent changing of clothing. Autonomic dysfunctions do occur in Parkinson's disease[54], but these do not explain the episodes of drenching sweats that can occur in some patients. It is not known whether this complication of levodopa is central or peripheral, but its occurrence in the presence of carbidopa strongly suggests that it is a central disorder. Although the receptors involved are not certain, one possibility is that it may be related to dopamine receptors in the hypothalamus. Although trials of β-blockers are recommended, they have been ineffective in my experience.

Akathisia

Akathisia, meaning inability to sit still, probably occurs more often in Parkinson's disease than is commonly recognized. It can be a sensory complaint of the disease itself and also an adverse effect from levodopa. Lang and Johnson[55] asked patients with Parkinson's disease specifically for complaints of restlessness and found that 86% did have this subjective complaint. Most patients with Parkinson's disease who complained of an inner feeling of restlessness did not overtly manifest any signs such as moving about. From Lang and Johnson's study it was not clear if akathisia represented an adverse effect from levodopa or was a feature of the disease. In most of their patients it appeared only after the introduction of antiparkinson drugs, but a small number had this symptom early in the course of Parkinson's disease, prior to receiving any medication. It is likely that other antiparkinson agents may also contribute to this complaint, for I have seen it in patients with idiopathic torsion dystonia after starting anticholinergic drugs. But levodopa clearly can cause it, since I have also seen patients with idiopathic torsion dystonia who developed akathisia after starting levodopa as the sole pharmacological agent.

In general, akathisia is most commonly encountered as a complication of dopamine receptor blocking drugs, predominantly the antipsychotics[56]. From these drugs, akathisia can appear as an acute symptom following introduction of the antipsychotic (referred to as acute akathisia) and the symptom is relieved by discontinuing the offending drug. Akathisia can also appear as a late complication of these drugs and remain persistent (referred to as tardive akathisia). Tardive akathisia occurs in association with tardive dyskinesia and tardive dystonia. Unfortunately, the mechanism of akathisia induced by neuroleptics is not clearly understood. Why both antidopaminergics and dopaminergics should produce akathisia remains a mystery. It seems reasonable to conclude that levodopa-induced akathisia is a central pharmacodynamic problem. Its treatment is to test benzodiazepines and β-blockers, and if these attempts fail, to reduce the dosage of levodopa if the symptoms are too pronounced.

Respiratory distress

Respiratory distress such as dyspnea can occur as a symptom of Parkinson's disease in some patients. We have encountered it also during the 'off' stage in a number of patients[57]. In addition, it can also occur as a complication of dystonia, usually peak-dose dystonia[58].

Pain

Pain and other sensory complaints are common symptoms of Parkinson's disease[59-61]. Usually these symptoms are controlled by treatment with levodopa. However, I have observed some patients with Parkinson's disease who developed sensory complaints, including pain, as a result of levodopa therapy. Often the pain is an accompaniment of 'off' and also peak-dose dystonia[35,36]. A rare patient may have sensory complaints from levodopa therapy, unaccompanied by dystonia. We have treated two of these patients with electroconvulsive therapy with good results (unpublished observations). If parkinsonian pain occurs during an 'off' or due to parkinsonism, one should increase medications to avoid 'offs'. If pain occurs during peak-dose dystonia, one needs to lower the dose. If pain is secondary to Sinemet or agonists, one needs to reduce or eliminate the causal agent. Occasionally, the ergot dopamine agonists, bromocriptine and pergolide, cause a burning pain with inflammatory skin on parts of the body, known as St. Anthony's fire. The agonist needs to be discontinued.

REFERENCES

1. Fahn, S. (1989). Adverse effects of levodopa in Parkinson's disease. In Calne, D.B. (ed.) *Drugs for the Treatment of Parkinson's Disease. Handbook of Experimental Pharmacology.* Vol. 88, pp. 385–409. (Berlin: Springer-Verlag)
2. Fahn, S. (1982). Fluctuations of disability in Parkinson's disease: pathophysiological aspects. In Marsden, C.D. and Fahn, S. (eds.) *Movement Disorders*, pp. 123–45. (London: Butterworth Scientific)
3. Marsden, C.D., Parkes, J.D. and Quinn, N. (1982). Fluctuations of disability in Parkinson's disease – clinical aspects. In Marsden, C.D. and Fahn, S. (eds.) *Movement Disorders*, pp. 96–122. (London: Butterworth Scientific)
4. Ballard, P.A., Tetrud, J.W. and Langston, J.W. (1985). Permanent human parkinsonism due to 1-methyl-4-phenyl-1,2,3,6-tetrahydropyridine (MPTP): seven cases. *Neurology*, **35**, 949–56
5. McDowell, F.H. and Sweet, R.D. (1976). The 'on–off' phenomenon. In Birkmayer, W. and Hornykiewicz, O. (eds.) *Advances in Parkinsonism*, pp. 603–12. (Basle: Editiones Roche)
6. Horstink, M.W.I.M., Zijlmans, J.C.M., Pasman, J.W., Berger, H.J.C., Korten, J.J. and Vanthof, M.A. (1990). Which risk factors predict the levodopa response in fluctuating Parkinson's disease. *Ann. Neurol.*, **27**, 537–43
7. Roos, R.A.C., Vredevoogd, C.B. and Vandervelde, E.A. (1990). Response fluctuations in Parkinson's disease. *Neurology*, **40**, 1344–6
8. Poewe, W.H., Lees, A.J. and Stern, G.M. (1986). Low-dose L-dopa therapy in Parkinson's disease: a 6-year follow-up study. *Neurology*, **36**, 1528–30
9. Muenter, M.D. and Tyce, G.M. (1971). L-dopa therapy of Parkinson's disease: plasma L-dopa concentration, therapeutic response, and side effects. *Mayo Clin. Proc.*, **46**, 231–9
10. Shoulson, I., Glaubiger, G.A. and Chase, T.N. (1975). 'On–off' response: clinical and biochemical correlations during oral and intravenous levodopa administration. *Neurology*, **25**, 1144–8
11. Hardie, R.J., Lees, A.J. and Stern, G.M. (1984). On–off fluctuations in Parkinson's disease. *Brain*, **107**, 487–506
12. Nutt, J.G. (1987). On–off phenomenon: relation to levodopa pharmacokinetics and pharmacodynamics. *Ann. Neurol.*, **22**, 535–40
13. Sage, J.I., Trooskin, S., Sonsalla, P.K. and Heikkila, R.E. (1989). Experience

with continuous enteral levodopa infusions in the treatment of 9 patients with advanced Parkinson's disease. *Neurology*, **39** (Suppl. 2), 60–3

14. Obeso, J.A., Vaamonde, J., Grandas, F., Luquin, M.R., Rodriguez, M. *et al.* (1989). Overcoming pharmacokinetic problems in the treatment of Parkinson's disease. *Movement Disorders*, **4** (Suppl. 1), S70–85

15. Pederzoli, M., Girotti, F., Scigliano, G., Aiello, G., Carella, F. and Caraceni, T. (1983). L-dopa long-term treatment in Parkinson's disease: age-related side effects. *Neurology*, **33**, 1518–22

16. Rinne, U.K. (1989). Early dopamine agonist therapy in Parkinson's disease. *Movement Disorders*, **4** (Suppl. 1), S86–94

17. Rinne, U.K. (1989). Lisuride, a dopamine agonist in the treatment of early Parkinson's disease. *Neurology*, **39**, 336–9

18. Blin, J., Bonnet, A.-M. and Agid, Y. (1988). Does levodopa aggravate Parkinson's disease? *Neurology*, **38**, 1410–16

19. Mouradian, M.M., Heuser, I.J.E., Baronti, F., Fabbrini, G., Juncos, J.L. and Chase, T.N. (1989). Pathogenesis of dyskinesias in Parkinson's disease. *Ann. Neurol.*, **25**, 523–6

20. Mouradian, M.M., Juncos, J.L., Fabbrini, G., Schlegel, J., Bartko, J.J. and Chase, T.N. (1988). Motor fluctuations in Parkinson's disease: central pathophysiological mechanisms, II. *Ann. Neurol.*, **24**, 372–8

21. Obeso, J.A., Grandas, F., Vaamonde, J., Luquin, M.R., Artieda, J., Lera, G., Rodriquez, L.M. and Martinez-Lage, J.M. (1989). Motor complications associated with chronic levodopa therapy in Parkinson's disease. *Neurology*, **39** (Suppl. 2), 11–19

22. Bush, D.F., Liss, C.L., Morton, A. and Sinemet CR Multicenter Study Group (1989). An open multicenter long-term treatment evaluation of Sinemet CR. *Neurology*, **39** (Suppl. 2), 101–4

23. Fahn, S. (1974). 'On–off' phenomenon with levodopa therapy in parkinson-ism: clinical and pharmacologic correlations and the effect of intramuscular pyridoxine. *Neurology*, **24**, 431–41

24. Clough, C.G., Bergmann, K.J. and Yahr, M.D. (1984). Cholinergic and dopaminergic mechanisms in Parkinson's disease after long-term L-dopa administration. *Adv. Neurol.*, **40**, 131–40

25. Frankel, J.P., Lees, A.J., Kempster, P.A. and Stern, G.M. (1990). Subcutane-ous apomorphine in the treatment of Parkinson's disease. *J. Neurol. Neurosurg. Psychiatr.*, **53**, 96–101

26. Rivera-Calimlin, L., Dujovne, C.A., Morgan, J.P., Lasagna, L. and Bianchine, J.R. (1970). L-dopa treatment failure: explanation and correction. *Br. Med. J.*, **4**, 93–4

27. Fahn, S. (1977). Episodic failure of absorption of levodopa: a factor in the

control of clinical fluctuations in the treatment of parkinsonism. *Neurology,* **27**, 390

28. Melamed, E., Bitton, V. and Zelig, O. (1986). Episodic unresponsiveness to single doses of L-dopa in parkinsonian fluctuators. *Neurology,* **36**, 100–3

29. Melamed, E. and Bitton, V. (1984). Delayed onset of responses to individual doses of L-dopa therapy. *Neurology,* **34** (Suppl. 2), 270

30. Duvoisin, R.C. (1974). Hyperkinetic reactions with L-dopa. In Yahr, M.D. (ed.) *Current Concepts in the Treatment of Parkinsonism,* pp. 203–10. (New York: Raven Press)

31. Horstink, M.W.I.M., Zijlmans, J.C.M., Pasman, J.W., Berger, H.J.C. and Vanthof, M.A. (1990). Severity of Parkinson's disease is a risk factor for peak-dose dyskinesia. *J. Neurol. Neurosurg. Psychiatr.,* **53**, 224–6

32. Muenter, M.D., Sharpless, N.S., Tyce, G.M. and Darley, F.L. (1977). Patterns of dystonia ('I-D-I' and 'D-I-D') in response to L-dopa therapy of Parkinson's disease. *Mayo Clin. Proc.,* **52**, 163–74

33. Nutt, J.G., Woodward, W.R. and Anderson, J.L. (1985). The effect of carbidopa on the pharmacokinetics of intravenously administered levodopa: the mechanism of action in the treatment of parkinsonism. *Ann. Neurol.,* **18**, 527–43

34. Lhermitte, F., Agid, Y. and Signoret, J.L. (1978). Onset and end-of-dose levodopa-induced dyskinesias. *Arch. Neurol.,* **35**, 261–2

35. Melamed, E. (1979). Early-morning dystonia: a late side effect of long-term levodopa therapy in Parkinson's disease. *Arch. Neurol.,* **36**, 308–10

36. Ilson, J., Fahn, S. and Cote, L. (1984). Painful dystonic spasms in Parkinson's disease. *Adv. Neurol.,* **40**, 395–8

37. de Yebenes, J.G., Vazquez, A., Martinez, A., Mena, M.A., del Rio, R.M. *et al.* (1988). Biochemical findings in symptomatic dystonias. *Adv. Neurol.,* **50**, 167–75

38. Friedman, J.H. and Lannon, M.C. (1990). Clozapine in idiopathic Parkinson's disease. *Neurology,* **40**, 1151–2

39. Pfeiffer, R.F., Kang, J., Graber, B., Hofman, R. and Wilson, J. (1990). Clozapine for psychosis in Parkinson's disease. *Movement Disorders,* **5**, 239–42

40. Wolters, E.C., Hurwitz, T.A., Mak, E., Teal, P., Peppard, F.R., Remick, R., Calne, S. and Calne, D.B. (1990). Clozapine in the treatment of parkinsonian patients with dopaminomimetic psychosis. *Neurology,* **40**, 832–4

41. Friedman, J.H., Feinberg, S.S. and Feldman, R.G. (1985). A neuroleptic malignantlike syndrome due to levodopa therapy withdrawal. *J. Am. Med. Assoc.,* **254**, 2792–5

42. Hirschorn, K.A. and Greenberg, H.S. (1988). Successful treatment of

levodopa-induced myoclonus and levodopa withdrawal-induced neuroleptic malignant syndrome: a case report. *Clin. Neuropharmacol.*, **2**, 278–81

43. Yahr, M.D. (1976). Evaluation of long-term therapy in Parkinson's disease: mortality and therapeutic efficacy. In Birkmayer, W. and Hornykiewicz, O. (eds.) *Advances in Parkinsonism*, pp. 444–55. (Basle: Editiones Roche)

44. Ehringer, H. and Hornykiewicz, O. (1960). Verteilung von Noradrenalin und Dopamin (3-Hydroxytryamin) im Gehirn des Menschen und ihr Verhalten bei Erkrankungen des extrapyramidalen Systems. *Klin. Wschr.*, **38**, 1238–9

45. Bernheimer, H., Birkmayer, W., Hornykiewicz, O., Jellinger, K. and Seitelberger, F. (1973). Brain dopamine and the syndromes of Parkinson and Huntington. *J. Neurol. Sci.*, **20**, 415–55

46. Calne, D.B., Stern, G.M., Laurence, D.R., Sharkey, J. and Armitage, P. (1969). L-dopa in postencephalitic parkinsonism. *Lancet*, **1**, 744–6

47. Duvoisin, R.C., Antunes, J.L. and Yahr, M.D. (1972). Response of patients with postencephalitic parkinsonism to levodopa. *J. Neurol. Neurosurg. Psychiatr.*, **35**, 487–95

48. Rinne, U.K., Koskinen, V. and Lonnberg, P. (1980). Neurotransmitter receptors in the parkinsonian brain. In Rinne, U.K., Klingler, M. and Stamm, G. (eds.) *Parkinson's Disease: Current Progress, Problems and Management*, pp. 93–107. (Amsterdam: Elsevier/North-Holland Biomedical Press)

49. Direnfeld, L.K., Feldman, R.G., Alexander, M.P. and Kelly-Hayes, M. (1980). Is L-dopa drug holiday useful? *Neurology*, **30**, 785–8

50. Weiner, W.J., Koller, W.C., Perlik, S., Nausieda, P.A. and Klawans, H.L. (1980). Drug holiday and management of Parkinson disease. *Neurology*, **30**, 1257–61

51. Narabayashi, H., Kondo, T., Yokochi, F. and Nagatsu, T. (1986). Clinical effects of L-threo-3,4-dihydroxyphenylserine in cases of parkinsonism and pure akinesia. *Adv. Neurol.*, **45**, 593–602

52. Klawans, H.L. (1986). Individual manifestations of Parkinson's disease after ten or more years of levodopa. *Movement Disorders*, **1**, 187–92

53. Hoehn, M.M. (1975). Levodopa-induced postural hypotension. *Arch. Neurol.*, **32**, 50–1

54. Goetz, C.G., Lutge, W. and Tanner, C.M. (1986). Autonomic dysfunction in Parkinson's disease. *Neurology*, **36**, 73–5

55. Lang, A.E. and Johnson, K. (1987). Akathisia in idiopathic Parkinson's disease. *Neurology*, **37**, 477–81

56. Fahn, S. (1984). The tardive dyskinesias. In Matthews, W.B. and Glaser, G.H. (eds.) *Recent Advances in Clinical Neurology*, Vol. 4, pp. 229–60. (Edinburgh: Churchill Livingstone)

57. Ilson, J., Braun, N. and Fahn, S. (1983). Respiratory fluctuations in Parkinson's disease. *Neurology,* **33** (Suppl. 2), 113
58. Braun, A.R., Tanner, C.M., Goetz, C.G. and Klawans, H.L. (1983). Respiratory distress due to pharyngeal dystonia: a side effect of chronic dopamine agonism. *Neurology,* **33** (Suppl. 2), 220
59. Snider, S.R., Fahn, S., Isgreen, W.P. and Cote, L.J. (1976). Primary sensory symptoms in parkinsonism. *Neurology,* **26**, 423–9
60. Koller, W.C. (1984). Sensory symptoms in Parkinson's disease. *Neurology,* **34**, 957–9
61. Goetz, C.G., Tanner, C.M., Levy, M., Wilson, R.S. and Garron, D.C. (1986). Pain in Parkinson's disease. *Movement Disorders,* **1**, 45–9

7

Aspects of levodopa pharmacokinetics and pharmacodynamics: bases of the modification of drug response during chronic treatment of Parkinson's disease

J.M. Cedarbaum and C.W. Olanow

INTRODUCTION: GENERAL PHARMACOLOGY OF LEVODOPA

Familiarity with the pharmacokinetics and pharmacodynamics of levodopa is essential in order to understand its mechanism of action in Parkinson's disease. In addition, this information is necessary in order to develop a conceptual framework for integrating the contribution of other antiparkinsonian agents into the overall management of the parkinsonian patient. Many of the shortcomings of chronic levodopa therapy arise from its particular pharmacokinetic properties. Continued treatment with levodopa, in the face of progressive degeneration of dopaminergic neurons, may alter the biological response to the drug[1] and patients with Parkinson's disease are living longer[2] due to the widespread use of levodopa and other symptomatic treatments. Consequently it is likely that we are seeing and treating a larger population of patients with advanced disease, whose nervous systems no doubt have undergone a greater degree of degeneration in both dopaminergic and non-dopaminergic systems than was seen in the pre-levodopa era. Physicians are thus faced with the challenge of achieving therapeutic results in these patients which are qualitatively and quantitatively similar to those achieved in early stages of the disease.

It is currently accepted that Parkinson's disease is a syndrome of dopamine deficiency in the brain. Dopamine itself does not cross the blood–brain barrier, and thus cannot be administered systemically to restore brain dopamine levels in Parkinson's disease patients. Its precursor amino acid levodopa, does, however, enter the brain from the circulation, where, even in advanced stages of the disease (see below), it is converted into dopamine. The metabolic pathways leading to the synthesis and breakdown of dopamine are illustrated in Figure 1. Levodopa is generated from the essential amino acid tyrosine by the enzyme tyrosine hydroxylase (TH). Dopamine is synthesized in both brain and periphery from levodopa by the action of the enzyme aromatic amino acid dopadecarboxylase (DDC) upon levodopa. In the normal brain, dopamine is synthesized in terminals of neurons of the substantia nigra which project to the caudate/putamen, is stored in vesicles, and then released. At the synapse, two types of dopamine receptors, termed D_1 and D_2, produce distinct postsynaptic effects, as detailed elsewhere in this volume. Once released, the action of dopamine is terminated either by re-uptake into the nerve terminal, where it is converted by monoamine oxidase (MAO) into dihydroxyphenylacetic acid (DOPAC), or into glial cells, where O-methylation by the enzyme catechol-O-methyltransferase (COMT) yields 3-methoxytyramine or 3-MT. COMT acting on DOPAC, or MAO acting on 3-MT produces homovanillic acid, or HVA, which is the normal end product of dopamine metabolism in the human brain.

Because it is an amino acid, and a homologue of the essential aromatic amino acids, levodopa has a short circulating half-life. In primates and in man, the half-life of levodopa has been variously estimated to be between 30 min and 1 hour (see ref. 3 for review). Levodopa is extensively metabolized[4], and, in addition, finds metabolic sinks in muscle[5,6], erythrocytes (J.M. Cedarbaum, unpublished observations), and in the formation of skin melanin, of which it is the principal building block[7].

Orally-administered levodopa encounters several barriers in its transit to the brain. The lining of the gastrointestinal tract is rich in both DDC[8] and COMT[9]. Thus, when administered alone, over 90% of levodopa is metabolized in a 'first pass' before ever reaching the brain[8]. In addition,

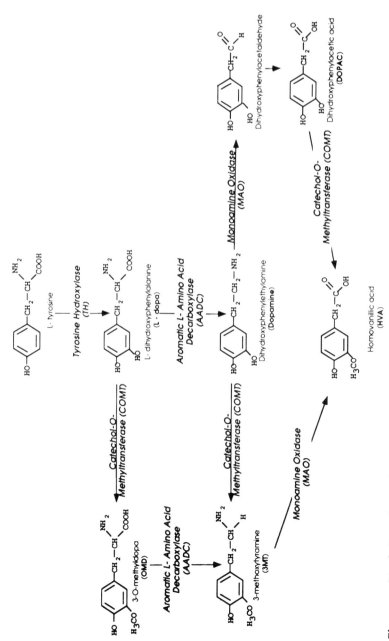

Figure I Metabolic pathways for the synthesis and metabolism of dopamine

the blood–brain barrier also contains DDC[10], although the role of cerebral capillary DDC in preventing the entry of levodopa into the brain remains uncertain. At both the gut and the blood–brain barrier level, levodopa must compete with other large neutral amino acids for access to the saturable large neutral amino acid (LNAA) carrier. The dietary LNAAs are normally present in much higher concentrations than levodopa[11]. The LNAA carrier at the blood–brain barrier appears to be more sensitive to the competing effect of other amino acids on levodopa transport than that in the gut, since orally administered amino acids can significantly reduce the effectiveness of intravenously administered levodopa[12]. However, fluctuations in plasma amino acids within the range of those occurring on a normal diet probably do little to alter levodopa flux into the brain[13]. Finally, it appears from evidence gathered in dogs, that the density of this carrier system is not uniform throughout the small intestine; levodopa absorption is much more efficient in the proximal third of the small bowel[14]. Thus variations in gastric emptying, which is not a uniform process, can greatly alter the rate of presentation of drug to the primary absorptive region of the gut, further complicating the process of gaining access to the circulation and to the brain[15]. Failure of absorption of individual doses of levodopa is probably the major mechanism underlying apparently 'drug-resistant' 'off' periods[16].

In current practice the oral bioavailability of levodopa is enhanced by co-administering an inhibitor of DDC, either carbidopa (in Sinemet®) or benserazide (in Madopar®)[17]. Use of a DDC inhibitor allows the attainment of plasma levodopa levels in the 'therapeutic' range despite administration of one-fourth to one-fifth of traditional levodopa doses. In addition, side-effects such as nausea, flushing and palpitations, which are caused by circulating dopamine, are markedly diminished. The fact that the elimination half-life of levodopa in plasma is only slightly prolonged by administration of a DDC inhibitor[18] emphasizes both the role of DDC as a first-pass metabolic pathway, and the importance of other metabolic pathways in the systemic clearance of the drug. Blockade of peripheral decarboxylation of levodopa does, however, have a downside in that more of the drug's metabolism is shunted into the COMT pathway, leading to formation of the metabolite 3-*O*-methyldopa (OMD). OMD accumulates in plasma due to its long half-life[19], reaching concentrations several-fold that of levodopa[20,21]. OMD, like levodopa, is an LNAA, and can compete with levodopa for uptake into the circulation and the brain[11].

Pharmacokinetic and pharmacodynamic problems with levodopa treatment manifest themselves as motor response fluctuations (RF) (Table 1). RF consist of alternating states of parkinsonism (the 'off' condition) and eumobility (the 'on' state). Patients' 'on' time is often complicated by the presence of involuntary movements or dyskinesias (Table 2). As defined in Tables 1 and 2, several varieties of both RF and dyskinesias are seen in Parkinson's disease patients. However, all forms of RF have in common the fact that the time course of alternation between the 'on' and 'off' conditions basically correlates with the availability of levodopa to the brain, as reflected in plasma levodopa levels[22-24]. Dyskinesias, on the other hand, are thought to reflect supersensitivity of postsynaptic dopamine receptors which arises as the result of chronic denervation[25,26].

Pharmacokinetic limitations upon the duration of effectiveness of levodopa were observed in initial clinical investigations[27]. In fact, the short duration of action of single intravenous doses of levodopa was cited as evidence against its potential utility[28]. As experience was gained with oral levodopa in the clinic, it became apparent that after 5 or so years of treatment, 50% or more of Parkinson's disease patients develop fluctuating responses to levodopa[24]. Several authors have correlated both the short duration of the clinical response, and the timing of dyskinesias

Table 1   Types of levodopa-related motor response fluctuations

'Wearing-off'	predictable loss of antiparkinsonian efficacy correlated with plasma half-life of drug
'On–off' or 'Yo–yo'	unpredictable, brittle pattern of motor fluctuations in which the state of mobility bears no apparent relationship to the timing of medication administration
'Diphasic' or 'D-I-D'	a pattern of unstable medication response characteristic of young-onset Parkinson's disease patients, in which motor improvement due to levodopa is bracketed by bursts of dyskinetic movements at the onset and end of the period of drug effect

Table 2   Patterns of levodopa and dopamine agonist-induced dyskinesia

Varieties of movements	
Dystonia	sustained, writhing or twisting movements produced by excessive, fluctuating muscle tonus
Chorea	fidgety, rapid distal dyskinesia which the patient may 'cover up' by merging it into a voluntary or habitual motion
Tics	rapid, suppressible, complex involuntary movements resembling fragments of purposeful behaviors
Myoclonus	lightning-like contractions of a group of muscles or portions of a single muscle
Temporal patterns	
Peak-dose	dyskinesias occurring at the peak of the antiparkinsonian effect of a dose of medication
Square-wave	dyskinesias occurring throughout the 'on' period
Beginning- and/or end-of-dose	dyskinesias (often dystonic) occurring at the beginning and end of the dose–response cycle

in these patients with the time course of the rise and fall of plasma levodopa levels.

Shoulson, Glaubiger and Chase were the first to demonstrate that continuous intravenous infusions of levodopa could stabilize plasma levodopa levels and thereby the clinical response of Parkinson's disease patients[23], a finding subsequently confirmed on multiple occasions[29,30]. As could be predicted on the basis of oral drug administration, though individual dose–response curves vary considerably, patients have relatively reproducible thresholds for turning 'on' and 'off'. Furthermore, the motor response appears to be 'all-or-nothing'. That is, higher plasma levodopa levels do not translate into quantitatively greater degrees of motor improvement. On the other hand, the *duration* of response does appear to be proportional to the dose[31].

The elimination kinetics of levodopa in patients with Parkinson's disease do not appear to change with the development of RF[32]. What does vary in Parkinson's disease patients with RF, however, is the half-life of the antiparkinsonian response itself. Chase and his co-workers have investigated this phenomenon by studying motor function in Parkinson's disease patients following the discontinuation of an intravenous levodopa infusion[1,33–35]. In patients with early disease who have never been treated, or in those with a stable response, clinical improvement far outlasts the falling levodopa level in plasma. In patients with clinically evident fluctuations, a clear fall-off in motor function which parallels the decline in plasma levodopa level is seen. In those patients with advanced disease who experience severe and abrupt ('on–off') responses to levodopa, the half-life of efficacy of the antiparkinsonian response may be shorter than the pharmacological half-life of the drug.

PHARMACOKINETIC BEHAVIOR OF LEVODOPA IN THE CNS COMPARTMENT

Observations such as those mentioned above have led to the following explanation for the emergence of RF. When parkinsonian symptoms develop, degeneration of presynaptic dopamine nerve terminals in the striatum although severe, is not complete. There is still sufficient reserve within the brain of the early Parkinson's disease patient that dopamine synthesized from levodopa can be stored, or taken back up into the presynaptic terminal and released for up to several hours after plasma levodopa levels have returned to baseline. Remaining dopamine nerve terminals are also able to compensate further by increasing the rate of dopamine synthesis[36,37]. Eventually degeneration of dopamine nerve terminals reaches a point where storage of neurotransmitter is inadequate and remaining compensatory mechanisms fail. Availability of dopamine in the brain must now passively follow plasma levodopa levels[38], although there is a lag between the rise in plasma levodopa following a dose and the onset of clinical effect[39].

We have recently demonstrated in living Parkinson's disease patients that the lag time to onset of antiparkinsonian effect of levodopa, as well as the duration of effect of a single dose of the drug on motor function, correlate closely with the time course of appearance and disappearance of levodopa and dopamine in the cerebrospinal fluid contained in the lateral ventricles of the brain[39,40]. Four patients, all approximately 1 year post adrenal medulla to caudate-nucleus autograft surgery, with indwelling Ommaya reservoirs in the right lateral ventricle, served as the study population. All four patients were continuing to experience RF; two had peak-dose dyskinesias and dystonias as well. Levels of levodopa in plasma and ventricular CSF were obtained, along with clinical ratings of motor function, at intervals following a single dose of Sinemet 25/250. The amount of levodopa in the central compartment was estimated to be about 10% of that in plasma. Peak CSF levodopa levels lagged behind those in plasma (Figure 2). The magnitude of the peak CSF level (C_{max}), however, correlated closely with that of the peak plasma level ($r = 0.98$). When change in motor score was plotted against plasma levodopa concentration, a counterclockwise hysteresis loop was generated (Figure 3), as previously reported by Nutt and Woodward[31]. Such curves are generally taken as indicative of a compartmental lag, reflecting either time taken for the drug to penetrate the active compartment, or time taken to generate an active metabolite from a prodrug. On the other hand, plots of CSF levodopa vs. change in motor score revealed a straight line, indicative of identity of the compartment under study with the active compartment (Figure 3).

Quite surprisingly, whereas curves of plasma levodopa vs. dyskinesia score yielded the expected counterclockwise hysteresis loop, plots of CSF levodopa vs. dyskinesia revealed a clockwise loop (Figure 4). Clockwise hysteresis loops suggest a receptor sensitization phenomenon, i.e. that the peak of the response lags behind the peak concentration of the drug in the effector compartment itself. This suggests that the receptor mechanisms underlying dyskinesia are qualitatively different from those which are responsible for the antiparkinsonian effects of levodopa. The shape of the curve yields no information as to precisely what that mechanism might be; possibilities include a distinct population of receptors, or a distinct intracellular response mechanism, perhaps one with feed-forward or self-amplifying properties, which operate differently from those underlying the classic motor response to the drug.

EFFECTS OF SUBSTANTIA NIGRA CELL LOSS AND DOPAMINERGIC DRUG TREATMENT ON DOPAMINE RECEPTORS

The development of drug-induced dyskinesia in Parkinson's disease has traditionally been attributed to postsynaptic dopamine receptor

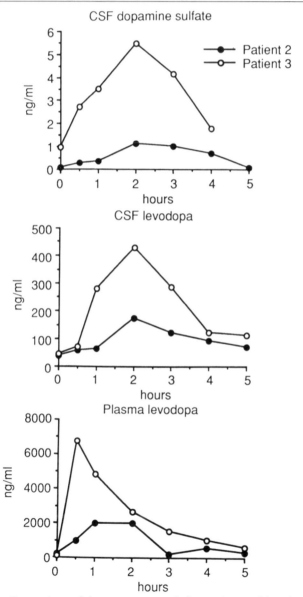

Figure 2 Comparison of the appearance and disappearance of levodopa in plasma (bottom panel) and of levodopa (middle panel) and dopamine (top panel) in ventricular cerebrospinal fluid (CSF) of two patients with advanced Parkinson's disease

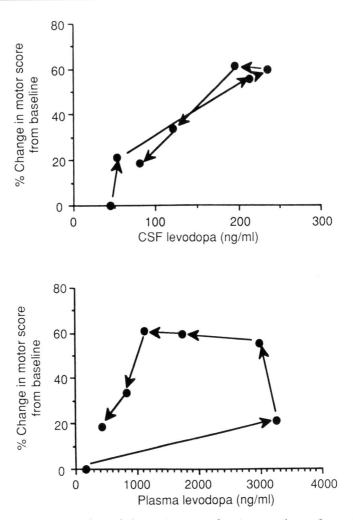

Figure 3 Hysteresis plots of change in motor function vs. plasma (bottom) and cerebrospinal fluid (CSF) (top) levodopa levels. Time vector is indicated by the arrows. Note counterclockwise loop in the bottom panel indicative of the compartmental lag time required for levodopa to enter the central nervous system

supersensitivity. Dopamine receptors become supersensitive following denervation which deprives them of their normal dopamine input[26]. Behavioral manifestations of supersensitivity in animal models are exaggerated if an agonist for the denervated receptor is given at intervals longer than its pharmacological half-life, and are reduced if the agonist

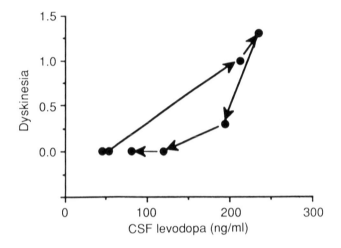

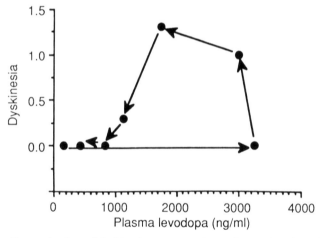

Figure 4 Hysteresis plots of dyskinesia scores vs. plasma (bottom) and cerebrospinal fluid (CSF) (top) levodopa levels. Note that the plot of cerebrospinal fluid levodopa vs. dyskinesia score yields a clockwise loop suggestive of an augmenting or sensitization of the receptor response underlying the phenomenon of dyskinesia

is given in a sustained, continuous fashion[41]. The former situation is essentially that achieved clinically in the management of Parkinson's disease with levodopa. We customarily give a drug with a short half-life of 1–2 h at intervals of 3, 4 or more hours. Each trough in plasma levodopa (and hence brain dopamine) concentration could be viewed as a mini-period of 'denervation', hence a renewed stimulus to the development of receptor supersensitivity. It is not inconceivable then, that repeating such cycles day-in and day-out for many years could result in permanent modification of the response to dopaminergic drugs. Such alterations might occur either at the level of the receptors themselves, or in second messengers or other mediators of the cellular response to dopamine.

Is there evidence that post-receptor changes might be involved in the generation of dyskinesia in Parkinson's disease? It certainly seems possible, although the answer to the riddle is far from simple. To begin with, let us consider the two major populations of dopamine receptors, D_1 and D_2. All our current selective dopamine agonists with antiparkinsonian efficacy in humans possess D_2 agonist activity. In primate models, selective D_1 agonists appear to be without effect[42], even though some studies showed some initial promise[43]. However, a modicum of D_1 agonism is needed for D_2 drugs to express their maximal antiparkinsonian efficacy in animals, as evidenced by the lack of efficacy of the D_2 receptor agonist bromocriptine when brain dopamine has been depleted by the administration of the TH inhibitor α-methyl-paratyrosine[44,45]. With our current drug armamentarium, this means that at least a small amount of levodopa must be given along with a D_2 agonist to provide some D_1 receptor stimulation. In selected patients, however, D_2 agonists, such as bromocriptine, can, if used as the major dopaminergic drug, achieve antiparkinsonian efficacy equivalent to that of levodopa, but with less dyskinesia[46]. Thus, D_1–D_2 receptor interactions may play a role in the genesis of dyskinesia.

An additional speculation is that the normal interactions between D_1 and D_2 receptors might break down in Parkinson's disease, and that this breakdown might be further affected by chronic levodopa administration. Recent evidence suggests that chronic levodopa administration to a dopamine-denervated striatum affects D_1 and D_2 receptors differentially, in a manner critically dependent upon the pattern and timing of levodopa administration[47-49]. Thus, continuous levodopa administration does not affect dopamine agonist induced rotation in rats bearing unilateral 6-hydroxydopamine lesions of the substantia nigra, whereas pulsatile administration sensitizes the response to D_2 receptor agonists and the mixed D_1–D_2 receptor agonist apomorphine, but downregulates purely D_1 receptor-mediated responses.

Behavioral evidence of dopamine receptor supersensitivity is given by an increase in B_{max}, an estimate of the number of receptor binding sites present in tissue[25]. In Parkinson's disease and in the 6-hydroxydopamine animal model of Parkinson's disease, depletion of dopamine in the striatum is followed by increases in the numbers of D_2 receptors which can be measured by *in vitro* binding assays, or of D_1 receptors as indicated in increased activity of dopamine-stimulated adenylcyclase activity, as well as by a number of other parameters of D_1 receptor function[50-54]. An increase in the level of D_2 receptor mRNA in the striatum has also been reported following dopaminergic denervation[55,56]. However, if *in vivo* administration of ligand is employed to assay receptor numbers, no increase in D_2 receptors can be found[57,58]. This suggests that, if extra dopamine receptors are being generated, they may not all be accessible to dopamine which is released into the synaptic cleft.

Finally, there are suggestions that, over the long term, adaptations in neuronal function take place. For example, initially after a 6-hydroxydopamine lesion, neurons of the caudate-putamen are found to fire at increased frequencies, suggesting removal of a tonic inhibition. Yet several weeks later, firing rates have returned to normal, even at a time when behavioral measures of receptor supersensitivity can still be elicited[59]. In intact rats, stimulation of both D_1 and D_2 receptors is necessary to inhibit spontaneous or glutamate-evoked unit activity of striatal neurons, but in rats having a 6-hydroxydopamine lesioned striatum, either a D_1 or D_2 agonist appears fully effective[60]. In addition, intracellular recording reveals that only in denervated striatum can D_2 agonists alone inhibit evoked activity in intrinsic striatal neurons[61]. Additionally, apomorphine-induced contralateral rotation, the behavioral hallmark of dopamine receptor supersensitivity, can still be elicited in 6-hydroxydopamine-treated animals who have been chronically treated with a dopamine receptor antagonist. In these animals, the increase in dopamine receptor number on the lesioned side is masked by an equivalent degree of 'supersensitivity' on the unlesioned side[62]. Yet the animals still behave as if an asymmetry in receptor function exists.

Observations such as these suggest that, with chronic dopamine denervation, alterations in neuronal signal transduction mechanisms must be occurring beyond the level of the receptors themselves. Recent application of molecular biological approaches has given some insight into what some of these changes might be, although our picture of molecular events in the dopamine-denervated, levodopa-treated striatum is far from complete at the present time. For example, transcription of mRNA for the proto-oncogene c-*fos*, a phenomenon which happens rapidly in neuronal nuclei following a variety of events and stimuli, is not activated in normal striatum following administration of levodopa or of dopamine agonists. Yet following destruction of the nigrostriatal pathway, either levodopa or a D_1-receptor agonist will activate the c-*fos* gene widely throughout the striatum[63–65]. D_2 receptor agonists, however, are totally without effect in this system, even at doses which produce contralateral rotation. Even though both the behavioral and the electrophysiological synergism between D_1 and D_2 receptors which is present in the intact striatum are disrupted in the presence of a 6-hydroxydopamine lesion, co-administration of D_1 and D_2 agonists produces a synergistic effect on c-*fos* expression. Thus the biological response represented by c-*fos* expression appears to be unrelated to the 'supersensitive' behavior elicited in the dopamine-depleted striatum[66].

The effect of chronic drug treatment on c-*fos* expression has yet to be determined. However, the effect of combined dopamine denervation and receptor stimulation has been examined in another system. Dopamine denervation produces an up-regulation of preproenkephalin messenger RNA in the striatum[67]. Enkephalins are preferentially expressed in medium spiny striatal neurons which project to the external globus pallidus and carry mostly D_2 receptors[68]. Prodynorphin and substance P gene expression, which are co-localized to GABAergic striatal neurons projecting to the internal globus pallidus and pars reticulata of the substantia nigra which are rich in D_1 receptors[68], are either slightly decreased or are unaffected by dopamine denervation. However, seven once-daily administrations of apomorphine, a mixed D_1-D_2 receptor agonist, markedly increases prodynorphin expression and normalizes expression of preproenkephalin[69]. Selective D_1 agonists elevate dynorphin and substance P expression in dopamine-depleted striatum, but do not affect enkephalin expression levels. The converse is true for D_2 receptor agonists[56] (see Table 3). This suggests that the outflow pathway from the striatum directly through the globus pallidus and pars reticulata to the thalamus is augmented, whereas the striatal–subthalamic–internal

Table 3 Some physiological changes in the basal ganglia with dopamine denervation

	Intact	Denervated	Lesion + drug
Number of D_1 receptors		normal	normal
Adenyl cyclase		increased	increased
Number of D_2 receptors		increased	normal
Inhibition of striatal neuronal activity	$D_1 + D_2$	either D_1 or D_2	not tested
c-*fos* expression	absent	absent	stimulatable by levodopa and D_1 (but not D_2) receptor agonists
Enkephalin mRNA		increased	normal
Dynorphin mRNA		normal to increased	greatly increased by repeated apomorphine

pallidal loop is suppressed when dopamine's influence in the striatum is diminished.

Engber and colleagues, using 2-deoxyglucose autoradiography, have recently demonstrated metabolic changes in striatal output nuclei and brain regions they innervate which are consistent with this proposal[49]. In their study, chronic levodopa treatment decreased metabolic activity in the D_1 receptor-mediated striatonigral and striatoentopeduncular (equivalent to the internal portion of the globus pallidus in man) pathway and increased glucose metabolism in the D_2 receptor-mediated striatopallidal–subthalamic pathway. This increase in glucose metabolic activity presumably reflects increased activity of inhibitory GABAergic and enkephalinergic terminals in the subthalamic nucleus. Decreased activity in the latter circuit, as reviewed by Crossman[70], is associated with the production of choreiform or ballistic involuntary movements.

An interesting additional finding in the study of Gerfen and co-workers[56] was that maximal D_1 receptor-mediated responses in lesioned striatum were attained with intermittent administration of a D_1 agonist, whereas maximal D_2 receptor-mediated responses were obtained with continuous, rather than pulsatile drug administration. Interestingly, depleting striatal dopamine with a 6-hydroxydopamine lesion increased levels of D_2 receptor message (an expected finding), but decreased D_1 receptor mRNA expression. Intermittent, but not continuous D_1 agonist administration increased D_1 receptor message levels in lesioned striatum, whereas continuous D_2 agonist administration was required to reduce D_2 receptor messages to pre-lesion levels. Engber and colleagues also demonstrated a dependency of changes in glucose metabolic activity in these pathways upon the pattern of levodopa administration[49]. Intermittent levodopa administration in their study led to more marked metabolic changes than did continuous administration. These findings confirmed and extended the results of Juncos[47] and of Susel[48] and their colleagues, again suggesting that the pattern and timing of drug administration can profoundly affect responses in both the normal and the dopamine-denervated nigrostriatal system.

Thus a complex picture emerges. Following depletion of striatal dopamine, both D_1 and D_2 receptors can independently elicit behavioral and electrophysiological responses which in the intact animal require concurrent activation of both receptor types; D_1 receptor activation stimulates c-*fos* expression, expression of both dopamine receptor and neuropeptide mRNAs is altered, and the balance of activity in the two parallel output pathways of the basal ganglia is altered. Therefore the aim of maximizing function in the parkinsonian patient should focus on restoring not just dopamine itself, but the normal physiological balance of neurotransmission in the extrapyramidal system.

Since the pattern of firing of substantia nigra dopamine neurons appears to vary only slightly in relation to ongoing motor activity[71], it has been assumed that striatal neurons are bathed in a continuous stream of dopamine. Concentrations of dopamine in the extracellular fluid of the brain are preserved to a remarkable extent, even in the face of massive degeneration of dopamine nerve terminals[37]. However, it may be expected that local regulatory influences may not be fully operative once dopamine depletion severe enough to result in parkinsonian symptoms develops. Dopamine derived from exogenously administered levodopa is not stored in vesicles and, to some extent, may not even be found in dopaminergic neurons in parkinsonian brain[72].

METHODS OF LEVODOPA ADMINISTRATION AND MOTOR RESPONSE

Paradigms in which the pattern of levodopa administration has been varied in attempts to provide more continuous, physiological levels of dopamine in the brain have confirmed in patients that the pattern and timing of drug administration can alter the response to levodopa. Thus Mouradian found that continuous intravenous levodopa administration to patients with RF resulted in reduced variability in motor function, and a shift to the left in the levodopa dose–response curve[73] which is more pronounced for production of dyskinesia than it is for the antiparkinsonian effect of the drug. When we administered levodopa continuously via duodenal infusion to a patient with RF, levodopa dose requirements gradually rose, and the patient never attained a full 'on' state. On the other hand, when the infusions were interrupted for just 8 h each night, drug requirements gradually diminished, so that after several months he experienced an excellent motor response for most of the day while taking just 70% of the maximal dose he received during the period of continuous infusion[74]. In fact, over the next year, his dose requirement continued to decline until he was using only 40% of his original levodopa dose (unpublished observations)! It is tempting to speculate that, in his case, with sustained levodopa administration during the day, D_2 receptor function was normalized as receptors were down-regulated, and D_1 receptors were up-regulated, thus restoring $D_1–D_2$ receptor interactions towards normal.

The above-cited data which indicate that chronic levodopa administration might alter the response of brain dopamine receptors to levodopa and dopamine-like drugs should not be interpreted to mean that chronic levodopa administration is deleterious to the Parkinson's disease patient. We were able to find no evidence that early initiation of levodopa therapy hastened the onset of dyskinesia, RF or dementia in our patient population[75]. In fact, delaying the initiation of levodopa therapy when the disease is first diagnosed may increase the predisposition of patients to develop dyskinesia[75–77] and RF[78]. In addition, the latency with which dyskinesias commence following the start of levodopa therapy is inversely proportional to the duration of disease at the time treatment was initiated[76]. These observations, taken together, suggest that as the period of dopamine depletion prior to beginning definitive symptomatic treatment gets longer, the greater chance there is that permanent receptor changes which predispose to the development of dyskinesia might take place.

A rational approach to maintaining the normal pattern of receptor responses in the parkinsonian striatum would be to attempt to emulate the relatively continuous pattern of dopamine release which is assumed to prevail in the normal brain, based on the relatively steady firing rates of midbrain dopaminergic neurons[79], and the lack of change in the firing rates of these cells in response to movement[71]. Since continuous intravenous administration of levodopa is cumbersome[30], a number of alternative approaches to providing sustained augmentation of striatal dopaminergic tone have been developed. Dopamine agonists which are available today have much longer pharmacological half-lives than does levodopa[80,81]. Agonists with differing degrees of selectivity at D_1 and D_2 receptors are being developed, and such development is to be eagerly awaited. Other approaches to providing sustained stimulation of brain dopamine receptors in Parkinson's disease include: drugs which extend the pharmacological half-life of levodopa or dopamine, such as inhibitors of the enzymes MAO-B[82-84] and COMT[85]; new levodopa formulations which provide the drug in a sustained-release form (reviewed in ref. 86); transplantation of adrenal medullary[87] or fetal brain tissue[88]; the use of anti-oxidant drugs[89] or, possibly someday, neurotrophic factors[90], and other agents which might prevent or arrest the degeneration of dopaminergic neurons.

REFERENCES

1. Mouradian, M.M. and Chase, T.N. (1988). Hypothesis: Central mechanisms and levodopa response fluctuations in Parkinson's disease. *Clin. Neurophar-macol.,* **11**, 378–85

2. Hoehn, M.M. (1983). Parkinsonism treated with levodopa: progression and mortality. *J. Neural Transmission,* **19**, 253–64

3. Cedarbaum, J.M. (1987). Clinical pharmacokinetics of antiparkinsonian drugs. *Clin. Neuropharmacokinet.,* **13**, 141–78

4. Calne, D., Karoum, F., Ruthven, C. and Sandler, M. (1969). The metabolism of orally administered L-dopa in parkinsonism. *Br. J. Pharma-col.,* **37**, 57–68

5. Ordonez, L.A., Romero, J.A. and Wurtman, R.J. (1972). Tissue distribution of L-dopa: evidence for a reservoir in skeletal muscle. *Fed. Proc.,* **31**, 589

6. Rose, S., Jenner, P. and Marsden, C.D. (1988). The effect of carbidopa on plasma and muscle levels of L-dopa, dopamine and their metabolites following L-dopa administration to rats. *Movement Disorders,* **3**, 117–25

7. Fitzpatrick, T.B., Miyamoto, M. and Ishikawa, K. (1967). The evolution

of concepts of melanin biology. *Arch. Dermatol.*, **96**, 295–323

8. Andersson, I., Granerus, A.K., Jagenburg, R. and Svanborg, A. (1975). Intestinal decarboxylation of orally administered L-dopa. *Acta Med. Scand.*, **198**, 415–20

9. Nissinen, E., Tuominen, R., Perhoniemi, V. and Kaakkola, S. (1988). Catechol-O-methyltransferase activity in human and rat small intestine. *Life Sci.*, **42**, 2609–14

10. Hardebo, J.E. and Owman, C. (1980). Barrier mechanism for neurotransmitter monoamines and their precursors at the blood–brain interface. *Ann. Neurol.*, **8**, 1–11

11. Wade, D.N., Mearrick, B.T. and Morris, J. (1973). Active transport of L-dopa in the intestine. *Nature*, **242**, 463–5

12. Nutt, J.G., Woodward, W.R., Hammarstad, J.P. and Carter, J.H. (1984). The 'on-off' phenomenon in Parkinson's disease: relation to levodopa absorption and transport. *N. Engl. J. Med.*, **310**, 483–8

13. Nutt, J.G., Woodward, W.R., Carter, J.H. and Trotman, T.L. (1989). Influence of fluctuations of plasma large neutral amino acids with normal diets on the clinical response to levodopa. *J. Neurol. Neurosurg. Psychiatr.*, **52**, 481–7

14. Sasahara, K., Nitani, T., Habara, T., Kojima, T., Kawahara, Y., Morioka, T. and Hakajima, E. (1981). Dosage form design for improvement of bioavailability of levodopa. V. Absorption and metabolism of levodopa in intestinal segments of dogs. *J. Pharm. Sci.*, **70**, 1157–60

15. Kurlan, R., Rothfield, K.P., Woodward, W.R., Nutt, J.G., Miller, C., Lichter, D. and Shoulson, I. (1988). Erratic gastric emptying of levodopa may cause 'random' fluctuations of parkinsonian mobility. *Neurology*, **38**, 419–21

16. Melamed, E., Bitton, V. and Zelig, O. (1986). Episodic total unresponsiveness to single doses of L-dopa in Parkinsonian fluctuators: a side-effect of long-term L-dopa therapy. *Neurology*, **36**, 100–3

17. Cedarbaum, J.M. and Schleifer, L.S. (1990). Drugs for Parkinson's disease, spasticity, and acute muscle spasms. In Gilman, A., Rall, T., Nies, A. and Taylor, P. (eds.) *Goodman and Gilman's The Pharmacological Basis of Therapeutics*, pp. 463–84. (New York: Pergamon Press)

18. Nutt, J.G., Woodward, W.R. and Anderson, J.L. (1985). The effect of carbidopa on the pharmacokinetics of intravenously administered levodopa: the mechanism of action in the treatment of parkinsonism. *Ann. Neurol.*, **18**, 537–43

19. Kuruma, I., Bartholini, G., Tissot, R. and Pletscher, A. (1971). The metabolism of L-3-O-methyldopa, a precursor of dopa in man. *Clin. Pharmacol. Therap.*, **12**, 678–82

20. Messiha, F., Hsu, T. and Bianchine, J. (1972). Peripheral aromatic L-aminoacids decarboxylase inhibitor in parkinsonism. I. Effect on O-methylated metabolites of 1-2-^{14}C-dopa. *J. Clin. Invest.*, **51**, 452–5

21. Muenter, M.D., Sharpless, N.S. and Tyce, G.M. (1972). Plasma 3-O-methyldopa in L-dopa therapy of Parkinson's disease. *Mayo Clin. Proc.*, **47**, 389–95

22. Muenter, M.D. and Tyce, G.M. (1971). L-dopa therapy of Parkinson's disease: plasma L-dopa concentration, therapeutic response and side effects. *Mayo Clin. Proc.*, **46**, 231–9

23. Shoulson, I., Glaubiger, G.A. and Chase, T.N. (1975). 'On–off' response: clinical and biochemical correlations during oral and intravenous levodopa administration in Parkinsonian patients. *Neurology*, **25**, 1144–8

24. Sweet, R.D. and McDowell, F.H. (1974). Plasma dopa concentrations and the 'on–off' effect after chronic treatment of Parkinson's disease. *Neurology*, **24**, 953–6

25. Creese, I., Burt, D.R. and Snyder, S.H. (1977). Dopamine receptor binding enhancement accompanies lesion-induced behavioral supersensitivity. *Science*, **197**, 596–8

26. Lee, T., Seeman, P., Rajput, A., Farlay, I.J. and Hornykiewicz, O. (1978). Receptor basis for dopaminergic supersensitivity in Parkinson's disease. *Nature*, **273**, 59–61

27. Cotzias, G.C., Papavasiliou, P.S. and Gellene, R.S. (1969). Modification of Parkinsonism – chronic treatment with L-dopa. *N. Engl. J. Med.*, **280**, 337–45

28. Birkmeyer, W. and Hornykiewicz, O. (1961). Der 1,3,5, dioxyphenylalanine (dopa), effect beider Parkinson akinese. *Wein Klin. Wochenschr.*, **73**, 787–8

29. Hardie, R.J., Lees, A.J. and Stern, G.M. (1984). On-off fluctuations in Parkinson's disease: a clinical and neuropharmacological study. *Brain*, **107**, 487–506

30. Quinn, N.P., Parkes, J.D. and Marsden, C.D. (1984). Control of on/off phenomenon by continuous intravenous infusion of levodopa. *Neurology*, **34**, 1131–6

31. Nutt, J.G. and Woodward, W.R. (1986). Levodopa pharmacokinetics and pharmacodynamics in fluctuating parkinsonian patients. *Neurology*, **36**, 739–44

32. Gancher, S.T., Nutt, J.G. and Woodward, W.R. (1987). Peripheral pharmacokinetics of levodopa in untreated, stable and fluctuating patients. *Neurology*, **37**, 940–4

33. Fabbrini, G., Juncos, J., Mouradian, M.M., Serrati, C. and Chase, T.N. (1987). Levodopa pharmacokinetic mechanisms and motor fluctuations in

Parkinson's disease. *Ann. Neurol.*, **21**, 370–6

34. Fabbrini, G., Mouradian, M.M., Juncos, J.L., Schlegel, J., Mohr, E. and Chase, T.N. (1988). Motor fluctuations in Parkinson's disease: central pathophysiological mechanisms, Part I. *Ann. Neurol.*, **24**, 366–71

35. Mouradian, M.M., Juncos, J.L., Fabrini, G. and Chase, T.N. (1987). Motor fluctuations in Parkinson's disease: pathogenetic and therapeutic studies. *Ann. Neurol.*, **22**, 475–9

36. Agid, Y., Javoy, F. and Glowinski, J. (1973). Hyperactivity of remaining dopaminergic neurons after destruction of the nigrostriatal dopaminergic system in the rat. *Nature New Biol.*, **245**, 150–1

37. Zigmond, M.E., Abercrombie, E.D., Berger, T.W., Grace, A.A. and Stricker, E.M. (1990). Compensations after lesions of central dopaminergic neurons: some clinical and basic implications. *Trends Neurol. Sci.*, **13**, 290–6

38. Spencer, S.E. and Wooten, G.F. (1984). Altered pharmacokinetics of L-dopa metabolism in rat striatum deprived of dopaminergic innervation. *Neurology*, **34**, 1005–8

39. Olanow, C.W., Gauger, L.L. and Cedarbaum, J.M. (1991). Temporal relationships between plasma and CSF pharmacokinetics of levodopa and clinical effect in Parkinson's disease. *Ann. Neurol.*, **29**, 556–9

40. Cedarbaum, J.M. and Olanow, C.W. (1991). Dopamine sulfate in ventricular cerebrospinal fluid and motor function in Parkinson's disease. *Neurology*, in press

41. Post, R.M. (1980). Intermittent versus continuous stimulation: effect of time on the development of sensitization or tolerance. *Life Sci.*, **26**, 1275–82

42. Nomoto, M., Jenner, P. and Marsden, C.D. (1985). The dopamine D_2 agonist LY141865, but not the D_1 agonist SKF 38393, reverses parkinsonism induced by 1-methyl-4-phenyl-1,2,3,6-tetrahydropyridine (MPTP) in the common marmoset. *Neurosci. Lett.*, **57**, 37–41

43. Temlett, J.A., Chong, P.N., Oertel, W.H., Jenner, P. and Marsden, C.D. (1988). The D_1 dopamine receptor partial agonist CY208-243 exhibits antiparkinsonian activity in the MPTP-treated marmoset. *Eur. J. Pharmacol.*, **156**, 197–206

44. Gershanik, O., Heikkila, R.E. and Duvoisin, R.C. (1983). Behavioral correlations of dopamine receptor activation. *Neurology*, **33**, 1489–92

45. Markstein, R. (1981). Neurochemical effects of some ergot derivatives: a basis for their antiparkinson actions. *J. Neural Transmission*, **51**, 39–59

46. Rinne, U.K. (1989). Early dopamine agonist therapy in Parkinson's disease. *Movement Disorders*, **4** (Suppl. 1), S86–S94

47. Juncos, J.L., Engber, T.M., Raisman, R., Susel, Z., Thibaut, F., Ploska, A., Agill, Y. and Chase, T.N. (1989). Continuous and intermittent levodopa

differentially affect basal ganglia function. *Ann. Neurol.,* **25**, 473–8
48. Engber, T.M., Susel, Z., Juncos, J.L. and Chase, T.N. (1989). Continuous and intermittent levodopa differentially affect rotation induced by D_1 and D_2 dopamine agonists. *Eur. J. Pharmacol.,* **168**, 291–8
49. Engber, T.M., Susel, Z., Kuo, S. and Chase, T. (1990). Chronic levodopa treatment alters basal and dopamine agonist-stimulated cerebral glucose utilization. *J. Neurosci.,* **10**, 3889–95
50. Ariano, M. (1988). Striatal D_1 dopamine receptor distribution following chemical lesion of the nigrostriatal pathway. *Brain Res.,* **443**, 204–14
51. Buonamici, M., Caccia, C., Carpentieri, M., Pegrassi, L. and Rossi, A.C. (1986). D_1 receptor supersensitivity in the rat striatum after unilateral 6-hydroxydopamine lesions. *Eur. J. Pharmacol.,* **126**, 347–8
52. Mishra, R.K., Wong, Y.W., Varmuzon, S.L. and Taft, L. (1978). Lesions and drug-induced supersensitivity and subsensitivity of caudate dopamine receptors. *Life Sci.,* **23**, 443–6
53. Guttman, M. and Seeman, P. (1985). L-dopa reverses the elevated density of D_2-dopamine receptors in Parkinson's disease striatum. *J. Neural Transmission,* **64**, 93–103
54. Raisman, R., Cash, R., Ruberg, M., Javoy-Agid, F. and Agid, Y. (1985). Binding of [³H]SCH 23390 to D_1 receptors in the putamen of control and parkinsonian subjects. *Eur. J. Pharmacol.,* **113**, 467–70
55. Mansour, A., Meador-Woodruff, J.H., Camp, D.M., Robinson, T.E., Bunzow, J., Van Tol, H., Cirelli, V., Akil, H. and Watson, S.J. (1990). The effects of nigrostriatal 6-hydroxydopamine lesions on dopamine D_2 receptor mRNA and opioid systems. In *International Narcotics Research Conference (INRC) '89,* pp. 227–30. (New York: Alan R. Liss Inc.)
56. Gerfen, C.R., Engber, T.M., Mahan, L.C., Susel, Z., Chase, T.N., Monsona, F.J. Jr. and Sibley, D.R. (1990). D_1 and D_2 dopamine receptor-mediated gene expression of striatonigral and striatopallidal neurons. *Science,* **250**, 1429–31
57. Bennett, J.P. Jr. and Wooten, G.F. (1986). Dopamine denervation does not alter *in vivo* ³H-spiperone binding in rat striatum: implications for external imaging of dopamine receptors in Parkinson's disease. *Ann. Neurol.,* **19**, 378–83
58. Leslie, C. and Bennett, J.P. Jr. (1977). Striatal D_1- and D_2-dopamine receptor sites are separately detectable *in vivo. Brain Res.,* **415**, 90–7
59. Siggins, G.R., Hoffer, B.J., Bloom, F.E. and Ungerstedt, U. (1976). Cytochemical and electrophysiological studies of dopamine in the caudate nucleus. In Yahr, M. (ed.) *The Basal Ganglia,* pp. 227–48. (New York: Raven Press)
60. Hu, X.T., Wachtel, S.R., Galloway, M.P. and White, F.J. (1990). Lesions

of the nigrostriatal dopamine projection increase the inhibitory effects of D_1 and D_2 dopamine agonists on caudate-putamen neurons and relieve D_2 receptors from the necessity of D_1 receptor stimulation. *J. Neurosci.*, **10**, 2318–29

61. Calabresi, P., Benedetti, M., Mercuri, B. and Bernardi, G. (1988). Depletion of catecholamines reveals inhibitory effects of bromocriptine and lysuride on neostriatal neurones recorded intracellularly *in vitro*. *Neuropharmacology*, **27**, 579–87

62. LaHoste, G.J., Andreini, M. and Marshall, J.F. (1990). The role of D_1/D_2 interaction and dopamine receptor density in behavioral supersensitivity to dopamine agonists. *Neurosci. Abs.*, **16**, 953

63. Robertson, G.S., Vincent, S.R. and Fibiger, H.C. (1990). Striatonigral projection neurons contain D_1 dopamine receptor-activated c-*fos*. *Brain Res.*, **523**, 288–90

64. Robertson, G.S., Gerrera, D.G., Dragunow, M. and Robertson, H.A. (1989). L-dopa activates c-*fos* in the striatum ipsilateral to a 6-hydroxydopamine lesion of the substantia nigra. *Eur. J. Pharmacol.*, **159**, 99–100

65. Robertson, H.A., Peterson, M.R., Murphy, K. and Roberston, G.S. (1989). D_1-dopamine receptor agonists selectively activate striatal c-*fos* independent of rotational behavior. *Brain Res.*, **503**, 346–9

66. Paul, M.L., Graybiel, A.M. and Robertson, H.A. (1990). Synergistic activation of the immediate-early gene c-*fos* in striosomes by D_1- and D_2-selective dopamine agonists. *Neurosci. Abs.*, **16**, 954

67. Normand, E., Popovici, T., Onteniente, B., Fellman, D., Piakier-Tonneau, P., Auffray, C. and Block, B. (1988). Dopaminergic neurons of the substantia nigra modulate preproenkephalin A gene expression in rat striatal neurons. *Brain Res.*, **439**, 39–46

68. Beckstead, R.M. (1988). Association of dopamine D_1 and D_2 receptors with specific cellular elements in the basal ganglia of the cat: the uneven topography of dopamine receptors in the striatum is determined by intrinsic striatal cells, not nigrostriatal axons. *Neuroscience*, **27**, 851–63

69. Li, S.J., Jiang, H.K., Stachowick, M.S., Hudson, P.M., Owyang, V., Nanry, K., Tolson, H.A. and Hong, J.J. (1990). Influence of nigrostriatal dopaminergic tone on the biosynthesis of dynorphin and enkephalin in rat striatum. *Mol. Brain Res.*, **8**, 269–75

70. Crossman, A.R. (1990). A hypothesis on the pathophysiological mechanisms that underlie levodopa- or dopamine agonist-induced dyskinesia in Parkinson's disease: implications for future strategies in treatment. *Movement Disorders*, **5**, 100–8

71. DeLong, M.R., Crutcher, M.D. and Georgropoulos, G. (1983). Relations between movement and single cell discharge in the substantia nigra of the

behaving monkey. *J. Neurosci.*, **3**, 1599–606

72. Melamed, E. (1988). Mechanism of action of exogenous L-dopa. Is it a physiological therapy for Parkinson's disease? In Jankovic, J. and Tolosa, E. (eds.) *Parkinson's Disease and Movement Disorders*, pp. 87–94. (Baltimore: Urban & Schwarzenberg)

73. Mouradian, M.M., Heuser, L.J.E., Baronti, F. and Chase, T.N. (1988). Modifications of central pharmacodynamics of levodopa by its continuous infusion. *Neurology*, **38** (Suppl. 1), 178

74. Cedarbaum, J.M., Silvestri, M. and Kutt, H. (1990). Sustained enteral levodopa infusion increases, whereas interrupted infusion decreases levodopa dose requirements. *Neurology*, **90**, 995–7

75. Cedarbaum, J.M., Gandy, S.E. and McDowell, F.H. (1991). 'Early' initiation of levodopa treatment does not promote the development of motor response fluctuations, dyskinesias or dementia in Parkinson's disease. *Neurology*, **41**, 622–9

76. Bergmann, K.J., Mendoza, M.R. and Yahr, M.D. (1986). Parkinson's disease and long-term levodopa therapy. *Adv. Neurol.*, **45**, 463–7

77. Blin, J., Bonnet, A.-M. and Agid, Y. (1988). Does levodopa aggravate Parkinson's disease? *Neurology*, **38**, 1410–16

78. Caraceni, T., Scigliano, G. and Mussicco, M. (1991). The occurrence of motor fluctuations in Parkinsonian patients treated long term with levodopa: role of early treatment and disease progression. *Neurology*, **41**, 380–4

79. Bunney, B.S., Walters, J.R., Roth, R.H. and Aghajanian, G.K. (1973). Dopaminergic neurons: Effect of antipsychotic drugs and amphetamine on single cell activity. *J. Pharmacol. Exp. Ther.*, **185**, 560–71

80. Goldstein, M., Lieberman, A., Lew, J.S., Asano, T., Rosenfeld, M.R. and Makman, M.H. (1980). Interaction of pergolide with central dopamine receptors. *Proc. Natl. Acad. Sci.*, **77**, 3725–8

81. Schran, H.F., Bhuta, S.I., Schwartz, H.J. and Thorner, M.O. (1980). The pharmacokinetics of bromocriptine in man. In Goldstein, M. (ed.) *Ergot Compounds and Brain Function: Neuroendocrine and Neuropsychiatric Aspects*, pp. 125–39. (New York: Raven Press)

82. Cedarbaum, J.M., Silvestri, M., Clark, M., Harts, A. and Kutt, H. (1990). Deprenyl, levodopa pharmacokinetics and modification of response fluctuations in Parkinson's disease. *Clin. Neuropharmacol.* **13**, 29–35

83. Elizan, T.S., Moros, D.A. and Yahr, M.D. (1991). Early combination of selegiline and low-dose levodopa as initial symptomatic therapy in Parkinson's disease. *Arch. Neurol.*, **48**, 31–4

84. Golbe, L.I. (1988). Deprenyl as symptomatic therapy in Parkinson's disease. *Clin. Neuropharmacol.*, **11**, 387–400

85. Cedarbaum, J.M., Leger, G. and Guttman, M. (1991). Reduction of

circulating 3-*O*-methyldopa by inhibition of catechol-*O*-methyltransferase with OR-611 and OR-462 in cynomolgus monkeys: implications for the treatment of Parkinson's disease. *Clin. Neuropharmacol.*, **19**, 330–42

86. Cedarbaum, J.M. (1990). Pharmacokinetic and pharmacodynamic considerations in the management of motor response fluctuations in Parkinson's disease. *Neurol. Clin. N.A.*, **8**, 31–48

87. Madrazo, I., Drucker-Colin, R., Diaz, V. *et al.* (1987). Open microsurgical autograft of adrenal medulla to the right caudate nucleus in two patients with intractable Parkinson's disease. *N. Engl. J. Med.*, **316**, 831–4

88. Lindvall, O., Rehncrona, S., Brundin, B., Gustavii, B., Astedt, B., Widner, H., Lindholm, T., Björklund, A., Leenders, K.L., Rothwell, J.C., Frackowiak, R., Marsden, C.D., Johnels, B., Steg, G., Freedman, R., Hoffer, B.J., Seiger, A., Bygdeman, M., Strömberg, I. and Olson, L. (1989). Human fetal dopamine neurons grafted into the striatum in two patients with severe Parkinson's disease: a detailed account of methodology and a 6-month follow-up. *Arch. Neurol.*, **46**, 615–33

89. Parkinson Study Group (1989). Effect of deprenyl on the progression of disability in early Parkinson's disease. *N. Engl. J. Med.*, **321**, 1364–71

90. Hyman, C., Hofer, M., Barde, Y.-A., Juhaz, M., Yancopoulos, G.D., Squinto, S.P. and Lindsay, R.M. (1991). BDNF is a neurotrophic factor for dopaminergic neurons of the substantia nigra. *Nature (London)*, **350**, 230–2

8

Dopamine agonists: historical perspective

A.N. Lieberman and M. Goldstein

INTRODUCTION

Levodopa, alone, or combined with a decarboxylase inhibitor, reverses most of the symptoms of Parkinson's disease. However, not all symptoms improve[1] and in many patients, improvement diminishes and becomes erratic (response fluctuation)[2]. The response fluctuations are usually associated with abnormal movements (dyskinesias)[2-4]. In addition, some patients also develop mental and autonomic disturbances[5,6]. Some symptoms reflect disease progression as patients live longer and exhibit symptoms not seen in the pre-levodopa era[6,7]. However, some symptoms reflect levels of levodopa higher than those produced endogenously[8]. Dopamine agonists have certain advantages over levodopa[9,10]. Agonists, unlike levodopa, do not have to be converted to dopamine by the failing nigrostriatal system; they can be given in small amounts; they diminish response fluctuations, and may improve symptoms not improved by levodopa. Moreover, because agonists decrease the requirement for levodopa less dopamine accumulates. Accumulated dopamine may undergo auto-oxidation and generate cytotoxic free radicals and increase the oxidative stress on the dopamine neurons. By reducing dopamine formation, agonists may protect the neurons from this oxidative stress[11-13].

The exogenous administration of levodopa does not mimic the endogenous production and delivery of dopamine[14-18] to the different subsets of dopamine receptors with different sensitivities and localizations on both pre- and postsynaptic neurons in the substantia nigra (SN) and the striatum[19-21]. Two main subtypes of dopamine receptor are recognized, one positively (D_1) and the other negatively (D_2) linked to adenylate cyclase. D_2 receptors appear to be on cholinergic and GABAergic striatal and on dopamine SN neurons[22,23]. D_1 receptors appear to be on striatal neurons, including those projecting to the SN pars reticulata. Using agonists or antagonists selective for either the D_1 or D_2 receptor has demonstrated that different behavioral, pharmacological and physiological effects are mediated by each of the receptors[20,21]. However, stimulation of the D_2 receptor is more closely associated with antiparkinsonian activity[19,24,25].

While many dopamine agonists have been developed, only three are widely used: bromocriptine (Parlodel®)[9], lisuride (Dopergin®)[26] and pergolide (Permax®)[27]. Apomorphine has limited use in selected patients. There are structural, biochemical and pharmacological differences between these agonists[19,24,25] and while most patients will respond to each of them[9,10,26-29], some patients respond better, or have fewer adverse effects, with a particular agonist.

It is convenient to consider the use of agonists in three situations: patients with early Parkinson's disease not on levodopa; patients with moderate Parkinson's disease on levodopa, with or without response fluctuations, and patients with advanced Parkinson's disease.

HISTORICAL OVERVIEW

Historically, agonists were first used in patients with moderate or advanced Parkinson's disease[9,10,26-29]. These patients had been on high doses of levodopa and were experiencing combinations of decreased efficacy, response fluctuations, freezing spells, falls, violent tremors, dyskinesias and mental change. While most symptoms resulted from disease progression, some symptoms resulted from the high pulsatile doses of levodopa. At the time it was thought agonists could replace levodopa and provide an antiparkinsonian therapy with fewer adverse effects[9,26-29]. It soon became apparent that the agonists could not replace levodopa, but by decreasing the dose of levodopa many of the adverse effects could be reduced. The success of agonists in decreasing the response fluctuations and dyskinesias[29-36] led to their being used before patients developed response fluctuations, and even earlier as monotherapy for newly diagnosed Parkinson's disease patients. Several studies demonstrated that as monotherapy the agonists had an antiparkinsonian effect that was less than that of levodopa, but which was not associated with fluctuations or dyskinesias[33-36]. Nonetheless, interest in the agonists as monotherapy waned until it was demonstrated that deprenyl (Eldepryl®), like the agonists, delays the need for levodopa in newly diagnosed Parkinson's disease patients. While there is controversy as to whether this results from a slowing of the progression of the disease or from a symptomatic effect of deprenyl, the delay is impressive[37-40].

AGONISTS AS ADJUNCTS TO LEVODOPA IN MODERATE PARKINSON'S DISEASE

It is convenient to examine first the use of agonists as adjuncts to levodopa in patients with response fluctuations. The initial benefit obtained in most patients on levodopa begins to wane between 2 and 5 years after starting treatment[1-3,6-8]. After several more years, disease severity is usually worse than before starting levodopa, but one-third of patients are still better than before levodopa. Usually, tremor, rigidity, handwriting and finger dexterity remain improved while postural reflexes, speech and gait worsen.

Several hypotheses have been proposed to explain this. Initially it was thought that compensation for the progressive SN dopamine neuron loss was achieved through an increased conversion of the exogenously administered levodopa to dopamine by the remaining SN neurons and by the development of supersensitivity of the postsynaptic striatal receptors[41,42]. It was also thought that compensation could be achieved through the conversion of levodopa to dopamine in striatal neurons which normally do not synthesize dopamine[14,16]. It is possible that as the disease progresses, levodopa no longer compensates for the resulting striatal dopamine deficiency because the remaining SN neurons are too few in number to generate enough dopamine[6,17]. The benefit that patients derive from the agonists which bypass the degenerating SN neurons and directly stimulate the striatal dopamine receptors supports this hypothesis. Negating this hypothesis is the observation that some severely incapacitated patients with marked degeneration of SN neurons respond as well as less incapacitated patients to levodopa. However, in most of these severely incapacitated patients the favorable response to levodopa is of short duration and it is probable that the favorable response is related more to postsynaptic receptor sensitivity than to dopamine synthesis and that this supersensitivity quickly disappears[29].

Another explanation for the decreased response to levodopa is degeneration of the striatal receptors. While some studies show a reduction in the number of striatal receptors, others do not[23,29]. The reduction in striatal receptors could also result from down-regulation of the receptors by chronic dopamine stimulation.

Another explanation for the decreased response to levodopa is the endogenous production of toxic metabolites[43]. This explanation has raised questions about when to start levodopa[7,8]. If toxic metabolites of levodopa are responsible for the loss of efficacy, then treatment with levodopa should be delayed until the patient has a level of disability that cannot be controlled with other drugs[8]. If not, then treatment with levodopa may begin sooner[7]. The experience with MPTP-induced Parkinson's disease where patients have a marked loss of SN neurons, quickly become disabled and rapidly lose their response to levodopa, supports disease severity as being more important than accumulation of toxic metabolites as the cause of the decreased response to levodopa. However, the acutely developing MPTP-induced Parkinson's disease may not be the model for the slowly evolving idiopathic Parkinson's disease.

Decreased levodopa efficacy is usually associated with response fluctuations and dyskinesias, but the mechanisms underlying these phenomena may be different[1,2]. Early in Parkinson's disease most patients maintain a smooth and prolonged response (several hours) to a single dose of levodopa[4,44]. This occurs despite a short half-life of levodopa (between 0.77 and 1.08 hours). It has been suggested that the long duration effect is secondary to the accumulation of a reservoir of dopamine in the striatum[17] or to the activation of a second messenger which drives behavior long after the eliciting signal has subsided[29]. Even after response fluctuations to a single dose of levodopa develop the long duration effect continues, as demonstrated by the additional deterioration that occurs 3–5 days after levodopa is stopped.

After 2–5 years of treatment most patients find that the beneficial effect of a single dose of levodopa 'wears off' before the next dose is due[44]. Eventually efficacy shortens so that a predictable 'wearing off' occurs several times a day. The emotional state of the patient also plays a role, as anxiety or distress often precipitate a temporary worsening of symptoms. A few patients experience unpredictable, random and abrupt loss of efficacy ('on–off' phenomenon). With the development of 'wearing off' phenomena, the clinical response becomes closely tied to the rise and fall in plasma levodopa levels.

It is probable that 'peripheral' pharmacokinetic mechanisms combined with a shorter central action of levodopa are responsible for the 'wearing off' phenomenon[18,45]. It is not known if chronic pulsatile levodopa treatment alters the peripheral handling of levodopa, or whether normal variations in peripheral absorption and metabolism become obvious only when the central effects of levodopa are shortened[15,16,18,45]. Additional mechanisms also must be considered since fluctuations are not completely eliminated by continuous infusion of levodopa. It has been suggested that short-term changes in the affinity state of dopamine receptors from high to low or vice-versa might account for some of the fluctuations. Receptor changes could be induced by rising or falling levels of dopamine[46].

A variety of abnormal movements and postures may occur in patients on levodopa. Peak-dose dyskinesias are abnormal movements occurring midway between levodopa doses. Some patients may develop dyskinesias throughout the dose interval[4,29]. The earlier that dyskinesias appear and the longer that they are present, the more sensitive patients become to them and the lower the dose of levodopa that they can tolerate. A few patients appear very sensitive to this effect. Such patients are best managed with agonists alone or with agonists and low doses of levodopa.

The abnormal movements may be choreatic, ballistic, athetotic, tic-like, dystonic or a combination[2,4]. Early morning dystonia, usually involving the feet also occurs during chronic levodopa treatment. However, unlike the dyskinesias, early morning dystonia occurs when the effects of levodopa are low and is relieved by another dose of levodopa or an agonist[47,48].

The dyskinesias and dystonias result from the effects of levodopa on the striatum. Although levodopa-induced dyskinesias are not restricted to Parkinson's disease, it appears that degeneration of the SN dopamine system predisposes to them[41]. It has been suggested that chronic levodopa or agonist treatment can induce postsynaptic hypersensitivity in some receptors. This contrasts with the better recognized downregulation of receptors which occurs with chronic treatment. If excessive dopamine activity induces dyskinesias, it is not known which dopamine receptors are responsible. Experience with dopamine agonists provides insight into this question[41]. The ergot agonists, such as bromocriptine and lisuride, stimulate D_2 receptors and antagonize D_1 receptors. Pergolide, like dopamine, stimulates both D_2 and D_1 receptors. Bromocriptine and lisuride induce the fewest dyskinesias, implying that D_1 agonism may be responsible for the dyskinesias. It has also been argued that it is the lower potency of the agonists compared to levodopa that accounts for the lower incidence of dyskinesias[25,29,41].

Earlier use of agonists

Because fluctuations and dyskinesias are reduced when levodopa is reduced and replaced with an agonist, it has been suggested that the agonists might be more effective if used earlier[34,35]. Increasing evidence supports using agonists earlier, before fluctuations or dyskinesias develop. Most of the studies combining an agonist with levodopa utilize bromocriptine. It is probable that similar results would be obtained with the other agonists. Bromocriptine used alone in levodopa-untreated patients results in few fluctuations or dyskinesias. However, the antiparkinsonian efficacy is less than that of levodopa[34,36]. The combination of low doses of levodopa (300–600 mg/day with a decarboxylase inhibitor) and low doses of bromocriptine (15–25 mg/day) provides an alternative to higher doses of levodopa[34–36]. Using this approach, several studies report a response equal to that obtained with higher doses of levodopa alone, with fewer fluctuations and dyskinesias even after 5 years[30–36].

Most investigators now advocate adding an agonist to levodopa soon after starting levodopa. The agonist is started in low doses of 1.0–2.5 mg/day for bromocriptine and 0.1–0.2 mg/day for pergolide and lisuride, and is built up gradually in increments of 1.0–2.5 mg/day each week to a maximum of 10–40 mg for bromocriptine. By using agonists in low doses and increasing the dose gradually, most adverse reactions are avoided. Such combined treatment in patients is as important as combination therapy in other conditions, such as hypertension, heart disease, diabetes and infection. With increasing Parkinson's disease, the dosage of the agonist increases[33]. This may mean that it is more difficult to stimulate the receptors or that tachyphylaxis develops.

LEVODOPA AND DOPAMINE AGONISTS IN ADVANCED PARKINSON'S DISEASE

Advanced Parkinson's disease in the levodopa–dopamine agonist era differs from advanced Parkinson's disease in the pre-levodopa era. In the pre-levodopa era, advanced Parkinson's disease patients had rigidity, tremor, bradykinesia and gait difficulty[49], while advanced Parkinson's disease patients on levodopa are not rigid, may not be bradykinetic and may be able to walk, but have postural instability and sustain serious falls. Some patients have violent tremors that are not responsive to levodopa or anticholinergics, some have autonomic insufficiency and many have mental changes. While these patients may also have response fluctuations and dyskinesias, the postural instability, autonomic insufficiency and mental changes dominate their lives. The pathophysiology of these symptoms differs from that of the fluctuations and dyskinesias[36].

Pathophysiology of advanced Parkinson's disease

In advanced Parkinson's disease, in addition to the loss of the SN neurons, changes also occur in the striatum and in its connections with the cortex and spinal cord. The striatum, the caudate nucleus and the putamen, receives its major input from the sensory and motor cortex via the corticostriatal tract[50,51]. Different portions of the tract project to the caudate nucleus or the putamen and different behaviors are associated with these two structures[20,21,50,51]. The caudate nucleus and its connections are involved in cognition and planning motor activity, while the putamen and its connections are involved in executing motor paradigms[50,51]. In Parkinson's disease, the putamen is more severely affected than the caudate.

The corticostriatal tract releases excitatory amino acids (glutamate and aspartate) that stimulate striatal N-methyl-D-aspartate (NMDA) receptors. The NMDA receptors may be on the axons of the corticostriatal tract or on striatal neurons. In the striatum the effects of the descending excitatory corticostriatal tract are modulated by an ascending inhibitory and excitatory dopamine nigrostriatal tract[50,52]. Neurons in the caudate nucleus and the putamen project to the internal and external segment of the globus pallidus (GPi, Gpe). The Gpe projects to the subthalamic nucleus (STN), which in turn projects to the Gpi. The GPi projects to the ventral lateral (VL) and ventral anterior (VA) nucleus of the thalamus. The VL and VA neurons project to the supplementary motor area. There is also a pathway from the striatum to the SN pars reticulata that acts as an inhibitory feedback control on the nigrostriatal dopamine pathway. The neurons in the caudate nucleus, putamen, pallium and thalamus are topographically arranged[21,50-52].

Differential interruption of the cortico-striato-pallido-thalamo-cortical loop, topographical distribution of neurons, differential loss of dopamine innervation to the caudate nucleus and the putamen, and intrinsic differences between the caudate nucleus and putamen may explain the heterogeneity of symptoms in advanced Parkinson's disease.

Thus, neurons governing axial movements are heavily represented in the striatum. These movements are more likely to be closely linked to dopamine activity. Neurons governing appendicular movements are heavily represented in the motor cortex. These movements are less likely to be linked to dopamine activity. This may explain, in part, why symptoms such as writing and finger dexterity remain improved while symptoms such as axial bradykinesia and gait deteriorate during chronic levodopa treatment[53]. Bradykinesia may result from disinhibition (excitation) of the neurons in the STN while dyskinesia may result from inhibition of these neurons. Severe tremor may result from disinhibition of the neurons in the VL thalamic nucleus[51,52]. The influence of dopamine, GABAergic, cholinergic and noradrenergic circuits in regulating the neurons in the thalamus may explain why levodopa, anticholinergic agents and beta blockers may at times be effective in controlling tremor.

Levodopa and postural instability

Postural instability, associated with a loss of righting reflexes, is responsible for the disabling falls that occur in some patients[50,51,54], and has several causes. Patients with postural instability may behave as though they have a proprioceptive loss which, by standard testing, they do not.

Proprioceptive fibers ascend from the dorsal root ganglia via the posterior columns to neurons in the contralateral nucleus gracilis. Fibers from the gracilis then ascend, via the medial lemniscus, to the VPL and VPM nuclei of the thalamus and then to the sensorimotor cortex. While most of the sensory input to the striatum is indirect, processed in the cortex and then relayed to the striatum, there is also a direct sensory input as collaterals from the medial lemniscus pass to the centrum medianum and then to the striatum. Thus, abnormalities in propriocep-tion beyond conscious perception may be partially responsible for postural instability.

The postural instability of Parkinson's disease also resembles that of cerebellar dysfunction, but is unassociated with titubation or dysmetria. While proprioceptive and cerebellar impairment may play a role, the postural instability of advanced Parkinson's disease, arises mainly from impairment of the brainstem nuclei that regulate extensor tone[54]. The extensor muscles that maintain posture are regulated by neurons in the spinal cord that are, in turn, regulated by neurons in the pedunculo-pontine nucleus (PPN), the pontine and medullary reticular formation (RF) and the vestibular nucleus (VN). In progressive supranuclear palsy (PSP), the loss of neurons in the PPN, RF and VN, results in postural instability. As these neurons are non-dopamine, the postural instability of PSP does not respond to levodopa. In advanced Parkinson's disease the postural instability is similar to, but less marked than, that in PSP[54].

In advanced Parkinson's disease, levodopa may aggravate postural instability. Thus, some Parkinson's disease patients may fall because of levodopa-induced dyskinesias, while some may fall because of levodopa-induced ataxia (without dyskinesias). The levodopa-induced ataxia may be associated with freezing spells, festination and forced running. In these instances the falls may lessen as levodopa is decreased and the patients become bradykinetic. Some of these patients have likened their situation to a car running downhill without brakes: slowing down lets them brake more easily. Other Parkinson's disease patients may fall when changing velocity or direction (i.e. while turning). In these patients turning is associated with freezing and festination, as if the underlying parkinsonism was unmasked by the act of turning. Some improve with a dopamine agonist or with small increases in levodopa. The complexity of falling becomes apparent when it is realized that the same symptoms, freezing and festination may indicate too much or too little dopamine.

In some patients falls may occur when the patient abruptly and unpredictably changes from an 'on' to an 'off'. Treatment of these falls consists of dampening the fluctuations by replacing as much levodopa as possible with an agonist. While in these patients it is impossible to replace levodopa completely, it may be possible to replace a third or half of it. Bromocriptine 10 mg (lisuride and pergolide 1 mg) substitutes for 50–100 mg of levodopa (with a decarboxylase inhibitor). The limiting factor in replacing levodopa with an agonist in these patients is the occurrence of mental changes.

Emotional upset, exercise, perceptual change (for example, approaching a door), all may influence the brainstem nuclei sufficiently to result in a fall. Such falls are even more difficult to treat. While treatment of postural instability is difficult, the condition is so disabling that more than sympathy is in order. The patient should be investigated, using high field (1.5 tesla) magnetic resonance imaging (MRI), for other causes of postural instability. Occasionally an unsuspected subdural hematoma, a consequence of the frequent falls, or normal pressure hydrocephalus will be discovered. The appearance of putaminal hypointensity on a T2 weighted MRI, or brainstem atrophy suggest levodopa unresponsiveness[55]. At this time, while no treatment is available, the patient and the family should be instructed to keep the patient in a wheelchair and walk only with support. In this situation the risk of a fall leading to a fractured skull, pelvis or hip, outweighs the benefits of mobility. It will be challenging to see whether this situation can be mitigated by neuroprotective treatment.

Mental changes in advanced Parkinson's disease

Mental disturbances including nightmares, visual hallucinations, confusion, paranaoia and personality changes occur during levodopa treatment[56-58]. These disturbances occur more frequently in patients with pre-existing cognitive impairment. While some patients progress almost predictably from sleep disturbances to visual hallucinations to psychosis, in others the psychosis appears without warning. In most instances the mental disturbances do not disappear promptly when levodopa is discontinued. This suggests a 'long-duration' non-motor effect of levodopa analogous to its 'long-duration' motor effect. Short duration changes in mood and behavior also occur and often are linked to the 'short-duration' motor responses[29]. The best explanation for the mental disturbances associated with levodopa is activation of dopamine receptors in mesolimbic and mesocortical systems. Activation of cholinergic serotonergic or noradrenergic neurons may also play a role. Mental disturbances occur more frequently with dopamine agonists than with levodopa.

The occurrence of mental changes in patients with advanced Parkinson's disease does not mean that levodopa or dopamine agonists have to be discontinued. An attempt should be made to correct any contributing abnormality such as dehydration, infection, acidosis, hypoxemia, hyponatremia, or hypo- or hyperthyroidism. All but essential medications should be stopped. Anxiolytics, hypnotics, anticholinergics and, if possible, antidepressants should be discontinued slowly, as abrupt stoppage results in agitation. Occasionally, drug holidays (temporary levodopa withdrawal) may be useful[59]. Levodopa withdrawal should only be done in a hospital with physicians familiar with the technique[59,60]. The emergence of a severe parkinsonian state with its attendant risks of aspiration and phlebitis, as well as a life-threatening malignant neuroleptic syndrome, are real possibilities. Psychiatric consultation should be obtained, as occasionally the maniacal agitation is an agitated depression that responds to antidepressants, or the dementia is the pseudodementia of depression that responds to antidepressants or electroconvulsive therapy. Occasionally, the psychotic behavior may respond to molindone (Mobane®) or clozapine (Clozaril®), antipsychotic agents without extrapyramidal side-effects.

Autonomic insufficiency

Patients with advanced Parkinson's disease exhibit a variety of symptoms of autonomic insufficiency. Indeed, the number and severity of the symptoms suggest that these patients suffer from multisystem atrophy[60-63]. While there are differences in the onset, rate of progression and responsiveness (or non-responsiveness) to levodopa between multisystem atrophy and advanced Parkinson's disease, the conditions resemble each other. The pathological substrate underlying both conditions is degeneration of dopamine and noradrenergic neurons in the hypothalamus, locus ceruleus, dorsal vagal nucleus and the sympathetic ganglia[61-63]. Autonomic symptoms such as orthostatic hypotension may be aggravated by dopamine agonists and, to a lesser extent, by levodopa. In the presence of orthostatic hypotension, levodopa should be given in small amounts to avoid the bolus effect of a single large dose, and dopamine agonists should not be given at the same time as levodopa. Dopamine agonists should be started before bed to minimize postural hypotension. An attempt should be made to correct contributing factors that aggravate orthostasis such as volume depletion (secondary to diuretics) or sympathetic blockade (secondary to β-blockers). The effective circulating fluid volume may be increased by wearing elastic stockings or using volume expanders such as fludrocortisone.

Other effects of anti-parkinsonian therapy

There are conflicting reports on the effects of levodopa and the dopamine agonists on the heart, and of their safety in patients with arteriosclerotic heart disease[64,65]. However, no causal relationship has been demonstrated between them and angina or arrhythmias.

Some patients on high doses of levodopa experience shortness of breath[66]. This is usually associated with response fluctuations and may be viewed as a 'dyskinesia' resulting from overstimulation of autonomic brainstem nuclei. These patients improve when levodopa is reduced. However, before assuming that the shortness of breath is a 'dyskinesia', the patient should be evaluated for cardiac and pulmonary disease. Rarely, patients with Parkinson's disease develop stridor secondary to vocal cord paralysis[67]. Such paralysis (more common in multisystem atrophy) does not respond to levodopa or dopamine agonists and requires tracheostomy.

Some patients on levodopa experience profuse sweating. This is usually associated with marked response fluctuations and may improve when agonists are substituted for levodopa. Patients on levodopa with a decarboxylase inhibitor who experience nausea and vomiting are likely to experience the same symptoms with a dopamine agonist. Nausea can be minimized by starting the agonist in a low dose, increasing the dose slowly and giving the agonist with food. If nausea and vomiting persist, the patient should be investigated for gastric or duodenal ulcer disease which can be aggravated by levodopa or dopamine agonists. Nausea and vomiting associated with levodopa or dopamine agonists usually responds to domperidone.

USE OF AGONISTS IN EARLY PARKINSON'S DISEASE

Studies demonstrating a neuroprotective effect of deprenyl in recently diagnosed levodopa-untreated patients has led to renewed interest in using dopamine agonists in these patients[37-40]. Several studies have demonstrated that bromocriptine also delays the need for levodopa, but as bromocriptine has antiparkinsonian activity, none of the studies claim a protective effect. In 13 studies, a total of 754 Parkinson's disease patients were placed on bromocriptine as monotherapy[68-80]. The mean age of the patients was 62 ± 4 years, mean Parkinson's disease duration was 2.5 ± 1.3 years, mean stage was 2.4 ± 0.3, and the mean dose of bromocriptine was 19 mg (range 10–70 mg). Among these patients, 344 (46%) improved.

Patients on bromocriptine did not require levodopa for 2.3 years (range 0.5–6.0 years). This compares favourably with deprenyl where patients did not require levodopa for 1.1 years (range 0.3–3.0 years). As the studies with bromocriptine were conducted independently of the studies with deprenyl, there were no direct comparisons. Bromocriptine, by stimulating the presynaptic nigrostriatal dopamine neurons, causes decreased firing of these neurons which, in turn, results in decreased dopamine turnover. Since the metabolism of bromocriptine does not, like dopamine, generate free radicals, bromocriptine may in this way delay disease progression.

In the future, the availability of selective D_1 and D_2 agonists may lead to new therapeutic strategies in which sequencing of these agonists will be important. Such combinations with deprenyl and with constant non-pulsatile levels of levodopa (such as those obtained with sustained release levodopa preparations) may provide the best long-term treatment.

REFERENCES

1. Marsden, C.D. and Parkes, J.D. (1977). Success and problems of long-term levodopa therapy in Parkinson's disease. *Lancet,* **1**, 345–9
2. Marsden, C.D. and Parkes, J.D. (1976). 'On–off' effects in patients with Parkinson's disease on chronic levodopa therapy. *Lancet,* **1**, 292–349
3. Fahn, S. (1974). 'On–off' phenomenon with levodopa therapy in Parkinsonism. *Neurology,* **24**, 432–41
4. Muenter, M.D., Sharpless, N.S. and Tyce, G.M. (1977). Patterns of

dystonia ('I-D-I' and 'D-I-D') in response to L-dopa therapy for Parkinson's disease. *Mayo Clin. Proc.,* **52**, 163–74

5. Lieberman, A., Dziatolowski, M. and Kupersmith, M. (1979). Dementia in Parkinson disease. *Ann. Neurol.,* **6**, 355–9

6. Lieberman, A.N. (1987). Update on Parkinson disease. *N.Y. State J. Med.,* **87**, 147–53

7. Markham, C.H. and Diamond S.G. (1981). Evidence to support early levodopa therapy in Parkinson disease. *Neurology,* **31**, 125–31

8. Lesser, R.P., Fahn, S. and Snider, S.R. (1979). Analysis of the clinical problems in parkinsonism and the complications of long-term levodopa therapy. *Neurology,* **29**, 1253–60

9. Lieberman, A.N. and Goldstein, M. (1985). Bromocriptine in Parkinson disease. *Pharmacol. Rev.,* **37**, 217–27

10. Lieberman, A.N., Goldstein, M. and Leibowitz, M. (1981). Treatment of advanced Parkinson disease with pergolide. *Neurology,* **31**, 675–82

11. Dexter, D.T., Carter, C. and Wells, F.R. (1989). Basal lipid peroxidation in substantia nigra is increased in Parkinson's disease. *J. Neurochem.,* **52**, 381–9

12. Jenner, P. (1989). Clues to the mechanism underlying dopamine cell death in Parkinson's disease. *J. Neurol. Neurosurg. Psychiatr.,* **52** (Suppl.), 22–8

13. Cohen, G. and Spina, M.B. (1989). Deprenyl suppresses the oxidant stress associated with increased dopamine turnover. *Ann. Neurol.,* **26**, 689–90

14. Melamed, E., Hefti, F. and Wurtman, R.J. (1980). Nonaminergic striatal neurons convert exogenous L-dopa to dopamine in Parkinsonism. *Ann. Neurol.,* **8**, 558–63

15. Melamed, E., Hefti, F. and Pettibone, D.J. (1981). Aromatic L-amino acid decarboxylase in rat corpus striatum: implications for action of L-dopa in Parkinsonism. *Neurology,* **31**, 651–5

16. Melamed, A., Globus, M. and Friedlender, E. (1983). Chronic L-dopa administration decreases striatal accumulation of dopamine from exogenous L-dopa in rats with intact nigrostriatal projections. *Neurology,* **33**, 950–3

17. Spencer, S.E. and Wooten, G.F. (1984). Altered pharmacokinetics of L-dopa metabolism in rat striatum deprived of dopaminergic innervations. *Neurology,* **34**, 1105–8

18. Nutt, J.G., Woodward, W.R. and Anderson, J.L. (1985). The effect of carbidopa on the pharmacokinetics of intravenously administered levodopa; the mechanism of action in the treatment of Parkinsonism. *Ann. Neurol.,* **18**, 537–43

19. Markstein, R. (1981). Neurochemical effects of some ergot derivatives: a basis for their antiparkinson actions. *J. Neural Transmission,* **51**, 39–59

20. Fuxe, K., Agnati, L.F. and Harfstrand, A. (1986). Heterogeneities in the

dopamine neuron systems and dopamine co-transmission in the basal ganglia and the relevance of receptor-receptor interactions. In Fahn, S., Marsden, C.D. and Jenner, P. (eds.) *Recent Developments in Parkinson's Disease,* pp. 17–32. (New York: Raven Press)

21. Graybiel, A.M. (1986). Dopamine-containing innervation of the striatum: subsystems and their striatal correspondents. In Fahn, S., Marsden, C.D. and Jenner, P. (eds.) *Recent Developments in Parkinson's Disease,* pp. 1–16. (New York: Raven Press)

22. Kebabian, J.W. and Calne, D.B. (1979). Multiple receptors for dopamine. *Nature (London),* **277,** 93–6

23. Reisine, T.D., Fields, J.Z. and Yamamura, H.J. (1977). Neurotransmitter receptor alterations in Parkinson's disease. *Life Sci.,* **21,** 335–44

24. Schwartz, R., Fuxe, K. and Agnati, L.F. (1978). Effect of bromocriptine on ³H spiroperidol binding sites in rat striatum – evidence for actions of dopamine receptors not linked to adenylate cyclase. *Life Sci.,* **23,** 465–70

25. Karobath, M. (1986). Dopamine agonists: new vistas. In Fahn, S., Marsden, C.D. and Jenner, P. (eds.) *Recent Developments in Parkinson's Disease,* pp. 175–82. (New York: Raven Press)

26. Lieberman, A., Goldstein, M. and Gopinathan, G. (1983). Further studies with lisuride in Parkinson's disease. *Eur. Neurol.,* **22,** 119–23

27. Lieberman, A., Goldstein, M. and Gopinathan, G. (1982). Further studies with pergolide. *Neurology,* **32,** 1181–4

28. Calne, D.B., Williams, A.C. and Neophytides, A. (1978). Long-term treatment of parkinsonism with bromocriptine. *Lancet,* **1,** 735–8

29. Lang, A.E. (1987). Manipulating the dopaminergic system in Parkinson's disease. *Pharmacol. Ther.,* **32,** 51–76

30. Godwin-Austen, R.B. and Smith, N.J. (1977). Comparison of the effects of bromocriptine and levodopa in Parkinson's disease. *J. Neurol. Neurosurg. Psychiatr.,* **44,** 4479–82

31. Gron, U. (1977). Bromocriptine versus placebo in levodopa treated patients with Parkinson's disease. *Acta Neurol. Scand.,* **56,** 269–73

32. Jansen, N.H. (1978). Bromocriptine in levodopa response losing parkinsonism: a double blind study. *Eur. Neurol.,* **17,** 92–9

33. Larsen, T.A., Newman, R. and Lewitt, P. (1984). Severity of Parkinson's disease and the dosage of bromocriptine. *Neurology,* **34,** 795–7

34. Rinne, U.K. (1987). Early combination of bromocriptine and levodopa in the treatment of Parkinson's disease: a 5-year follow-up. *Neurology,* **37,** 826–8

35. Rascol, A., Montastruc, J.L. and Rascol, O. (1984). Should dopamine agonists be given early or late in the treatment of Parkinson's disease? *J. Neurol. Sci.,* **11** (Suppl. 1), 229–38

36. Lieberman, A., Gopinathan, G. and Neophytides, A. (1986). Management of levodopa failures: the use of dopamine agonists. *Clin. Neuropharm.*, **9** (Suppl. 2), S9–S21

37. Tetrud, J.W. and Langston, J.W. (1989). The effect of deprenyl (Selegiline) on the natural history of Parkinson's disease. *Science*, **245**, 519–22

38. The Parkinson Study Group (1989). Effect of deprenyl on the progression of disability in early Parkinson's disease. *N. Engl. J. Med.*, **321**, 1364–71

39. Elizan, T., Yahr, M. and Moros, D. (1989). Selegiline use to prevent progression of Parkinson's disease: Experience in 22 *de novo* patients. *Arch. Neurol.*, **46**, 1275–9

40. Myllyla, V.V., Sotaniemi, D.A. and Tuominen, J. (1989). Selegiline as primary treatment in early phase Parkinson's disease – an interim report. *Acta Neurol. Scand.*, **126**, 177–82

41. Boyce, S., Rupniak, N.M.J. and Steventon, M.J. (1990). Differential effects of D_1 and D_2 agonists in MPTP treated primates: functional implications for Parkinson's disease. *Neurology*, **40**, 923–33

42. Zigmond, M.J., Acheson, A.L. and Stachowiak, M.K. (1984). Neurochemical compensation after partial injury of the nigrostriatal bundle in an animal model of preclinical parkinsonism. *Arch. Neurol.*, **41**, 856–61

43. Gervas, J.J., Muradas, V. and Bazan, E. (1983). Effects of 3-O-M-dopa on monoamine metabolism in rat brain. *Neurology*, **33**, 278–82

44. Melamed, E., Britton, V. and Zellig, O. (1986). Episodic unresponsiveness to single doses of L-dopa in parkinsonian fluctuations. *Neurology*, **36**, 100–3

45. Nutt, J.G., Woodward, W.R. and Hammerstad, J.P. (1984). The 'on-off' phenomenon in Parkinson disease: relation to levodopa absorption and transport. *N. Engl. J. Med.*, **310**, 483–8

46. Goldstein, M., Lieberman, A. and Meller, E. (1985). A possible molecular mechanism for the antiparkinson action of bromocriptine in combination with levodopa. *Trends Pharmacol. Sci.*, **6**, 436–7

47. Kidron, D. and Melamed, E. (1987). Forms of dystonia in patients with Parkinson disease. *Neurology*, **37**, 1009–11

48. Poewe, W.H., Lees, A.J. and Stern, C.M. (1988). Dystonia in Parkinson's disease: clinical and pharmacological features. *Ann. Neurol.*, **23**, 73–8

49. Lieberman, A. (1974). Parkinson's disease: a clinical review. *Am. J. Med. Sci.*, **267**(2), 66–80

50. Alexander, G.E., DeLong, M.R. and Strick, P.L. (1986). Paralleled organization of functionally segregated circuits linking basal ganglia and cortex. *Annu. Rev. Neurol. Sci.*, **9**, 357–81

51. Miller, W.C. and DeLong, M.R. (1988). Parkinsonian symptomatology, anatomical and psychological analysis. *Ann. N.Y. Acad. Sci.*, **55**, 287–311

52. Bergman, H., Wichmann, T. and DeLong, M.R. (1990). Reversal of

experimental parkinsonism by lesions of the subthalamic nucleus. *Science,* **249**, 1436–8

53. Weinrich, M., Kuch, K. and Garcia, F. (1988). Axial versus distal motor impairment in Parkinson disease. *Neurology,* **38**, 540–5

54. Hirsch, E.C., Graybiel, A.M. and Duyckaerts, C. (1987). Neuronal loss in the pedunculopontine segmental nucleus in Parkinson disease and in progressive supranuclear palsy. *Proc. Natl. Acad. Sci. USA,* **84**, 5976–80

55. Drayer, B.P. (1987). Magnetic resonance imaging and brain iron: implications in the diagnosis and pathochemistry of movement disorders and dementia. *Barrow Neurol. Inst. Q.,* **3**, 15–30

56. Damasio, A.R., Lobo-Antunes, J. and Macedo, C. (1971). Psychiatric aspects in parkinsonism treated with L-dopa. *J. Neurol. Neurosurg. Psychiatr.,* **34**, 502–7

57. Rinne, J.O., Rummukainen, J. and Puljarvi, L. (1989). Dementia in Parkinson disease is related to neuronal loss in the medial substantia nigra. *Ann. Neurol.,* **26**, 47–50

58. Perry, R.H., Irving, D. and Blessed, G. (1990). Senile dementia of Lewy body type. *J. Neurol. Sci.,* **95**, 119–39

59. Weiner, W.J., Koller, W.C. and Perlik, S. (1980). Drug holiday and management of parkinson disease. *Neurology,* **30**, 1257–61

60. Mayeux, R., Stern, Y. and Mulvey, K. (1985). Reappraisal of temporary levodopa withdrawal (drug holiday) in Parkinson disease. *N. Engl. J. Med.,* **313**, 724–8

61. Spokes, E.G.S., Bannister, R. and Oppenheimer, D. (1979). Multiple system atrophy with autonomic failure. *J. Neurol. Sci.,* **43**, 59–82

62. Hartog Jager, W.A.D. and Bethlem, J. (1960). The distribution of Lewy bodies in the central nervous system in idiopathic paralysis agitans. *J. Neurol. Neurosurg. Psychiatr.,* **23**, 283–9

63. Rajput, A.H. and Rozdilsky, B. (1976). Dysautonomia in parkinsonism: clinicopathological study. *J. Neurol. Neurosurg. Psychiatr.,* **39**, 1092–100

64. Leibowitz, M., Lieberman, A. and Goldstein, M. (1981). Cardiac effects of pergolide. *Clin. Pharm. Therapy,* **30**, 718–23

65. Tanner, C.M., Chablani, R. and Goetz, C.G. (1985). Pergolide mesylate: lack of cardiac toxicity in patients with cardiac disease. *Neurology,* **35**, 918–21

66. Hovestadt, A., Bogaard, J.M. and Meerwaldt, J.D. (1989). Pulmonary function in Parkinson disease. *J. Neurol. Neurosurg. Psychiatr.,* **52**, 329–33

67. Plasse, H.M. and Lieberman, A.N. (1981). Bilateral vocal cord paralysis in Parkinson disease. *Arch. Otolaryngol.,* **107**, 252–3

68. Nakanishi, T., Iwata, M. and Goto, I. (1989). Second interim report of the nationwide collaborative study on the long-term effects of bromocriptine in

the treatment of parkinsonian patients. *Eur. Neurol.,* **29** (Suppl. 1), 3–8

69. Hely, M.A., Morris, J. and Rail, D. (1989). The Sydney Multicentre Study of Parkinson's disease: a report on the first 3 years. *J. Neurol. Neurosurg. Psychiatr.,* **52**, 324–8

70. UK Bromocriptine Research Group (1989). Bromocriptine in Parkinson's disease: a double-blind study comparing 'low-slow' and 'high-fast' introductory dosage regimens in *de novo* patients. *J. Neurol. Neurosurg. Psychiatr.,* **52**, 77–82

71. Libman, I., Gawell, M. and Riopelle, R. (1989). A comparison bromocriptine (Parlodel) and levodopa-carbidopa (Sinemet) for treatment of 'de novo' Parkinson's disease patients. *Can. J. Neurol. Sci.,* **14**, 576–80

72. Alberts, M.J., Stajich, J. and Olanow, C.W. (1987). A randomized blinded study of low-dose bromocriptine versus low-dose carbidopa/levodopa in untreated Parkinson's patients. In Fahn, S., Marsden, C.D., Calne, D. and Goldstein, M. (eds.) *Recent Developments in Parkinson's Disease.* Vol. II, pp. 201–8. (Florham Park, NJ: MacMillan Healthcare Information)

73. Rascol, A., Guiraud, B. and Montastruc, J.L. (1979). Long-term treatment of Parkinson's disease with bromocriptine. *J. Neurol. Neurosurg. Psychiatr.,* **42**, 143–50

74. Montastruc, J.L., Rascol, O. and Rascol, A. (1989). A randomised controlled study of bromocriptine versus levodopa in previously untreated Parkinsonian patients: a 3 year follow-up. *J. Neurol. Neurosurg. Psychiatr.,* **52**, 773–5

75. Rinne, U.K. (1987). Early combination of bromocriptine and levodopa in the treatment of Parkinson's disease: A 5-year follow up. *Neurology,* **37**, 826–8

76. Staal-Schreinemachers, A.L., Wesseling, H. and Kamphuis, D.J. (1986). Low-dose bromocriptine therapy in Parkinson's disease: double-blind, placebo-controlled study. *Neurology,* **36**, 291–3

77. Stern, G. and Lees, A. (1987). Long-term effects of bromocriptine given to *de novo* patients with idiopathic Parkinson's disease. *Adv. Neurol.,* **45**, 525–7

78. Teychenne, P., Bergsrud, D. and Elton, R. (1986). Bromocriptine: long-term low-dose therapy in Parkinson's disease. *Clin. Neuropharmacol.,* **9**, 138–45

79. Tolosa, E., Blesa, R. and Bayes, A. (1987). Low-dose bromocriptine in the the early phases of Parkinson's disease. *Clin. Neuropharmacol.,* **10**, 169–74.

80. van der Drift, J.H.A. (1986). Low-dosage treatment in *de novo* patients with Parkinson's disease: a prospective study. *Adv. Neurol.,* 45

9

Dopaminergic agonists in the treatment of Parkinson's disease

C.G. Goetz

INTRODUCTION

Although levodopa is still considered the major therapeutic agent for the treatment of Parkinson's disease symptoms, it is not an ideal drug for several reasons. First, levodopa has no activity at dopamine receptors, and its efficacy depends on enzymatic conversion to dopamine by dopadecarboxylase. As Parkinson's disease advances and the population of dopaminergic cells projecting to the striatum progressively declines, the activity of this enzyme diminishes[1]. Furthermore, the progressive decrease in brain dopadecarboxylase that occurs in Parkinson's disease is not uniform anatomically but occurs predominantly in the nigrostriatal system. Therefore, in Parkinson's disease, the converting enzyme is preferentially depleted in the specific area where it is most needed.

The half-life of levodopa is exceedingly short and at least some of the motor oscillations seen so frequently in advanced Parkinson's disease patients treated with levodopa appear to relate to fluctuations in circulating drug levels[2]. Additionally, levodopa lacks specificity. Since it is converted directly to dopamine, all dopaminergic receptor populations will be activated by its use. Furthermore, levodopa is also an intermediate in the synthesis of norepinephrine, and its ingestion may potentiate general catecholaminergic and possibly serotonergic function as well. Finally, the increased normal metabolism of dopamine that results from levodopa ingestion generates hydrogen peroxide and hydroxyl free radicals which may further damage already compromised cellular function.

Dopamine agonists, drugs that directly stimulate dopamine receptors, have been developed in an attempt to address several of these levodopa limitations. By acting at the postsynaptic dopamine receptors of the striatum, agonists bypass the degenerating presynaptic neuron from the substantia nigra and act independently of the synthetic dopaminergic enzyme system. Agonists have long half-lives, and because they do not increase the level of dopamine itself, they have the potential to be highly specific to subpopulations of dopamine receptors and to be devoid of properties related to norepinephrine and serotonin. Finally by lowering the turnover rates of dopamine, agonists could theoretically generate less hydrogen peroxide and free radicals and help to protect dopaminergic cells.

Numerous dopaminergic agonists have been tested in the treatment of Parkinson's disease in its various clinical stages during the last 15 years. Only bromocriptine and pergolide, however, are currently available in the United States. Several other agonists have been abandoned in the United States because of toxicity, including lergotrile (hepatitis), and mesulergine, and ciladopa (tumors in experimental animals). Other agents including CQA 206-291 (Sandoz) and SND-919 (Boehringer Ingelheim) are currently being evaluated in the US.

In most clinical trials with agonists, investigators have studied either patients with early disease and mild disability or those with severe functional compromise. Mildly affected patients are usually defined as Hoehn and Yahr Stage I and II (without postural reflex compromise) and those with severe disease are usually Stage IV (significant balance difficulty and falling). Stage III patients (mild postural abnormalities) are variably included in either study group and Stage V (inability to stand independently) patients are rarely included in any study.

BROMOCRIPTINE

Chemistry and agonist properties

Bromocriptine mesylate (Parlodel®) is an ergot alkaloid that has a low affinity for α-adrenergic receptors. It is a potent D_2 dopamine agonist and a mild D_1 receptor antagonist. It is absorbed rapidly from the gastrointestinal system and over 90% undergoes first-pass hepatic metabolism. Its plasma half-life is 7 hours, approximately 4 times that of levodopa and 2 times that of carbidopa/levodopa[3].

Early or mild Parkinson's disease

Monotherapy

A wide range of bromocriptine doses were studied in the early open-label trials of bromocriptine. Techenynne and colleagues[4] introduced the concept of low-dose bromocriptine where doses less than 10 mg/day were reported to be effective in controlling parkinsonian symptoms. Most other studies focused on moderate (10–30 mg/day) or high dosages (greater than 40 mg/day)[5-7]. Calne and colleagues[8] found that the daily required dosage of bromocriptine correlated with disease severity but that no patient groups were regularly helped by low dosages. The general practice of treatment with 10–30 mg/day has evolved in most subsequent studies of monotherapy with bromocriptine. Although short-term efficacy has been shown at these doses, long-term efficacy is limited and Rinne[9] found that most patients eventually required levodopa as an adjunct.

The incidence of adverse reactions with bromocriptine monotherapy was low and even absent in some studies. Rascol and co-workers used a mean dose of 56.5 mg/day bromocriptine and reported that no patients developed dyskinesia, dystonia or motor fluctuations after 4–8 years of treatment[5]. Lees and Stern similarly showed a low incidence of adverse effects in previously untreated Parkinson's disease patients[10].

Because of obvious concerns about selection bias in open-label trials with retrospective analyses, prospective randomized studies comparing levodopa and bromocriptine followed. In a 21-week study of 84 patients, divided into bromocriptine monotherapy or carbidopa/levodopa mono-therapy, the two groups had equivalent efficacy[11]. Olanow studied 60 previously untreated patients for a mean of 80 weeks. At 6 months, patients on carbidopa/levodopa (mean dose 360.1 mg/day) had equivalent efficacy with those on bromocriptine (mean dose 13.1 mg/day). Thereafter, however, efficacy was better in the levodopa group. Adverse motor reactions occurred only in the levodopa group with dyskinesia in one patient, peak-dose dystonia in seven patients and motor fluctuations in three[7]. Montastruc, Rascol and Rascol[6] followed patients over 3 years, 13 on levodopa alone (mean dose, 444 mg/day) and 15 on bromocriptine alone (mean dose, 50 mg/day). Although the efficacy was equivalent, motor side-effects were more frequent in the levodopa group. Psychosis (one patient) and poor efficacy (three patients) limited bromocriptine use. As a group, these studies suggest that monotherapy with bromocriptine can be effective in the first months of therapy, although after 6 months, efficacy may decline. Motor side-effects are consistently less frequent with bromocriptine than with levodopa.

Bromocriptine in conjunction with levodopa

The superior efficacy of levodopa and the reduced side-effects of bromocriptine suggested that combined therapy early in the disease could give maximal benefit. Rinne's pioneer work with this strategy has since been replicated and widely adopted in clinical practice in the US. After starting treatment with levodopa, he supplemented with bromocriptine rather than increasing levodopa further[11]. He found the efficacy of this combination to be superior to that of bromocriptine alone and equal to that achieved with levodopa. Motor fluctuations and dyskinesias were less frequent with combination therapy than with levodopa alone and benefits lasted for 5 years of follow-up[12]. Although this study is often cited, methodologically, it has been criticized; the three groups were not randomized and the levodopa data were in fact derived from historically matched controls. A randomized double-blind multicenter study from Japan included 702 patients, 286 assigned to bromocriptine (mean daily dose, 15 mg), 216 patients to bromocriptine plus carbidopa/levodopa (mean, 15 mg/day and 360 mg/day respectively), and 200 assigned to carbidopa/levodopa alone (mean, 360 mg/day). These data, summarized by Lieberman, mimicked Rinne's findings and indicated that combined bromocriptine plus carbidopa/levodopa resulted in motor improvement better than that seen with bromocriptine alone and fewer motor fluctuations or dyskinesias than seen with carbidopa/levodopa alone[13].

Advanced disease

Bromocriptine has been studied in advanced Parkinson's disease patients in both open-label and double-blind protocols. In these studies, bromocriptine was added to levodopa therapy as adjunct therapy. Lieberman and colleagues[14] examined 66 such patients with increasing disability despite treatment with levodopa. A total of 45 patients were able to tolerate at least 25 mg/day of bromocriptine and in these patients, levodopa dose was reduced by a mean of 10% and could be eliminated in seven patients; significant improvement occurred in rigidity, tremor, bradykinesia and postural reflex impairment, as well as overall disability; in 12 patients, follow-up data were obtained one year thereafter and in eight, bromocriptine remained effective. In a later publication[15], the same investigators reported that with time a progressive waning of efficacy developed with bromocriptine, although many patients remained improved or stable for at least 2 years. The mean dose of the first study was 45 mg/day, and 50 mg/day in the second group.

Other groups have demonstrated similar findings and documented not only global improvement but also fewer motor fluctuations and more frequent 'on' time with bromocriptine addition[16,17]. Kartzinel and colleagues[18] performed a double-blind study of bromocriptine and placebo as additions to levodopa therapy in eight patients and found overall improvement in the bromocriptine–levodopa group. Rigidity and tremor were better improved than balance. Hoehn and Elton[19] studied patients with a wide variety of disability and found that lower doses (maximal, 20 mg/day) still improved motor function, although improvement was most significant in the milder cases. Only two of six patients at Hoehn and Yahr Stage IV improved more than 30%, whereas two-thirds of patients at Stages II or III had more than 30% improvement.

Glantz and colleagues[20] investigated the effect of bromocriptine on motor fluctuations unrelated to the time or dose of levodopa (classic 'on–off'). A total of 23 patients were studied prospectively and 39% showed a reduced severity and frequency of unpredictable fluctuations.

In numerous studies, as the dosage of bromocriptine was increased, the dose of levodopa was decreased with improved or maintained efficacy. However, a common observation is that patients cannot completely stop their levodopa when bromocriptine is added and cessation of levodopa will result in a drastic increase in parkinsonism[21]. This observation suggests that anti-parkinsonian effects are not purely related to D_2 agonist effects and that mild D_1 stimulation effected by dopamine itself is still necessary for optimal benefit. Almost all long-term studies have demonstrated that the beneficial effects of bromocriptine eventually waned. It is not clear whether this decline is due to progression of the Parkinson's disease itself or whether there is definite pharmacological tolerance to the drug.

Toxicity

Significant side-effects, often necessitating discontinuation of bromocriptine, have been reported in up to 36% of patients with advanced Parkinson's disease[15]. With lower doses, only 15% of patients experienced side-effects severe enough to require drug withdrawal[19]. Orthostatic hypotension is the most important side-effect of bromocriptine in the early phase of drug introduction. Patients may become dizzy and even faint. In the various series reported above, orthostatic hypotension, lightheadedness or syncope was detected in approximately 33% of patients. Usually, once the patient received the drug for several doses, this effect waned. Nausea and vomiting, presumably due at least in part to bromocriptine's direct stimulation of the dopaminergic receptors in the area postrema of the medulla occurred in 20–30% of patients in early studies. Other less frequent complaints or complications include burning dysesthesias that may relate to vasoconstrictive properties of ergot drugs, gastric hemorrhage, skin rash (livedo reticularis) of the lower legs, rarely hepatitis or exacerbation of angina pectoris[14,19]. In the latter case, it is not clear whether the angina related to vascular effects of the bromocriptine or whether the improved motor function of patients on bromocriptine permitted their increased activity that unmasked underlying cardiac dysfunction.

In contrast to the studies of early monotherapy or combined therapy with levodopa in mildly disabled patients, neurologic and mental side-effects were reported with considerable frequency in studies of advanced patients. Involuntary movements, specifically chorea, increased in Lieberman's group as a whole and in 40% in another study[14,16]. Besides chorea, peak dose dystonia and myoclonus can also occur. Mental changes included agitation, confusion, depression, insomnnia, nightmares and hallucinations. These effects, occurring in 10–30% of patients, were the most frequent cause of discontinuation of the drug[19]. The use of low-dose bromocriptine significantly decreased the prevalence of this side-effect[19]. As a rule, it has been suggested that bromocriptine is associated with more psychiatric disturbance, but less dyskinesia than levodopa[22].

PERGOLIDE

Chemistry and receptor agonist profile

Pergolide mesylate was developed as a second ergot preparation to treat Parkinson's disease. It is considered approximately ten times more potent than bromocriptine and the usual total daily dose is 1–4 mg. It is a semisynthetic ergoline derivative and differs from bromocriptine in that it has a longer half-life and has D_1 agonist properties[22]. It reaches peak concentration in the plasma within 1–3 hours and a single dose is cleared completely within 7 days[23].

Early or mild Parkinson's disease

Monotherapy

Extensive monotherapy studies have not been performed. In a 3-month open-label evaluation of pergolide in ten previously untreated patients, Rinne found that a mean dose of 2.6 mg/day pergolide improved all features of Parkinson's disease, with tremor being most affected. He felt that this degree of improvement however was less than that seen with levodopa alone[24].

In a study of more advanced patients previously treated with levodopa and sometimes with bromocriptine, Maer and co-workers found that monotherapy with pergolide had equivalent efficacy to levodopa, with a longer duration of action. This study however lasted only 2 weeks and extrapolation of the data to chronic patient care is limited[25].

Pergolide in conjunction with levodopa

Similarly to bromocriptine, pergolide has been administered along with low-dose carbidopa/levodopa in an attempt to maximize efficacy and reduce motor fluctuations. These studies have been less numerous and not randomized double-blind controlled in design, but suggest similar results to those seen with bromocriptine[26,27].

163

Advanced disease

Like bromocriptine, pergolide has been studied as an adjunct to levodopa, and has significantly abated Parkinsonian disability in patients with advanced Parkinson's disease. Kurlan and colleagues[28] studied 11 patients, all with advanced (Stage IV) disease, and demonstrated a 68% increase in mobile 'on' time. Like bromocriptine, however, improvement was not indefinitely maintained and by 6 months the improvement was only 30%; improvement had disappeared by 18 months. They found that partial but temporary restoration of mobility was achieved by switching some patients to alternate day therapy with pergolide and daily therapy with levodopa. Similarly, in 17 patients with advanced Parkinson's disease studied, Lieberman and colleagues[29] reported that patients initially responded with 60% group improvement in global disability. By 2 years, although still 20% less disabled than at study entry, patients found that the effect of pergolide had significantly waned. Similar patterns of improvement with pergolide have been reported by others[30-32]. We[30] studied 22 patients for 1 year and showed statistically significant improvement in global disability and gait difficulties with pergolide; maximal improvement was seen at 6 months and then slightly waned. No added improvement was seen, in spite of dosage adjustment, after 6 months of therapy. In those patients with motor fluctuations, improvement was maintained for the full year and in two patients, the problem resolved. No patient developed new motor fluctuations while receiving pergolide. Jankovic[31] found even after 2 years that the amount of mobile 'on' time remained 63% greater than before pergolide therapy.

Tanner and colleagues reported follow-up data on 17 patients in an open-label study where they found that pergolide plus carbidopa/levodopa treatment maintained patients at equivalent disability over 4 years compared with baseline on carbidopa/levodopa alone. There was also increased quantity of 'on' time. Previously developed hallucinations and chorea remained unchanged, sleep disruption improved and dystonia increased[33].

Most studies lasting longer than a few months were open-label. In one 6-month double-blind study of pergolide vs. placebo as adjunctive therapy to carbidopa/levodopa, Jankovic and Gorman found that significant improvement occurred with pergolide[34].

Toxicity

Pergolide is associated with side-effects that are similar in frequency and type to bromocriptine[14,16]. Early in its study, questions of cardiac toxicity were raised and this point delayed the more wide use and availability of this drug. To settle this controversy, Tanner and colleagues[35] administered pergolide for 1 year to six patients with stable heart disease and monitored their neurological and cardiac disabilities. Improvement was noted in all patients and cardiac status never worsened. They concluded that pergolide was a safe and effective therapy for parkinsonian patients, even when they have a stable cardiac disease. The other systemic side-effects of pergolide are similar to those seen with bromocriptine therapy. Hepatotoxicity and pleural thickening should be regarded as potential side-effects of this drug. Neurological side-effects include chorea, dystonia and myoclonus, and these abate with lower doses of the drug. Mental changes including agitation, depression, insomnia, hallucinations and psychotic behavior may occur early in therapy or after several months. Stern and colleagues[36] specifically studied neurobehavioral deficits in patients before and while receiving chronic pergolide and found no significant change in mental abnormalities related to pergolide.

COMPARISONS BETWEEN THE TWO AGONISTS

It is of clinical and economic importance to know whether one of these two agents is in fact superior to the other. Only a few studies have specifically addressed the relative safety and efficacy of bromocriptine and pergolide. Because bromocriptine was available several years before pergolide, most patients who have received both drugs received bromocriptine first, when they were younger and when their disease was less advanced. In a short-term study, LeWitt and co-workers[37] compared the two drugs in nine patients with mild parkinsonism and 15 with advanced disease, in a double-blind cross-over study; they found that the two drugs were equivalent and could not favor one over the other for efficacy or side-effect profile. Lieberman and colleagues[15] treated 25 patients chronically with bromocriptine, then pergolide. They favored pergolide, since it maintained its efficacy longer than bromocriptine, even though the pergolide was used later in the disease course. Goetz and colleagues[17] conducted a 5-year study where ten patients who initially responded to bromocriptine remained on this drug until efficacy waned (mean, 29 months); they then switched to pergolide and were followed for the same duration as their former bromocriptine exposure. Three conclusions were made: first, after 5 years of agonist therapy with levodopa, patients were improved compared to their disability at study entry; second, although peak efficacy was equivalent between the two drugs, pergolide remained effective longer than bromocriptine in these patients; third, in spite of having failed to continue responding to bromocriptine, these patients all promptly responded to a second agonist. This last observation suggests that all agonists are not identical and offers hope to patients whose response to one agonist has waned. Whether the patients who switched to pergolide and had improved efficacy will be able to again return to bromocriptine with renewed function has yet to be studied. In a related study, the same investigators examined a group of advanced Parkinson's disease patients switched from pergolide to bromocriptine. Patients maintained their clinical status after the switch, but did not improve further[38].

APOMORPHINE

Apomorphine is in fact the oldest of the available agonists, but has not been extensively used as an oral adjunct to levodopa therapy nor as monotherapy in Parkinson's disease. Its highly potent emetic qualities have limited its use primarily to study conditions. The drug has both D_1 and D_2 agonist functions and is highly hydrophilic. It can be used subcutaneously, orally and, theoretically, has applicability to other routes of administration.

In open-label studies, apomorphine was an effective anti-parkinsonian therapy as monotherapy or as an adjunct to levodopa[39]. In patients with other forms of parkinsonism or with other movement disorders, Cotzias and colleagues showed that responses to apomorphine and to levodopa were always similar qualitatively[40]. Looking at selective features of parkinsonism, Braham and co-workers found that apomorphine was highly effective in reducing parkinsonian tremor that was not responsive to levodopa[41]. The prominent emetic qualities of the drug prevented effective early double-blind studies, but when domperidone was developed and given along with apomorphine, Corsini and colleagues found all patients studied improved transiently, with a mean improvement of 43.3%. The improvement however lasted only 40 minutes[42].

Because of its very short activity and rapid onset of action, apomorphine has not been viewed as a practical therapy for regular management of Parkinson's disease. Rather, these qualities have suggested its applicability as 'rescue' therapy for patients with severe Parkinson's disease who develop occasional end-of-dose loss of efficacy or unpredictable motor fluctuations ('on–off'). Hardie and co-workers found that in eight patients who experienced 22 'off' episodes and received apomorphine 1 mg subcutaneously within 10 minutes of switching 'off' 20 episodes were effectively reversed and the others mildly reversed. With placebo used in 39 episodes, no 'off' episode was effectively reversed. Another agonist, lisuride, was tried in 35 'off' episodes but only clearly reversed the 'off' in 16 instances[43]. Such experiences have been reproduced and extended to include successful control of severe tremor in patients by continuous subcutaneous infusions of apomorphine[44–46]. Additionally, acute motor responses to apomorphine administration have been used as a putative means of predicting long-term response to dopaminergic drugs and could be useful in separating dopa-responders from non-responders prior to commitment to long-term drug trials[47].

MK-458 (4-PROPYL-9-HYDROXYNAPHTHOXAZINE, PHNO)

This novel and potent D_2 receptor agonist is a naphthoxazine compound structurally unrelated to ergoline or apomorphine classes of dopamine agonists. In animal models it is well absorbed after transdermal, subcutaneous and oral administration[48]. It has minimal or no D_1 receptor activity. The drug has been studied for anti-parkinsonian efficacy in short- and long-acting preparations. In an open-label evaluation of both drug forms in small numbers of patients, Muenter and co-workers found that the short-acting formulation produced a 3–4 hour therapeutic effect in most patients and the long-acting preparation lasted up to 10 hours[49]. As adjunct therapy to levodopa, MK-458 (mean dose, 8.1 mg/day) was studied in advanced Parkinson's disease patients by Lieberman and colleagues who found that levodopa could be reduced by 41% (mean)[50]. In both cited studies, dyskinesias were prominently absent as a side-effect of this drug. Similar efficacy was documented by Wooten and colleagues[51]. In our center, we studied MK-458 in a double-blind placebo-controlled evaluation in eight patients without levodopa therapy. Five received MK-458 during the double-blind period and the three others received MK-458 in open-label after completion of the double-blind period. The mean dose of MK-458 was 27.8 mg/day (standard deviation (SD), 14.3), and patients received the drug for a mean duration of 11.5 weeks (SD 3.2). We did not find significant improvement with the drug (Table 1). Behavioral aberrations occurred in 63% of patients (hallucinations in three patients and somnolence in two).

Although this drug will not be further developed, its high solubility offers prospects not afforded by many other preparations. The development of intraventricular or intrathecal pump therapy with agonists in Parkinson's disease patients will require compounds with similar high potency and high solubility. Improved selectivity to reduce toxicity is a future aim in the design of such drugs.

CQA 206-91 (N, N-DIETHYL-N'-[(8α)-1-ETHYL-6-METHYLERGOLINE-8-yl] SULFAMIDE HYDROCHLORIDE)

CQA 206-291 (CQA) is an ergoline derivative that has both dopamine antagonistic and agonistic properties. It appears to be a weak presynaptic dopaminergic receptor antagonist initially, with potent D_1 and D_2 agonist

Table 1 Response of eight patients to MK-458 as measured on the New York University Parkinson's Disease Scale (NYUPDS), Northwestern University Disability Scale (NUDS) and the Hoehn and Yahr Scale

Measure	Baseline		MK-458		
	Mean	(SD)	Mean	(SD)	p
NYUPDS	5.38	(0.92)	5.12	(1.89)	NS
NUDS	6.75	(1.58)	5.75	(1.39)	NS
Hoehn and Yahr	2.50	(0.53)	2.5	(0.53)	NS

effects later[52]. In an open–label, single-dose study of six Parkinson's disease patients withdrawn from levodopa therapy, CQA was found to have dose related anti-parkinsonian effects[53]. In a multi-center study using CQA as a monotherapy in 36 *de novo* Parkinson's disease patients, as well as an added treatment to 36 patients receiving levodopa preparations, Rascol and colleagues found CQA to be an effective anti-parkinsonian treatment[54]. The major side-effects encountered by these investigators included gastrointestinal distress, new or worsening dyskinesias, ortho-static hypotension, and confusion. In our center, we studied CQA in a double-blind placebo-controlled evaluation of 16 patients receiving levodopa therapy. Twelve patients received CQA, while four received placebo. There were no differences between the groups at baseline for age, duration of Parkinson's disease, Sinemet dose, Hoehn and Yahr stage, or disability measures from the Unified Parkinson's Disease Rating Scale (UPDRS). The mean duration of the double-blind period was 9.87 (SD 3.14) weeks, with CQA doses ranging between 15 mg and 30 mg q.d. Although there was no significant difference in the presence or number of side-effects for each group, the most common side-effects for the CQA group included gastrointestinal distress (three patients), dyskinesias (two patients), confusion (two patients), hallucinations (two patients), and dizziness (two patients). Single patient reports of headache, depression, muscle ache, and constipation also occurred. One patient in the placebo group reported multiple side-effects, including dyskinesias, confusion, hallucinations, and dystonia. Unlike the results of the study of Rascol and colleagues, we were unable to document any significant differences in post-study Hoehn and Yahr stage, Schwab and England Activities of Daily Living (ADL) scale, or UPDRS disability measures for the CQA group in comparison to the placebo control group (Table 2).

FUTURE PERSPECTIVES

The identification of different types of dopamine receptors, depending on their linkage to enzymes or their anatomic location, offers the biochemist the opportunity to design agonists to stimulate one popu-lation preferentially. Future drugs with high specificity may enhance the efficacy and also diminish the likelihood of toxic side-effects. Because

Table 2 Response to CQA 206-291 vs. placebo (mean followed by SD)

Measure	CQA		Placebo		p
Hoehn and Yahr	2.79	(0.89)	2.50	(0.58)	0.61
Schwab and England	72.50	(20.17)	80.00	(4.08)	0.95
UPDRS mentation	1.75	(3.11)	2.00	(4.00)	0.88
UPDRS ADL ('on')	12.67	(9.16)	10.50	(4.36)	0.81
UPDRS ADL ('off')	14.08	(9.24)	18.00	(12.54)	0.50
UPDRS motor	17.42	(7.69)	12.25	(3.50)	0.11

of their high potency and long half-lives, agonists may be feasible drugs for the development of alternate delivery systems, such as pumps or chemical implants. The new emphasis of drug trials for measuring prevention of disease raises the possibility that agonists could be studied for long-term effects on natural history of Parkinson's disease in appropriately designed protocols. The observation that at least four agonists with anti-parkinsonian efficacy were developed but later abandoned because of toxicity demonstrates that specificity and selectivity of these drugs are still not highly developed.

REFERENCES

1. Hornykiewicz, O. (1982). Brain neurotransmitter changes in Parkinson's disease. In Marsden, C.D. and Fahn, S. (eds.) *Movement Disorders, Neurology*, Vol. 2, pp.41-58. (London: Butterworth Scientific)
2. Nutt, J.G., Woodward, W.R., Hammerstad, J.P., Carter, J.H. and Anderson, J. (1983). Do the pharmacokinetics of L-dopa explain the on-off phenomenon? *Neurology*, **33** (Suppl. 2), 91
3. Olanow, C. (1988). Dopamine agonists in early Parkinson's disease. In Stern, M.B. and Hurtig, H.I. (eds), *The Comprehensive Management of Parkinson's Disease*, pp. 89-100. (New York: PMA Publishing Co.)
4. Teychenne, P.F., Bergsrud, D., Racy, A., Elton, R.L. and Vern, B. (1982). Bromocriptine: low-dose therapy in Parkinson's disease. *Neurology*, **32**, 577-83
5. Rascol, A., Montastruc, J.L., Guiraud-Chaumeil, B. and Clanet, M. (1982). Bromocriptine as the first treatment of Parkinson's disease: long-term results. *Rev. Neurol.*, **138**, 401-8

6. Montastruc, J.L., Rascol, O. and Rascol, A. (1989). A randomised controlled study of bromocriptine versus levodopa in previously untreated parkinsonian patients: a 3-year follow-up. *J. Neurol. Neurosurg. Psychiatr.*, **52**, 773–5

7. Olanow, C.W. (1988). Single-blind double observer-controlled study of carbidopa/levodopa vs. bromocriptine in untreated Parkinson patients. *Arch. Neurol.*, **45**, 206

8. Calne, D.B., Burton, K., Beckman, J. and Martin, W.R. (1984). Dopamine agonists in Parkinson's disease. *Can. J. Neurol. Sci.*, **11** (Suppl. 1), 221–4

9. Rinne, U.K. (1985). Combined bromocriptine–levodopa therapy early in Parkinson's disease. *Neurology*, **35**, 1196–8

10. Lees, A.J. and Stern, G.M. (1981). Sustained bromocriptine therapy in previously untreated patients with Parkinson's disease. *J. Neurol. Neurosurg. Psychiatr.*, **44**, 1020–3

11. Gawell, M.J., King, D.B., Libman, I., McLean, D.R., Paulseth, R., Raphy, B., Riopelle, R.J. and Bouchard, S. (1988). Bromocriptine in *de novo* Parkinson's disease patients. *Arch. Neurol.*, **45**, 206

12. Rinne, U.K. (1987). Early combination of bromocriptine and levodopa in the treatment of Parkinson's disease: 2–5 year follow-up. *Neurology*, **37**, 826–8

13. Lieberman, A.N. (1988). Dopamine agonists: new perspectives. *Neuro. View*, **4**, 1–20

14. Lieberman, A.N., Kupersmith, M., Casson, I., Durso, R., Foo, S.H., Khayali, M., Tartaro, T. and Goldstein, M. (1979). Bromocriptine and lergotrile: comparative efficacy in Parkinson disease. *Adv. Neurol.*, **24**, 461–73

15. Lieberman, A.N., Neophytides, A., Leibowitz, M., Gopinathan, G., Pact, V., Walker, R., Goodgold, A. and Goldstein, M. (1983). Comparative efficacy of pergolide and bromocriptine in patients with advanced Parkinson's disease. *Adv. Neurol.*, **37**, 95–108

16. Caraceni, T., Giovannini, P., Parati, E., Scigliano, G., Grassi, M.P. and Carella, F. (1984). Bromocriptine and lisuride in Parkinson's disease. *Adv. Neurol.*, **40**, 531–5

17. Goetz, C.G., Tanner, C.M., Glantz, R.H. and Klawans, H.L. (1985). Chronic agonist therapy for Parkinson's disease: a five-year study of bromocriptine and pergolide. *Neurology*, **35**, 749–51

18. Kartzinel, R., Shoulson, I. and Calne, D.B. (1976). Studies with bromocriptine: Double-blind comparison with levodopa in idiopathic Parkinsonism. *Neurology*, **26**, 511–3

19. Hoehn, M.M.M. and Elton, R.L. (1985). Low dosages of bromocriptine added to levodopa in Parkinson's disease. *Neurology*, **35**, 199–206

20. Glantz, R.H., Goetz, C.G., Nausieda, P.A., Weiner, W.J. and Klawans, H.L. (1981). The effect of bromocriptine on the on–off phenomenon. *J. Neural Transmission,* **52**, 41–7

21. Weiner, W.J. and Lang, A.E. (1989). Parkinson's disease. *Movement Disorders: A Comprehensive Survey,* pp. 23–115. (Mount Kisco, NY: Future Publishing Company)

22. Kartzinel, R., Perlow, M. and Teychenne, P. (1975). Bromocriptine and levodopa in parkinsonism. *Lancet,* **2**, 473–6

23. Rubin, A., Lemberger, L. and Dhahir, P. (1981). Physiologic disposition of pergolide. *Clin. Pharmacol. Ther.,* **30**, 258–65

24. Rinne, U.K. (1983). New ergot derivatives in the treatment of Parkinson's disease. In Calne, D.B., McDonald, R.J., Horowski, R. and Wuktke, W. (eds.) *Lisuride and other Dopamine Agonists,* pp. 431–42. (New York: Raven Press)

25. Mear, J.Y., Barroche, G., Smet, Y., Weber, M., Lhermitte, F. and Agid, Y. (1984). Pergolide in the treatment of Parkinson's disease. *Neurology,* **34**, 983–6

26. Tanner, C.M., Goetz, C.G., Glantz, R.H., Glatt, S.L. and Klawans, H.L. (1982). Pergolide mesylate and idiopathic Parkinson's disease. *Neurology,* **32**, 1175–9

27. Rinne, U.K. (1986). Dopamine agonists as primary treatment in Parkinson's disease. *Adv. Neurol.,* **45**, 519–23

28. Kurlan, R., Miller, C., Levy, R., Macik, B., Hamill, R. and Shoulson, I. (1985). Long-term experience with pergolide therapy of advanced parkinsonism. *Neurology,* **35**, 738–42

29. Lieberman, A.N., Goldstein, M., Leibowitz, M., Gopinathan, G., Neophytides, A., Hiesiger, E., Nelson, J. and Walker, R. (1983). Long-term effects of pergolide. *Neurology,* **33** (Suppl. 2), 112

30. Goetz, C.G., Tanner, C.M., Glantz, R.H. and Klawans, H.L. (1983). Pergolide in Parkinson's disease. *Arch. Neurol.,* **40**, 785–7

31. Jankovic, J. (1985). Long-term study of pergolide in Parkinson's disease. *Neurology,* **35**, 296–9

32. Tanner, C.M., Goetz, C.G., Glantz, R.H., Glatt, S.L. and Klawans, H.L. (1982). Pergolide mesylate and idiopathic Parkinson disease. *Neurology,* **32**, 1175–9

33. Tanner, C.M., Goetz, C.G., Glantz, R. and Klawans, H.L. (1986). Pergolide mesylate: four years experience in Parkinson's disease. *Adv. Neurol.,* **45**, 547–9

34. Jankovic, J. and Orman, J. (1986). Parallel double-blind study of pergolide in Parkinson's disease. *Adv. Neurol.,* **45**, 551–3

35. Tanner, C.M., Chablani, R., Goetz, C.G. and Klawans, H.L. (1985).

Pergolide mesylate: lack of cardiac toxicity in patients with cardiac disease. *Neurology,* **35**, 918–21

36. Stern, Y., Mayeux, R., Ilson, J., Fahn, S. and Cote, L. (1984). Pergolide therapy for Parkinson's disease: neurobehavioral changes. *Neurology,* **34**, 201–4

37. LeWitt, P.A., Ward, C.D., Larsen, T.A., Raphaelson, M.I., Newman, R.P., Foster, N., Dambrosiam, J.M. and Calne, D.B. (1983). Comparison of pergolide and bromocriptine therapy in parkinsonism. *Neurology,* **33**, 1009–14

38. Goetz, C.G., Shannon, K.M., Tanner, C.M., Carroll, V.S. and Klawans, H.L. (1989). Agonist substitution in advanced Parkinson's disease. *Neurology,* **39**, 1121–2

39. Duby, S.E., Cotzias, C.G., Papavasiliou, P.S. and Lawrence, W.H. (1972). Injected apomorphine and orally administered levodopa in parkinsonism. *Arch. Neurol.,* **27**, 474–80

40. Cotzias, G.C., Papavasiliou, P.S., Fehling, C., Kaufman, B. and Mena, I. (1970). Similarities between neurological effects of L-dopa and of apomorphine. *N. Engl. J. Med.,* **282**, 31–3

41. Braham, J., Sarova-Pinhas, I. and Goldhammer, Y. (1970). Apomorphine in parkinsonian tremor. *Br. Med. J.,* **3**, 768

42. Corsini, G.U., Del Zompo, M., Gessa, G.L. and Mangoni, A. (1979). Therapeutic efficacy of apomorphine combined with an extracerebral inhibitor of dopamine receptors in Parkinson's disease. *Lancet,* **1**, 954–6

43. Hardie, R.J., Lees, A.J. and Stern, G.M. (1984). On–off fluctuations in Parkinson's disease: a clinical and neuropharmacological study. *Brain,* **107**, 487–506

44. Stibe, C., Lees, A. and Stern, G. (1987). Subcutaneous infusion of apomorphine and lisuride in the treatment of parkinsonian on–off fluctuations. *Lancet,* **1**, 871

45. Stibe, C.M.H., Lees, A.J., Kempster, P.A. and Stern, G.M. (1988). Subcutaneous apomorphine in parkinsonian on–off oscillations. *Lancet,* **1**, 403–6

46. Poewe, W., Kleedorfer, B. and Gerstenbrand, F. (1988). Subcutaneous apomorphine in Parkinson's disease. *Lancet,* **1**, 943

47. Bonuccelli, U., Piccini, P., Del Cotto, P., Nocchiero, A., Corsini, G.U. and Muratorio, A. (1990). Apomorphine as a diagnostic tool for Parkinson's disease. Presented at the *42nd Annual Meeting of the American Academy of Neurology,* May, Miami Beach, Florida, USA

48. Jenner, P., Marsden, C.D., Nomoto, M. and Stahl, S. (1986). Antiparkinsonian activity of (+)- PHNO in the MPTP-treated marmoset following subcutaneous infusion or skin application. *Br. J. Pharmacol.,* **89**, 626

49. Muenter, M.D., Ahlskog, J.E., Bell, G. and McManis, P. (1988). PHNO [(+)-4-propyl-9-hydroxynaphthoxazine]: a new and effective anti-Parkinson's disease agent. *Neurology*, **38**, 1541–5

50. Lieberman, A., Chin, L. and Baumann, G. (1988). MK458, a selective and potent D$_2$ receptor agonist in advanced Parkinson's disease. *Clin. Neuropharm.*, **11**, 191–200

51. Wooten, G.F., Turk, M.F., Bennett, J.P. and Trugman, J.M. (1988). Treatment of Parkinson's disease with MK-458. Presented at the *American Academy of Neurology Annual Meeting*, April, Cincinnati, Ohio, USA

52. Jaton, A., Enz, A., Vigouret, J., Pfaffle, P. and Markstein, R. (1987). CQA 206-291, an ergot derivative with biphasic dopaminergic action. *Experientia*, **43**, 705

53. Temlett, J., Quinn, N., Marsden, C., Lataste, X. and Jaton, A. (1989). The antiparkinsonian activity of CQA 206-291, a new D$_2$ dopamine receptor agonist. *Clin. Neuropharm.*, **12**, 55–9

54. Rascol, O., Fabre, N., Teravainen, H., Poewe, W., Lucking, C., Rinne, U., Dupont, E., Hirt, D., Hoyer, M. and Lataste, X. (1988). CQA 206-291: a novel dopamine agonist in the treatment of Parkinson's disease. Presented at the *9th International Symposium on Parkinson's Disease*, June, Jerusalem

IO

Neural grafting for Parkinson's disease

J.H. Kordower, D.L. Felten and D.M. Gash

INTRODUCTION

Parkinson's disease is a neurodegenerative disorder characterized by bradykinesia, muscular rigidity, resting tremor and postural disturbances. A major contributing factor to the pathological features of Parkinson's disease is the progressive loss of dopaminergic neurons in substantia nigra pars compacta, with a resultant dopaminergic denervation of the striatum to which it projects. Although compensatory physiological responses to partial loss of dopaminergic neurons, such as enhanced synthesis and secretion of dopamine by the remaining neurons and postsynaptic dopamine receptor upregulation, may occur and forestall the onset of symptoms, the ultimate decompensation from loss of the nigrostriatal projections must be approached therapeutically.

Early efforts to treat Parkinson's disease were confined to symptomatic relief only, or in isolated cases, to ablative stereotaxic procedures to interrupt the resultant disinhibition of the pallido–thalamo–cortical connections to lower motoneurons. These approaches were neither curative nor widely successful. The advent of pharmacological replacement therapy with the use of levodopa heralded a new era of chemically specific replacement for depleted neurotransmitters involved in characteristic symptoms of neurological disease. With subsequent refinement of therapeutic regimens of levodopa by the addition of a peripheral decarboxylase inhibitor to permit better access of levodopa into the brain, pharmacological therapy became tolerable and efficacious. Extended therapy, however, often diminished in efficacy and produced disabling side-effects. The development of specific dopamine agonists that bypass the presynaptic dopaminergic terminals altogether added a new tool for pharmacological therapy, but also showed the same difficulty of diminished efficacy over time in many patients. Thus with pharmacological replacement or agonist therapy, both dopamine synthesis or direct dopamine receptor stimulation have proven to be inadequate strategies in permanently ameliorating the symptoms of Parkinson's disease in many patients over time.

In the past 15 years, the field of neural transplantation has been transformed from a tool to study central nervous system regeneration to a strategy for the treatment of neurological disease. The use of grafting procedures in experimental animal models of Parkinson's disease raised the possibility of directly replacing lost dopamine through implantation of dopamine-secreting cells into the striatum. Hundreds of patients with Parkinson's disease have received intrastriatal neural implants of adrenal medulla and many have received fetal ventral mesencephalon grafts, in an attempt to repopulate the brain with a source of dopamine-secreting cells. The results from these studies have been controversial. Interpreting the data from these clinical trials has often been complicated by the lack of appropriate control groups, and by difficulty in determining the influence of continued pharmacotherapy and intensive rehabilitative efforts in postoperative motor performance.

As these clinical trials have progressed, our understanding of the scope of neural graft function has matured. In some experimental, and possibly clinical, situations, neural implants can provide functional re-innervation of the dopamine-depleted striatum. It is also now well accepted that implants can provoke significant responses in the host brain as well as provide new populations of neurons. In this regard, neural grafts can liberate trophic molecules which have been shown to rescue neurons normally destined to die following experimental lesions. Furthermore, transplants can up-regulate transmitter synthesis or induce sprouting from residual neuronal populations. How these new concepts of graft function will alter the manner in which neural implants are applied as a therapeutic strategy for neurological disease remains to be determined.

The intense interest in this area has led to a plethora of books[1-4] and reviews[5-11] devoted to this topic. Some excellent reviews have detailed the studies using fetal ventral mesencephalon as donor material (see ref.

9). While these studies are reviewed in this chapter, we have chosen to focus on the potential role of trophic phenomena resulting from neural implants as they relate to nigrostriatal function and Parkinson's disease. It is our aim to present both positive and negative facets of the 'trophic factor hypothesis' and hope this information stimulates further deliberation of its merits as it relates to this novel treatment strategy for Parkinson's disease.

FETAL VENTRAL MESENCEPHALIC IMPLANTS

More experimental data are available on implants of fetal mesencephalic neurons into parkinsonian animals than for any other transplant system under study. This is due mainly to the fact that the major symptomatology in Parkinson's disease (bradykinesia and rigidity) results principally from a striatal dopamine insufficiency secondary to the degeneration of substantia nigra pars compacta neurons. The degeneration seen within the substantia nigra can easily be mimicked acutely in non-humans, producing characteristic abnormalities in motor function which then are used as indices of graft function. In rodents, unilateral injections of 6-hydroxydopamine (6-OHDA) into the ventral mesencephalon produce extensive lesions of the substantia nigra and ventral tegmental area[12]. Rats spontaneously rotate towards the side of the lesion. Amphetamine administration will exacerbate this asymmetry in nigrostriatal function and increase the rate of circling due to the release of dopamine. Dopamine agonists, such as apomorphine, reverse the direction of rotation by preferentially stimulating supersensitive dopaminergic receptors on the lesioned side. In addition to circling behavior, unilateral nigrostriatal lesioned rats demonstrate sensory neglect on the side contralateral to the lesion[13], and bilaterally lesioned rats demonstrate hoarding behavior[14] and ingestive abnormalities[15].

Using this model system, two groups of investigators have provided a substantial data base which demonstrates the ability of fetal mesencephalic neurons to serve as a donor source for transplantation[16-32]. At the University of Lund, Björkland and Stenevi[16,17] first demonstrated that implants of fetal ventral mesencephalon could survive implantation and innervate the denervated striatum. A combined Karolinska (Olson and Seiger) and United States (Perlow, Freed, Hoffer, and Wyatt) effort soon replicated and extended this initial finding, and provided the landmark demonstration that neural grafts could reverse motor asymmetries seen in nigrostriatal lesioned rats[18]. Studies aimed at characterizing these effects soon followed. Both solid grafts placed into preformed cavities[22] and cells injected in suspensions[24] were found to be viable methods of implantation. Following intraparenchymal transplantation, up to two-thirds of the striatum can be re-innervated in an organotypic fashion by allografts of fetal tissue[19,20,23]. The dense dopaminergic fibers extending from the graft represent preferential innervation, since cholecystokinin-containing ventral mesencephalic neurons do not innervate the striatum *in situ* or following implantation[25]. Host neurons and the transplanted neurons make numerous reciprocal synaptic contacts as well[27]. Fetal dopaminergic implants are active metabolically and demonstrate electrophysiological characteristics similar to those seen by substantia nigra neurons *in situ*[29]. The increase in dopamine receptor density in lesioned animals returns to baseline levels following striatal re-innervation by transplanted cells[30].

The behavioral characteristics of animals receiving fetal dopamine-containing grafts were also further elucidated. The benefits of fetal dopaminergic implants appear to be permanent since no return of motor dysfunction was seen for up to 2 years following implantation[19]. The effects upon rotation appear dependent upon the continued presence of the donor tissue since lesion of the graft returns motor dysfunction. The functionality of the implants was also found to be site-specific: grafts must re-innervate the dorsal caudoputamen to affect rotation behavior[20], and in contrast, graft innervation of the ventrolateral striatum ameliorates deficits in sensory function without affecting rotation[21]. Furthermore, hoarding behavior and aphagia are unaffected by these implants regardless of innervation patterns[14,15].

In addition to fetal allografts, xenografts of embryonic cells have been demonstrated to be a structurally and functionally competent source of donor material when grafted into immunosuppressed or immunologically deficient hosts[31–34]. Both mouse-to-rat and human-to-rat grafts survive implantation and reverse the lesion-induced motor dysfunction in lesioned animals. In general, the structural and functional characteristics of human-to-rat xenografts are similar to those seen with rat allografts. Dopamine is released from the implanted tissue, the graft is electrically active, and synaptic contacts are made between the graft and host. It appears, however, that the donor tissue dictates the pace and the limits of the implants' structural and functional characteristics. While fetal allografts can re-innervate two-thirds of the rodent striatum, human fetal nigral dopamine neurons, which contain the genetic message to send out longer processes, can re-innervate the entire striatum[31,33,34]. Furthermore, the initiation of functional recovery is protracted with human fetal tissue grafts which parallels the prolonged rate of development of human embryonic cells[31,33].

While the 6-OHDA model of Parkinson's disease in rodents is extremely useful in grafting studies, as in most model systems it has significant limitations. Other approaches to investigating the properties of implants are needed and they have been provided, in part, by the discovery of the neurotoxin N-methyl-4-phenyl 1,2,3,6-tetrahydropyridine (MPTP). MPTP is a toxic compound which causes parkinsonism in humans[35] and a parkinsonian syndrome in non-human primates[36,37]. Using MPTP to develop a primate model of Parkinson's disease has permitted experiments to determine if dopaminergic implants have similar functional and structural qualities following transplantation into monkeys. These experiments allowed for the testing of lesioned and subsequently grafted animals with a more sophisticated motor circuitry and an immune system with 'outbred' characteristics similar to humans. Furthermore, issues of 'scaling-up' from rodents to humans could be tested in larger non-human species which could serve as an intermediate model prior to human studies (see ref. 5 for further discussion). A number of groups have now established that allografts of fetal ventral mesencephalic neurons can survive implantation into MPTP-treated monkeys and partially re-innervate the host striatum[38-41]. Human-to-monkey xenografts have been reported to survive in MPTP-treated monkeys as well[42]. With monkey allografts, dopamine levels and turnover are increased proximal to the implant site[40,43]. While initial reports suggested that exceptionally large numbers of neurons can survive in monkeys, the numbers may have been seriously overstated by including a large endogenous striatal population of tyrosine hydroxylase-containing neurons in the cell counts[44]. Additional experiments suggest that the overall survival may be more modest[45]. In general, the survival and organotypic innervation patterns of fetal ventral mesencephalic cells appear better with younger fetuses, although surviving cells have been observed using older donors as well[39]. MPTP-induced akinesia, hypokinesia, rigidity, and tremor have all been reportedly ameliorated following fetal mesencephalic implants in monkeys[38–40].

ADRENAL CHROMAFFIN CELL IMPLANTS: AN EXAMINATION OF CELL SURVIVAL

Fetal ventral mesencephalic neurons survive extremely well following striatal implantation. They provide a dense organotypic innervation pattern to the denervated striatum, increase striatal dopamine levels to within normal limits, and consistently reverse the motor dysfunction seen in experimental parkinsonism. In spite of these facts pointing to fetal tissue as the best source of cells, the social, ethical, and practical issues surrounding the use of fetal tissues for transplantation have led researchers to seek non-fetal sources of dopaminergic cells for implantation. Cells derived from sympathetic ganglia[46], the carotid body[47], and tumor lines such as the PC-12 cells[48–51] have all been grafted into rodent models of Parkinson's disease with limited success. The most thoroughly tested catecholamine-producing cell type has been the chromaffin cell of the adrenal medulla, which is the only paraneural catecholamine cell source which has been transplanted clinically.

The initial rationale for using adrenal chromaffin cells as a donor source for neural grafting stems from the fact that these cells normally synthesize and secrete catecholamines. When dissected free from the overlying adrenal cortex, the chromaffin cells are released from the corticosteroid-mediated inhibition and down-regulate the synthesis of phenylethanolamine N-methyl transferase (PNMT). The dense core vesicles within chromaffin cells undergo morphologic changes and the cell shifts its catecholamine synthesis towards a greater production of dopamine and norepinephrine.

Freed and co-workers[52–54] were the first to demonstrate that grafts of adrenal medulla placed into the rat lateral ventricle, juxtaposed to the denervated striatum, survived, produced catecholamines, and attenuated the drug-induced motor assymmetries displayed by unilateral nigrostriatal-lesioned rats[55–57]. Grafted chromaffin cells maintained their endocrine phenotype and did not extend processes into the host neuropil. This led to the interpretation that these cells were functioning in a paracrine fashion, serving as an intraventricular biological pump of dopamine.

Grafts of chromaffin cells, both solid pieces and suspensions, placed into the striatal parenchyma, have met with inconsistent success. In lesioned rodents, many studies have reported functional benefits from such implants. The behavioral effects were neither as great in magnitude nor as long-lived as seen with fetal implants[57]. The survival of adrenal chromaffin cells grafted within the striatum has generally been poor in rodents[47,60], or monkeys with experimental parkinsonism[58-61] and in humans with idiopathic Parkinson's disease[62-68]. In one rodent study, fluorescent chromaffin cells could only be visualized for up to 400 min following implantation[57]. The chromaffin cell survival curve paralleled the time course of behavioral recovery. Other studies in rats have reported a significant attenuation of experimental parkinsonism for up to a few months following adrenal grafting. However, often fewer than 100 surviving adrenal chromaffin cells are found following sacrifice[47]. Similarly, poor survival of intrastriatally implanted adrenal medullary cells has been reported in Rhesus monkeys[58], Cebus monkeys[59,60] and Fasicularis monkeys[61]. In our studies using young adult Cebus monkeys, both stereotaxic and open microsurgical implantation techniques were utilized, since these procedures were reported as being successful in clinical trials[59,60]. Surviving chromaffin cells could only be observed in two of seven Cebus monkeys. An intense reactive gliosis was observed at the implant site and numerous macrophages filled the implant cavity. Of the few chromaffin cells which could be identified at the electron microscopic level, most appeared to be in the process of degeneration.

The human adrenal transplant cases which have undergone postmortem evaluations also have had poor chromaffin cell survival within the striatum[62-68]. Most of these cases clipped the implant to the head of the medial edge of the caudate nucleus to provide the graft with access to the nutritive environment of the lateral ventricle. In spite of this fact, only three[65,66,68] of the seven published autopsy cases[62-64,67] were able to identify a surviving implant. Of these three reports, only one could demonstrate a few cells which still synthesized tyrosine-hydroxylase (TH)[68], the rate limiting step for synthesis of dopamine and other catecholamines.

Although chromaffin cell survival has been poor within the striatum, these cells can survive well within other regions of the neuraxis. For instance, Sagen and co-workers[69] have consistently observed large chromaffin cell implants within the periaqueductal gray in intact rats.

Similarly, excellent survival of these cells can be observed within the hippocampus of rats[70] and within the cortex of non-human primates[58,71]. These data suggest that the environmental milieu of the implant, and not factors intrinsic to the chromaffin cells, determine the viability of a chromaffin cell implant. It is important to note that the hippocampus and cerebral cortex are sites with high levels of endogenous nerve growth factor (NGF)[72]. It is well known that exposure of adrenal chromaffin cells to NGF in culture, supports their survival, increases catecholamine production, and induces extensive neurite outgrowth from these cells (see reviews[7,8]) Indeed, adrenal medullary implants placed into the NGF-rich hippocampus display a neuronal-like morphology[70]. In contrast, the striatum, which contains low levels of NGF[72] appears to have difficulty supporting these implants. The seminal study of Strömberg and colleagues[73] took advantage of NGF's trophic and tropic influences on adrenal chromaffin cells by pretreating the cells with NGF prior to implantation, and then infusing NGF proximal to the implant site. This treatment dramatically enhanced the survival of the chromaffin tissue. Many of the surviving cells were morphologically differentiated for at least 3 months. Importantly, the chromaffin cells were able to attenuate the drug-induced motor asymmetries displayed by unilateral nigrostriatally lesioned rats for at least 1 year. It should be noted that the interpretation of NGF's effects on adrenal chromaffin cells has recently been questioned, because grafts of non-chromaffin tissue plus NGF have been reported to ameliorate apomorphine-induced rotation[74].

Our laboratories have attempted to increase the survival of grafted adrenal chromaffin cells by co-grafting them with biological sources of NGF. Our initial experiment[75] co-grafted chromaffin cells with a C6 glioma cell line (Figure 1, Table 1) that produces an NGF-like molecule[76,77]. Prior to implantation, the glioma cells were rendered amitotic with retinoic acid treatment. Anatomically, the co-graft increased the survival of adrenal chromaffin cells almost fourfold. Proximal to the implant, striatal dopamine levels were greatest in the co-graft condition compared with single grafts of either C6 glioma or adrenal medulla. Importantly, chromaffin cells in the co-graft condition displayed a greater and more sustained functional response than rats receiving adrenal medulla implants alone. These data demonstrate that co-grafts of biological sources of NGF can exert structural and functional

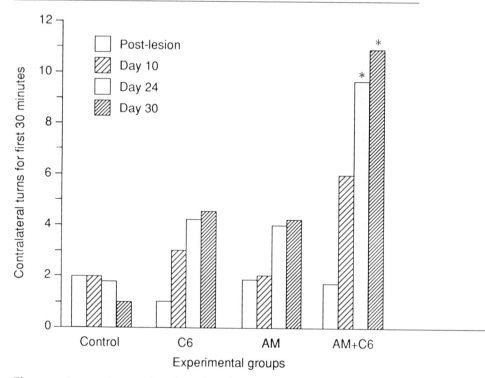

Figure 1 Increase in contralateral rotations (a measure of functionality) in unilateral nigrostriatal lesioned rats following single grafts of adrenal medulla (AM), C6 glioma (C6), or co-grafts of both tissues (AM + C6). Note that co-grafted rats displayed an enhanced recovery relative to either single graft group. (*denotes $p < 0.05$). (Modified from Bing and colleagues[75])

Table 1 Number of surviving cells (mean ± SEM). Interestingly, co-grafted rats displayed greater numbers of surviving C6 glioma cells, indicating that the medullary tissue has a trophic influence upon the glioma cells. (Modified from Bing and colleagues[75])

Group	Adrenal chromaffin cells	C6 glioma cells
Co-graft (n = 7)	399 ± 126.8★	3062 ± 892.2★
Adrenal medulla graft (n = 15)	116 ± 36.7	N/A
C6 glioma graft (n = 5)	N/A	1483 ± 762.8

★$p < 0.05$

trophic influences on adrenal medullary grafts in a manner similar to that seen with NGF infusions.

While useful for experimentation, it is obvious that grafts containing C6 gliomas will not have clinical utility. Therefore, similar studies were carried out using transected peripheral nerve as the co-graft donor tissue. The choice of peripheral nerve was predicated upon the observation that, following transection, the Schwann cells which ensheath the nerve begin the *de novo* production of NGF[78]. These Schwann cells also synthesize other trophic and tropic factors such as ciliary neuronotropic factor, laminin, brain derived neuronotropic factor and fibroblast growth factor (FGF)[79-81]. The potential that these factors might act in an additive or synergistic fashion increased our enthusiasm for this approach. A pilot experiment in rodents demonstrated that sciatic nerve/adrenal medulla co-grafts enhanced the survival of the chromaffin cells and potentiated the rotational response seen in lesioned rats following amphetamine administration[82]. It appears that these trophic effects were mediated specifically by factors released from the Schwann cells, since co-grafts containing optic nerve, which are ensheathed by oligodendroglia and not Schwann cells, were without effect.

A recent study by Date and co-workers[83] confirmed some of these observations. Mice were treated with MPTP and then received either single grafts containing adrenal medulla or sciatic nerve/adrenal medulla co-grafts. Mice receiving implants of adrenal medulla alone averaged only 85 surviving tyrosine-hydroxylase(TH)-immunoreactive chromaffin cells. In contrast, co-grafted mice averaged 214 surviving chromaffin cells, many of which displayed long neuritic processes.

The data gathered in rodent studies led to a series of *in vitro* and *in vivo* experiments carried out in aged hemiparkinsonian Rhesus monkeys to assess the potential of transected sural nerve to serve as a growth factor source[71]. We selected the sural nerve since it is easily resected surgically, with a sensory innervation pattern restricted to the lateral aspect of the foot and little toe. After 3 days in culture with autologous sural nerve, Rhesus adrenal chromaffin cells sent out long neuritic processes in a manner indistinguishable from that seen following NGF exposure, indicating that Schwann cells were releasing NGF-like factors. We then tested whether the trophic factors from the peripheral nerve would alter the survival and morphological characteristics of Rhesus adrenal cells following co-grafting. Monkeys received intrastriatal autografts of either adrenal medulla (*n* = 3) or sural nerve (*n* = 3) alone or a cograft (*n* = 3) of both donor tissues. Three months following grafting, implants of adrenal chromaffin cells alone survived well (Figure 2). The enhanced survival seen in this study relative to our previous one using Cebus monkeys[59,60] may be the result of a combination of factors including the species, age and immune status of the monkeys, the method of MPTP infusion, or the fact that a silver tissue carrier was not used in this latter study to hold the adrenal medullary tissue. Even with this better survival of adrenal cells alone, up to 67 000 chromaffin cells survived when adrenal cells were co-grafted with sural nerve (Figure 2). This enhanced graft viability is even more impressive in light

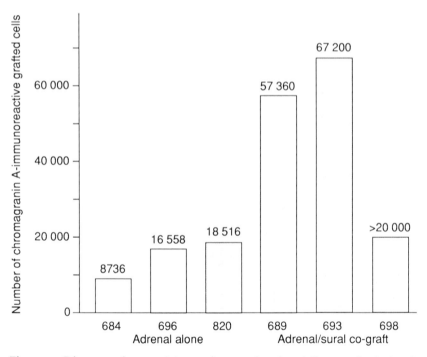

Figure 2 Rhesus monkeys receiving sural nerve adrenal medulla co-grafts displayed greater numbers of chromaffin cells surviving in the striatum than monkeys receiving single grafts of adrenal medulla. Only 20 000 surviving cells could be counted for monkey 698 since much of this transplant site was removed for ultrastructural analysis. The ultrastructural analysis revealed numerous healthy chromaffin cells as well. (Modified from Kordower *et al.*[69])

of the fact that the implants were matched for volume; thus one-third to one-half fewer chromaffin cells were implanted in the co-graft condition. Many of the implanted cells around the periphery of the surviving clusters were morphologically differentiated and extended long neuritic processes. Synaptic contacts, presumably from host axons, were found in apposition to grafted adrenal cells as well. The Schwann cells survived well in the brain and were seen migrating within the striatal parenchyma. They continued to express the receptor for NGF for at least 3 months which, along with the sustained neurite extension displayed by many of the grafted chromaffin cells, suggests that the Schwann cells may be providing a continuous source of NGF during this period.

A marked difference between the co-grafts and the single adrenal cell implants was the relative health of the implant site. Even in monkeys with large single grafts of adrenal medulla, numerous hemosiderin-containing macrophages were evident within the graft site. In contrast, co-grafted animals displayed healthy implants with limited astrocytic infiltration and few macrophages. It is interesting to note that, although few in number, macrophages were still found in all co-grafted animals. Macrophages and microglia secrete interleukin-1β[84–88] which has been demonstrated to increase NGF production 11-fold from transected peripheral nerves[89]. Indeed, it appears to be the macrophage infiltration following peripheral nerve injury which sparks the NGF-mediated regeneration in the peripheral nervous system. Thus a limited number of macrophages present near peripheral nerve/adrenal medulla co-grafts could potentiate the trophic effect provided by the Schwann cells.

Enhanced chromaffin cell survival in co-grafted monkeys has recently been replicated and extended by Bakay and co-workers[90] who observed up to 4000 surviving grafted chromaffin cells in hemiparkinsonian Rhesus monkeys, but over 40 000 surviving cells in sural nerve/adrenal medulla co-grafted animals. In addition, these co-grafted animals performed better than their adrenal alone-grafted counterparts in an arm-reaching task, providing a correlation between enhanced graft survival and functional improvement. Taken together, data gathered in rodents, non-humans, primates, and humans demonstrate that adrenal chromaffin cells generally survive poorly within the striatal parenchyma. Good survival has been achieved, however, in multiple non-human species by infusing NGF or by co-grafting adrenal chromaffin cells with NGF (and/or other trophic factor) producing cells.

ADRENAL CHROMAFFIN CELL IMPLANTS: THE CASE FOR HOST-DERIVED SPROUTING

In the search for surviving chromaffin cells using immunocytochemistry for TH, a number of investigators studying rodent and non-human primate models of Parkinson's disease observed an enhanced network of host-derived striatal TH-immunoreactive fibers following chromaffin cell implantation. These data have led to the 'trophic factor hypothesis' of graft function. Stated in its most liberal form, this hypothesis postulates that graft-mediated functional recovery is not due to dopamine secretion from the implanted cells, but rather to augmentation of remaining host mesostriatal dopaminergic systems. These effects may be mediated by diffusible molecules expressed by cells of the host immune system following damage and/or from the grafted cells. Many studies carried out in non-dopaminergic systems have demonstrated that grafts can modify host neurocircuitry, probably by trophic mechanisms[91,92]. Red nucleus neurons destined to die following axotomy are rescued following fetal spinal cord implants placed into the lesion cavity[93]. Similarly, the reversal of neurohypophysectomy-induced diabetes insipidus by intraventricular anterior hypothalamic transplants appears to be due to the rescue of axotomized vasopressinergic neurons within the supraoptic nucleus and not to the few magnocellular neurons contained within the transplant[94]. Nucleus basalis neurons, which shrink following cortical ablation, recover to normal size following cortical transplants[95]. The fact that the cognitive deficits observed following frontal cortex ablations are resolved within only 4 days of fetal cortical grafting[96] or cultured astrocyte implantation[97], further illustrates the ability of grafts to modify the host nervous system.

In many of these experimental situations, the factors mediating the observed effects remain to be elucidated. However, the lack of clear mechanisms of action does not mitigate the validity of the phenomenon nor does it designate these effects as 'non-specific'. We consider each of these effects as 'specific' but whose biological underpinnings still remain to be clarified. One drawback of the trophic factor hypothesis is that it has become a 'catch-all' explanation for poorly understood phenomena. For the hypothesis to have real value, its use in this manner must be avoided. While additional examples of the nervous system's ability to respond in a trophic fashion are welcome as additional phenomenology,

187

studies elucidating the mechanisms by which the nervous system responds in a trophic fashion following neural grafting are needed to uncover the breadth and detail of these phenomena.

Bohn and co-workers[98] were the first to demonstrate the trophic effects of adrenal medulla implants on the dopaminergic nigrostriatal system. They observed that intrastriatal implants of adrenal chromaffin cells survived poorly in MPTP-treated mice. However, an enhanced dense network of TH-immunoreactive fibers was seen in the striatum ipsilateral to the transplant. A similar trophic response has been discerned by Date and co-workers[99] in MPTP-treated mice with poorly surviving adrenal medullary allografts and xenografts. This finding indicates that elements within the host brain are capable of promoting a regenerative response. However, these studies, and others which will be described shortly, also suggested that the presence of adrenal cells augmented the trophic effect.

Two groups working with parkinsonian monkeys soon followed the original report with similar observations. Our group, as well as Bankiewicz and his colleagues, implanted adrenal medullary tissue into the denervated striatum either with[100] or without[101,102] a silver tissue carrier. Both groups observed a dense TH-immunoreactive fiber network both proximal to the implant and along the mesostriatal pathways (Figures 3a and b). Furthermore, both groups demonstrated that control implants or cavitations placed in the caudate nucleus were similarly able to induce enhanced TH-immunoreactivity in the striatum. In one study[100], the extent of this response appeared to correlate with the amount of damage to the caudate nucleus. Using an open microsurgical procedure, there was limited and circumscribed damage to the caudate nucleus engendered by the trocar passing into the parenchyma. Under these conditions, the enhanced TH fiber network was only observed within the caudate nucleus and proximal internal capsule. In contrast, the stereotaxic approach using a silver tissue carrier invoked significant damage to the caudate nucleus and provoked a greater inflammatory response in the perigraft region. Monkeys receiving such an implant displayed an enhanced TH fiber plexus along the entire nigrostriatal pathway ipsilateral to the implant.

The phenomena observed in the two primate groups may be qualitatively different (see below). However, these studies make the important observation that an up-regulation of host dopaminergic tone can occur in primates following transplantation. Indeed, two recent case

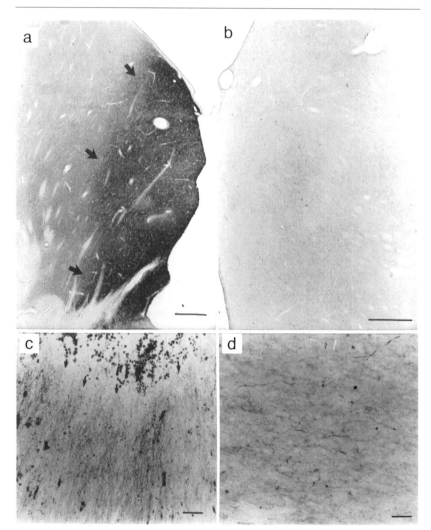

Figure 3 Following adrenal grafting, an enhanced network of TH-immunoreactive fibers is seen within the ipsilateral caudate nucleus in primates. (a) and (b) are low magnification photomicrographs demonstrating the enhanced TH-immunoreactivity in an adrenal grafted non-human primate ipsilateral to the implant (arrows in (a)) relative to the contralateral side (b); host TH-immunoreactive fiber staining within the caudate nucleus (c) proximal and (d) distal to a human adrenal medullary implant for Parkinson's disease. Note the increase in TH-fiber density and the streaming of fibers in the human case up towards the overlying implants site relative to the density and pattern of fiber staining distal to the graft within the same caudate nucleus. The graft/host interface in (c) is demarcated by the macrophages which were present at the graft site (arrows). (Scale bars (a), (b) = 500 μm; (c),(d) = 50 μm)

studies have suggested that such an effect can occur in humans as well. Hirsch and co-workers[63] observed an enhanced TH-immunoreactive fiber plexus proximal to a degenerated transplant site in a patient with Parkinson's disease who received an adrenal medullary implant. Kordower and colleagues[68] recently discerned a similar phenomenon in a patient with few surviving TH-immunoreactive chromaffin cells (Figures 3c and d). In this case report, the patient survived for 30 months following implantation, suggesting that the graft-induced modification of the host nigrostriatal system can be sustained long-term. Additionally, this case report reflects the first patient with a striatal graft who has come to autopsy and showed a sustained improvement following the transplant. Although case reports need to be interpreted cautiously, the human cases provide further evidence that adrenal grafts (or the damage induced by the graft procedure) can modulate the host dopaminergic system.

While the number of studies continues to grow supporting the 'trophic factor hypothesis' explanation of adrenal graft action, a critical analysis remains to be carried out with regards to this theory. Some aspects of the hypothesis which need more detailed scrutiny include:

(1)   The authenticity of trophic effect following adrenal grafting;

(2)   The mechanism(s) of trophic action;

(3)   The definition of a 'trophic effect';

(4)   Conditions under which the trophic effect can occur;

(5)   Functionality of the trophic effect;

(6)   Relevance of the trophic effect for the treatment of Parkinson's disease.

This list is not intended to be comprehensive but serves as a basis for others to expand upon.

The authenticity of trophic effect following adrenal grafting

One weakness of many studies describing the graft-mediated increase in host TH-immunoreactivity is the lack of quantification of this response. Such quantification is often difficult in non-human primates where, due to practical considerations, the numbers of animals in experimental and control groups tend to be relatively small. However, sample size is less of a problem in mouse studies. MPTP damages nigral neurons in mice and lowers striatal dopamine levels, although lesioned animals tend to recover over time.

Felten and co-workers[83] recently evaluated the trophic response to adrenal medullary implants using this model system. Mice treated with MPTP received either no transplant, a sham implant, an adrenal medulla implant, or a sciatic nerve/adrenal co-graft (Table 2). In this study, sham-implanted animals displayed a statistically significant increase in TH-immunoreactivity compared with non-implanted mice. Mice receiving adrenal chromaffin cell allografts displayed even greater striatal fiber densities than either the sham-implanted or non-implanted mice. This increase in TH-fiber innervation was accompanied by a 31% increase in striatal dopamine levels relative to sham-grafted animals. Interestingly, the most dense TH-fiber innervation was observed in co-grafted animals which contained the greatest number of surviving adrenal chromaffin cells. This suggests that, in addition to the damage induced by the transplant procedure, the implant material containing chromaffin cells, Schwann cells and fibroblasts provided additional trophic influences upon the host nigrostriatal system. Thus, the morphological changes seen within the striatum of MPTP-treated mice reflect statistically significant increases in TH and dopamine synthesis following

Table 2   Enhanced TH-immunoreactive fiber optical densities following grafts of adrenal medulla or adrenal medulla/sciatic nerve co-grafts. The areas measured are the four consecutive regions adjacent to the edge of the graft or needle tract. Values are expressed as mean $\pm$ SEM and are expressed as μm^2/total field view ($232.25 \times 232.25\ \mu m$). (Table modified from Date and colleagues[83])

Distance from graft or needle tract (μm)	Sham graft ($n = 5$)	Adrenal graft ($n = 5$)	Adrenal sciatic co-graft ($n = 5$)
0–232.25	583 ± 67	$3897 \pm 213\star$	$5046 \pm 605\star\dagger$
232.25–464.50	555 ± 49	$2056 \pm 189\star$	$3244 \pm 211\star\dagger$
464.50–696.75	489 ± 65	$1469 \pm 173\star$	$1633 \pm 201\star$
696.75–929.0	521 ± 77	$989 \pm 81\star$	$972 \pm 101\star$

$\star$Significantly different from sham operated group ($p < 0.01$); $\dagger$significantly different from adrenal graft group ($p < 0.01$)

implantation. However, it is important to note that the enhanced TH-immunoreactive fibers in the striatum of MPTP-lesioned mice, following adrenal grafts and co-grafts, occurred only in young mice. The host TH fiber response was greatly reduced with similar grafts in 12-month-old C57B1/6 mice. Similar quantitative analyses carried out in young and aged primates could greatly advance the 'trophic factor hypothesis'.

The mechanism(s) of trophic action

Little is known about the cell types and molecules responsible for the enhanced TH-immunoreactivity seen following adrenal grafting. Since damage alone can lead to an enhanced TH-immunoreactive fiber network, diffusible substances from the host organism released upon central neural system damage must be capable of mediating these effects. In rodent and primate adrenal grafting experiments, inflammatory and scavenger cells are the primary cell type within the perigraft region. Blood-borne macrophages, which scavenge non-viable chromaffin cells, secrete factors such as interleukin 1 (IL-1) which may mediate, in part, the trophic effect. Other candidates include microglia which are prominent in the perigraft region. Indeed, implants of microglia can induce a sprouting response in MPTP-treated monkeys (K. Bankiewicz, personal communication).

While the presence of surviving adrenal cells is not necessary for the induction of a dopaminergic trophic effect, as stated earlier it appears that the medullary tissue may secrete factors which can enhance the trophic response. Two studies have correlated the density of graft-induced striatal TH-immunoreactive profiles in the striatum with the number of surviving chromaffin cells. As discussed above, a TH-immunoreactive trophic effect is potentiated when cell size is enhanced by co-grafting adrenal chromaffin cells with a peripheral nerve[83]. Conversely, if graft survival is diminished by implanting chromaffin cells derived from allogenic or xenogenic donors, the graft-induced increase in TH-immunoreactivity is attenuated[99]. These data suggest that both host non-neuronal cells and adrenal chromaffin cells operate concurrently in eliciting a trophic response from host nigrostriatal neurons.

While the cell types involved in the trophic effect remain to be elucidated, so too are the molecules responsible for producing these effects. Two groups have examined the potential role of fibroblast growth factor (FGF) in nigrostriatal regeneration. FGF accumulates within the central nervous system at the site of focal brain damage[103]. Thus FGF is in a position to mediate the changes in TH-immunoreactivity following control implants or caudate cavitations. Following MPTP administration in mice, the elimination of TH-fiber staining within the caudoputamen can be reversed by intrastriatal administration of FGF[104,105]. The return of TH-fiber immunoreactivity is similar to that seen following adrenal cell grafting. Indeed, neither FGF infusion[104] nor adrenal cell grafting[106] augments TH staining in aged mice, further suggesting that these manipulations may act through similar mechanisms. Potentially, the fibroblasts within the adrenal medulla which are grafted along with the chromaffin cells could mimic the pharmacological administration of FGF. The correlation of enhanced graft survival with enhanced host-derived fiber innervation[83] would support this view. Alternatively, FGF and adrenal grafts could be producing similar effects through independent mechanisms. FGF also could act upon nigral neurons via multiple mechanisms. It could provide trophic influences directly on nigral neurons or could act as a mitogen for glial cells which in turn influence dopaminergic neurons[107–109]. Clearly, further studies are needed which directly aim at elucidating the underlying mechanisms of the trophic responses observed following adrenal cell grafting.

The definition of a 'trophic effect'

Throughout this and other manuscripts, the terms trophic response, sprouting, and TH up-regulation have often been used interchangeably. The studies documented above, describing changes in striatal TH-immunoreactivity following cavitation or adrenal medullary transplantation, all appear similar at face value. However, there is a question as to whether the changes in immunohistochemical profiles reflect actual sprouting (defined as the generation of new neural processes) or an up-regulation of TH synthesis in existing (but down-regulated) dopaminergic processes. Data exist to suggest that both phenomena can occur under different experimental circumstances. The best evidence for an actual sprouting of new neurites comes from the studies of Bankiewicz and co-workers[61,101,102]. Grafts placed into the head of the caudate nucleus in hemiparkinsonian monkeys induce an increase in TH-immunoreactivity in the perigraft region. These fibers can be traced to the more ventrally located nucleus accumbens and it has been hypothesized that these new processes are branches from the mesolimbic system. Indeed, the cells of origin, the ventral tegmental area (A10), are relatively spared following an intracarotid MPTP infusion and are thus available for up-regulation (Figure 4a). The fiber bundle streaming from the nucleus accumbens follows an atypical route which has not been described in normal monkeys via either immunohistochemical[110] or histofluorescent procedures[111]. This fact, along with the finding that these novel processes are immunoreactive for the GAP-43 protein (K. Bankiewicz, personal communication), suggests that an actual sprouting of new TH-immunoreactive processes can occur.

These findings appear different from what has been observed in partially lesioned MPTP-treated Cebus monkeys (Figure 4b) and mice. In our non-human primate studies[100], grafts of adrenal medulla were placed towards the body of the caudate nucleus, in a more caudal location than in Rhesus monkeys which demonstrated the sprouting response from the nucleus accumbens. As in the Bankiewicz study, an enhanced TH-immunoreactive fiber network was seen in the perigraft region within the caudate nucleus. In contrast, however, a fiber system originating from the nucleus accumbens was not observed. Rather, an enhanced TH-fiber system could be observed along the entire mesolimbic and nigrostriatal pathway as far caudally as the midbrain. This invigorated dopaminergic pathway was followed in sequential sections coursing along the natural path of the nigrostriatal system in these monkeys. Additional experiments have revealed that similar findings could be observed in adrenal grafted monkeys, sacrificed only a few days following implantation (Hansen and colleagues, unpublished data). It is extremely unlikely that new dopaminergic processes could grow through the midbrain and diencephalon to terminal zones within the caudate nucleus, especially within such a short time frame. These findings strongly suggest that an up-regulation of TH-synthesis, rather than a sprouting of new neural elements, is occurring under these conditions.

A similar effect probably occurs in MPTP-treated mice. It is important to note that MPTP induces a biochemical lesion resulting in a dopamine insufficiency, rather than the death of dopaminergic neurons of the substantia nigra pars compacta, in young mice[112]. The level of MPTP toxicity differs among mouse species, but the degree of structural damage to nigral neurons appears to be relatively minor. Grafting studies using this model system have not demonstrated an atypically oriented fiber bundle such as that originating from the nucleus accumbens. Taken together, these data also suggest that for the most part the enhanced TH-immunoreactivity seen following adrenal grafting in MPTP-treated mice is also the result of an up-regulation of dopamine synthesis and not a sprouting of new dopaminergic fibers. However, in sites very close to an adrenal graft or co-graft, the density of TH-positive fibers is greater than the density of TH-positive fibers in controls[99], raising the possibility that a limited sprouting of dopaminergic fibers may occur immediately adjacent to the graft in young mice.

TH-immunoreactive trophic effect: when can it occur?

The prospect of modifying host nigrostriatal function via neural grafting is a relatively new concept; originating with the report by Bohn and co-workers in 1986[98] and being further advanced with the non-human primate studies in the late 1980s. The question arises as to why this phenomenon was not described earlier when the demonstration of functional grafts spurred a renaissance in the field of neural transplantation. One explanation may be that most studies carried out in the early 1980s used fetal tissue as donor material and fetal tissue may not induce such an effect. A more likely explanation is that the discovery and characterization of the dopaminergic trophic response was dependent on the evolution of new animal models of Parkinson's disease.

The initial studies examining the neuroanatomical and functional correlates of dopaminergic grafts relied almost exclusively on the rotational model of Ungersted[12] in which injections of 6-hydroxydopamine were made unilaterally into the rat ventral mesencephalon or medial forebrain bundle. This lesion results in the destruction of more than 95% of the dopaminergic neurons within the substantia nigra *and* ventral tegmental area. As detailed above, the trophic effect following neural grafting can take two forms: an actual sprouting of new neural elements derived from the intact dopaminergic neurons of the mesolimbic system; or an upregulation of residual dopaminergic neurons

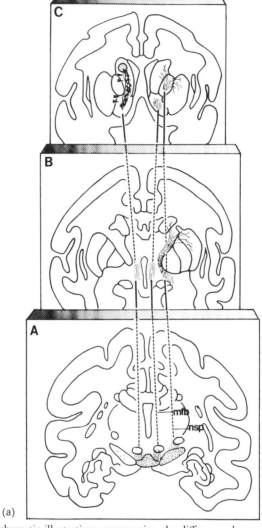

(a)

Figure 4 Schematic illustrations representing the differences between (a) TH-'sprouting' as described by Bankiewicz and colleagues[101,102] and (b) TH-'upregulation' as described by Fiandaca and co-workers[100]. (a) 'Sprouting' is seen in hemiparkinsonian Rhesus monkey where the substantia nigra is devastated ipsilateral to the lesion but the adjacent ventral tegmental area is intact (panel A). While the nigrostriatal pathway (nsp) is lesioned, the medial forebrain bundle (mfb) appears normal until the rostral telencephalon where fibers continue past their homotypic zones of intervention within

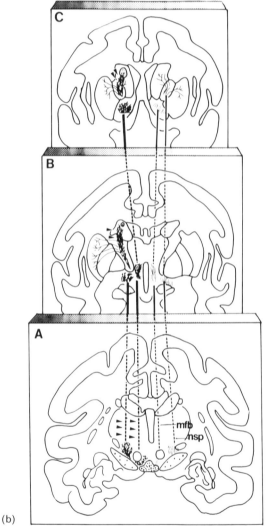

(b)

the nucleus accumbens and stream dorsally towards the graft (stippled area) taking a novel dopaminergic route (arrows, panel C). (b) In our systemically MPTP-treated Cebus monkeys, there was a reduced complement of substantia nigra neurons bilaterally (panel A). With upregulation, an enhanced TH-fiber network can be seen in the nsp and mfb as far caudally as the midbrain (arrows, panel A). These enhanced TH-fiber bundles follow the normal mesostriatal pathway (panel B) until they hyperinnervate the perigraft region (stippled area, panel C) within the partially lesioned substantia nigra. It is of note that, in both cases, the trophic effect depends upon the existence of viable dopaminergic neurons within the ventral mesencephalon. Since the rodent 6-hydroxydopamine (6-OHDA) model produces a comprehensive lesion of these cells, no neurons were available in earlier studies to respond to the implant and/or striatal damage and initiate a trophic response. In fact, the trophic response has only been observed in select animal models of Parkinson's disease. In each of these models, residual neurons remain within the ventral mesencephalon in a manner analogous to early stages of idiopathic Parkinson's disease. The trophic effect was first observed in the MPTP-treated mouse[98] where the lesion in young adult mice does not destroy the neurons of the substantia nigra but reduces their ability to synthesize dopamine. Therefore, the cells needed to manifest a trophic response are present and available for trophic stimulation. In aged mice, MPTP is more damaging to the neurons[112] and thus the trophic effect is reduced greatly[99].

A sprouting response has also been observed in monkeys rendered hemiparkinsonian via intracarotid infusion of MPTP. In this model system, the substantia nigra is lesioned to a degree comparable to that seen in 6-OHDA-lesioned rats. However, unlike 6-OHDA-lesioned rats, adjacent ventral tegmental area neurons are relatively spared. Again, neurons are available in the hemiparkinsonian monkey to effect a trophic response. Indeed, the dopaminergic sprouting response observed in this model appears to originate from the nucleus accumbens, a normal target region of ventral tegmental area neurons.

Lastly, an up-regulation of TH synthesis has been observed in monkeys following systemic MPTP administration[100]. However, these animals sustained only partial ($\approx$ 50%) lesions of the substantia nigra, maintaining a population of substantia nigra neurons to respond to trophic influences. Other non-human primate studies which use more intensive dosing regimes induce more comprehensive lesions of the ventral mesencephalon and do not report a sprouting or up-regulation of dopaminergic fibers (see, for example, reference 39).

Information derived from autopsy studies of parkinsonian patients who have undergone adrenal medullary transplants also supports the contention that the status of residual dopaminergic neurons within the ventral mesencephalon determines whether a sprouting response can occur. To date, seven transplant patients have undergone postmortem analysis[62-68]. Of these cases, the only two in which a trophic response has been observed are the two patients with a significant population of viable neurons remaining within the ventral mesencephalon[63,68]. The other cases report few residual melanin-containing neurons within the substantia nigra. These data indicate that if enhancing host dopaminergic activity through trophic mechanisms becomes a goal of neural transplantation, then patients with significant populations of residual ventral mesencephalic neurons will be the only reasonable recipients of such grafting procedures.

Can the trophic effect restore function?

To date, a limited data base exists regarding the ability of the trophic phenomenon to ameliorate experimental parkinsonism. This is due partly to the fact that the trophic response has not been readily observed in the unilateral nigrostriatal lesioned rat model of Parkinson's disease, the most favored experimental paradigm for study. The trophic phenomenon has been observed in young MPTP-treated mice. However, these mice do not readily exhibit behavioral deficits similar to those observed in Parkinson's disease[112]. Thus studies assessing the functional correlates of graft-induced trophic responses have been limited to experiments employing non-human primates. Again, the expense and practical difficulties of working with monkeys, combined with the inherent behavioral variability displayed by monkeys has limited the number of published reports using non-human primates.

However, a number of patterns are beginning to emerge. Among them is the concept that dopaminergic neurons contained within the graft are not a prerequisite for functional recovery. As established by Bankiewicz and co-workers[101,102] (Table 3), cavitation of the caudate nucleus, implants of control tissues, and grafts of adrenal medulla all appear to be capable of reversing, to varying degrees, MPTP-induced parkinsonism in non-human primates. Although the most complete functional recovery is seen with fetal central nervous system neurons (either dopaminergic or non-dopaminergic), a comparable attenuation of MPTP-induced motor dysfunction is seen with adrenal grafting or caudate cavitation alone[102]. In contrast, they have found that hemiparkinsonian monkeys with a surviving transplant but without a

Table 3 Effectiveness of graft strategies in reversing apomorphine-induced rotation in hemiparkinsonian monkeys. (Data adapted from Bankiewicz *et al.*[101,102])

Strategy	Result
Fetal monkey dopaminergic neurons	almost complete recovery
Fetal monkey non-dopaminergic neurons	almost complete recovery
Adrenal medullary allografts★	approximately 50% recovery
Adrenal medullary autografts★	approximately 50% recovery
Cavitation of caudate nucleus★	approximately 50% recovery
Stereotaxic adrenal autograft	no recovery
No surgical procedure	no recovery

★open microsurgical approach

sprouting response (due to atraumatic stereotaxic implantation) did not recover[101]. Thus it would appear that the presence of a surviving adrenal graft does not alone lead to functional recovery, while functional recovery can occur in monkeys with graft-induced sprouting but no surviving adrenal cells.

A case study of a patient receiving an adrenal medullary autograft further suggests that a trophic response can mediate functional recovery[68]. This patient demonstrated significant benefit from the transplant for up to 18 months following surgery. At the time of his death 30 months following grafting, he had returned to preoperative levels of function. However, this state may still be considered an improvement, given that the natural course of Parkinson's disease would probably have resulted in greater disability over the 30-month period if the operation had not been performed. At autopsy, only a few surviving TH-immunoreactive cells were observed within the graft site. However, a dense host-derived TH-immunoreactive fiber network was observed ventral to the implant (Figure 3) and on both lateral borders. While case reports need to be interpreted cautiously, these findings, along with the data generated in non-human primates, provide preliminary evidence that trophic effects exerted by adrenal medullary implants upon host dopaminergic neurons can have functional consequences. Additional data, however, are required to expand the existing data base and confirm these observations.

Is the trophic effect relevant for the treatment of Parkinson's disease?

Although structural changes in the nigrostriatal and mesolimbic pathways, and correlative functional changes in motor performance, can be observed in humans and non-humans, it is still unclear whether this effect is a worthwhile approach for clinical treatment. Parkinson's disease is most commonly a disease of the elderly, but aged MPTP-treated mice, even at a relatively modest 12 months of age, do not exhibit a trophic response to adrenal medullary grafting like their younger counterparts[106]. Autopsy cases which have demonstrated a trophic effect were of Parkinson's disease patients who were diagnosed early in life[63,68]. Whether this effect is applicable to an aged primate population still remains to be determined.

By definition, animal models of Parkinson's disease are approximations of the disease process. The MPTP-treated monkey, which is arguably the best animal model for Parkinson's disease, differs from idiopathic Parkinson's disease in ways which significantly impact upon neural transplant therapy. MPTP treatment produces acute damage while Parkinson's disease is a slow neurodegenerative process. MPTP-treated monkeys exhibit greater reductions of dopamine levels within the caudate nucleus compared with the putamen[43]. The reverse is true for idiopathic Parkinson's disease in which dopamine levels within the caudate nucleus can be near normal, while levels within the putamen are reduced by greater than 70–80%[113,114]. This information, combined with the fact that the putamen is more heavily interpolated into cortical–striatal–thalamic motor ciruitry than the caudate, has led to the hypothesis that this structure should be the site of neural grafting for Parkinson's disease[115]. The studies observing the trophic response utilized caudate nucleus implant sites and thus do not address the major locus of dopamine insufficiency in Parkinson's disease. It is questionable whether some forms of the trophic phenomenon could be generated following putamenal transplants. The sprouting of new dopaminergic fibers following neural grafting appears to be branches from the mesolimbic pathway[101,102]. Experimentally, these neurites can be seen coursing dorsally from the nucleus accumbens and entering the caudate nucleus from its ventral aspect. For a similar effect to occur following putamenal grafting, these fibers would need to take a longer and more lateral course, passing through the white matter fiber bundle comprising the internal capsule, or traversing through the striatal islands which are imbedded in the internal capsule. It remains to be determined whether these fibers can construct this passage through these physical barriers.

If not, the second approach for increasing dopaminergic tone through trophic mechanisms focuses on up-regulating TH-synthesis within the putamen. Since this process can follow the natural nigrostriatal pathway, the distance and mechanical constraints which may limit the sprouting effect would not be problematic. While the sprouting effect puts greater demands on ventral tegmental area neurons, a neuronal population less involved in the pathogenesis of Parkinson's disease than the substantia nigra pars compacta, trophic influences that enhance activity of nigrostriatal neurons are increasing the metabolic level of function within the very neurons being attacked by the disease process. A significant limiting factor in evaluating the merits of this approach is the fact that we still do not know why nigral neurons die in Parkinson's disease. Is it due to the lack of an endogenous trophic factor? If so, then adrenal grafting could potentially supply this factor, and an up-regulation of dopaminergic function could indeed be beneficial for the patient in the long-term. However another, less optimistic, scenario exists. It is possible that those nigral neurons forced to up-regulate their activity become even more susceptible to damage. It has been hypothesized that the degeneration of substantia nigra neurons is partly due to the production of free radicals, as a by product of catecholamine synthesis, which, under disease conditions, can not be cleared or prevented by endogenous scavenger mechanisms[116,117]. Can these host dopaminergic neurons, which are already under neurodegenerative duress, withstand this additional challenge? Will the increased demand upon these neurons ultimately potentiate nigrostriatal degeneration and thus accelerate the disease process? These issues need to be considered before clinical transplant strategies are aimed at optimizing trophic influences on host dopaminergic systems.

CLINICAL NEURAL TRANSPLANTATION

In 1982, two patients with Parkinson's disease were the first to receive autografts of adrenal medulla placed into the head of the right caudate nucleus in an attempt to reverse their motor disability[118]. After a brief period of benefit which may have been the result of dying chromaffin cells releasing catecholaminergic stores, both patients returned to their preoperative parkinsonian level of function. A positive note was the fact that the implant procedure did not have any adverse effects upon either patient suggesting that, at the very least, further clinical trials could be carried out safely. Two years later, two additional patients underwent putamenal autografts of adrenal medullary tissue[115]. As discussed above, the putamen is more involved in motor control than the caudate nucleus since it receives a greater innervation from motor cortex[119]. Furthermore, the putamen displays a greater dopamine insufficiency in Parkinson's disease[113,114]. These patients also did not benefit significantly from the implant.

Clinical transplant studies in the United States did not begin until a report by Madrazo and colleagues, suggesting that adrenal medullary autografts could dramatically reduce parkinsonian symptoms[120]. This study reported two patients who received an adrenal medullary autograft, using an open microsurgical approach which clipped the graft to the ependyma of the right caudate nucleus. These patients were reported to show a striking improvement in their parkinsonian signs. Interestingly, the unilateral implant reportedly produced bilateral benefit. The papers that followed from this group reported similar effects with greater numbers of patients[121]. Some of these patients were considered to be sufficiently improved to be removed from antiparkinsonian medication. These findings induced other centers in the United States and around the world to initiate neural grafting programs[122-129]. Reports from groups in China, Spain and Cuba were similarly encouraging[122,130,131]. Many of these patients had extended hospital stays and thus there was no way to assess the potential beneficial effects of intensive postoperative attention and therapy these patients received. None of the centers in the United States[122-129], however, were able to replicate the effects of Madrazo and colleagues. In addition, some centers experienced rates of morbidity and mortality which were unacceptable. Hallucinations and delusions resembling schizophrenia were often seen following transplantation (see, for example, ref. 128). This effect may have been the result of graft-related stimulation of the mesolimbic dopaminergic systems. Some complications were the result of removing the adrenal gland via a transabdominal, rather than a retroperitoneal, approach (for example, ref. 127). These results were viewed as disappointing in light of the significant benefits reported by Madrazo. By 1990, virtually every center in the United States had stopped performing adrenal medullary implants and this flurry of clinical trials was, in general, deemed a failure. While adrenal cell grafting clearly did not have the impact of levodopa upon the clinical management of Parkinson's disease, a careful scrutiny of the clinical data indicates that adrenal autografts were, however, able to modestly improve motor function in some patients, with the most consistent behavioral effect being a reduction in 'off' time (Table 4). It is important to note that even patients who initially responded well to the adrenal autograft tended to lose benefit from the procedure and returned to baseline level by 18 months following transplantation[129].

Experimental data gathered in mice, rats, and monkeys have clearly established that exposing chromaffin cell grafts to NGF, either by infusion[73] or co-grafting with an NGF-producing cell source[71,75,83], can augment graft viability and function. Based on these and other data, Olson and co-workers[132] grafted six pieces of autologous adrenal medulla to the putamen of a patient with Parkinson's disease. The grafts were arranged so that they surrounded a cannula which continuously delivered mouse βNGF (total dose 4 mg) over a 1-month period. After an initial period of worsening (1 month), this patient displayed steady and significant improvement of bradykinesia and rigidity. Electrophysiological measures of motor readiness potentials also improved, while some measures of gross and fine motor function remained unchanged. Tremor was a minor symptom preoperatively and was not assessed post-transplantation. Since various centers have used different testing criteria, it is difficult to determine whether the magnitude of the effect seen in this patient is greater than responding patients who received adrenal chromaffin cells alone or fetal mesencephalic implants. What is significant, however, is the fact that continued improvement in this patient was reported for 14 months[132] and has been sustained for 18 months (B. Hoffer, personal communication). In contrast, the benefit seen in those patients who responded to adrenal medulla grafts without NGF usually disappeared within 18 months after surgery[129].

What mechanisms underly the modest benefits reported in adrenal medulla-grafted cases of patients without NGF supplementation? Potentially, the chromaffin cells could be secreting dopamine. However, every patient who has received an adrenal autograft and subsequently been

Table 4 Patients with adrenal medullary autografts: American studies. Disease severity is as measured on the Hoehn and Yahr scale

Reference	n	Age of patients (years)	Duration of Parkinson's disease (years)	Disease severity*	Benefits
Allen et al.[127]	18	35–69	5–25	2–4	decreased tremor, improvements in bradykinesia, dexterity, speech, stability, posture and gait
Goetz et al.[123,124]	19	53 ± 8	13 ± 7	4	increased 'on' time, decreased 'off' time (improved quality of life measures)
Jancovic et al.[62]	3	43–59	12–21	2–4	increased quality of 'on' time, decreased severity of 'off' time, decreased tremor, and improved gait
Kelly et al.[126], Ahlskog et al.[125]	8	38–58	8–23	3–4	one patient moderately improved and three patients mildly improved at 1 year, decrease in the severity and duration of bradykinesia
Apuzzo et al.[128]	8	39–68	5–15	2–4	four of eight patients showed sustained (1 year) mild to moderate improvements in their clinical symptoms
Olanow et al.[129]*					a follow-up of the patients described by Goetz et al.[123,124]. Pattern of improvement seen at 12 months had deteriorated by 18 months

*Same demographics as Goetz et al. 1989, 1990 except for the death of one patient

analyzed histologically at autopsy has had no or minimal surviving adrenal chromaffin cells[62-68]. This is true for patients who have[68] and have not[62-67] responded to the procedure. Although parkinsonian adrenal glands demonstrate intense catecholamine histofluorescence (B. Hoffer, personal communication), levels of dopamine are reportedly low in patients with Parkinson's disease[133] and thus it is questionable whether sufficient dopamine levels could be secreted from the chromaffin cells even if they survived well. The surgical procedure may have enhanced the efficacy of levodopa by causing a breakdown of the blood–brain barrier within the striatum and giving the drug better access to its site of action. If some chromaffin cells do survive they will be invested with a fenestrated vasculature (see reviews 6–10), again giving levodopa a more focal entry to the striatum.

Alternatively, a trophic effect resulting from the implant may underlie the behavioral changes. Indeed, many graft recipients improve bilaterally following a unilateral transplant. Furthermore, autopsy on two graft recipients has demonstrated an enhanced TH-immunoreactivity in the perigraft region in a manner similar to that seen in experimental animals[63,68]. Lastly, the possibility of a placebo effect cannot be ignored. Placebo effects can be very powerful and the magnitude of the beneficial effects displayed by some transplant patients are sufficiently modest to consider that a placebo effect may be participating in the behavioral changes observed. Placebo effects are usually not long-lived, however, and the fact that some patients improved for over a year suggests that factors related to the transplant procedure are also mediating functional recovery.

Experimental evidence clearly demonstrates the superiority of fetal ventral mesencephalic neurons relative to adrenal chromaffin cells as a donor tissue for transplantation. Although social and ethical issues have slowed clinical trials in Parkinson's patients using fetal neuron transplants, a number of groups recently have initiated fetal grafting programs. Lindvall and co-workers[134-136] have published their findings on three patients with fetal mesencephalic grafts taken from early (7–9 weeks) gestational donors. Grafts were either placed into the putamen or into both the putamen and caudate nucleus. A patient with the implant in the putamen has demonstrated significant improvement following transplantation, which was correlated with enhanced fluorodopa uptake within the putamen on the grafted side[136]. The increased fluorodopa uptake is suggestive of graft survival; however other interpretations, including a trophic response to the implant by host dopaminergic systems have been proposed[137,138]. Others have recently reported success with fetal transplants. Freed and co-workers[139] have reported one patient receiving a fetal implant. Six months following transplantation, this patient has displayed a significant improvement in motor function as measured by standard tests and by a home computer test measuring finger dexterity. While encouraging, the magnitude of benefit achieved by these patients is comparable to that seen following adrenal grafting. Whether motor function in these patients continues to improve and is sustained over time remains to be determined.

Technical and theoretical questions remain to be resolved for the optimal effect of fetal grafting to be achieved. One problem may be getting large numbers of fetal neurons to survive. It has been estimated that only 1–2% (100–200 cells) of grafted dopaminergic neurons need to survive to induce a 50% reduction in amphetamine-induced rotation in rats[140]. While up to 25 000 neurons have been estimated to survive following grafting into immunosuppressed rats[140], such survival has not been achieved in non-human primates[36–39]. Experimentally, embryos are removed via Caesarean section and the tissue is easily dissected, optimizing the initial yield of donor cells. In contrast, following human suction abortion, small embryos are often fractured and the ventral mesencephalon is difficult to locate and dissect. Under these conditions, it is imperative that the dissection is carried out by an investigator who is both experienced in tissue dissection and has extensively practised this particular dissection from aborted embryos. Even with a precise dissection, it is as yet unclear what percentage of dopaminergic neurons will survive in humans. Can fetuses be pooled in humans for a single graft recipient? Lindvall and co-workers are testing this possibility[136]. If pooled fetuses can be used clinically, then tissue storage procedures will have great value. Collier and co-workers have demonstrated the ability to cryopreserve rat, monkey and human fetal dopaminergic cells[141]. These cells can be transplanted successfully although the grafts appear less vigorous than fresh tissue implants. Human fetal ventral mesencephalon can also be stored for up to 4 days in a hibernation medium. Following transplantation into immunosuppressed rats, these cells survive well, can migrate for short distances in the host brain, and innervate the host striatum in an organotypic pattern[142] (see Figure 5).

Another issue in need of resolution is the potential need for immuno-suppression. Human fetal allografts placed into rats clearly enjoy immunological privilege to the extent that large healthy grafts can easily be achieved. In primates, the data are less clear. Sladek and co-workers have described healthy fetal nigral allografts. However, many of these transplants have fewer than 300 surviving cells[45]. Some groups have demonstrated relatively small implants following fetal grafting in non-human primates (for example, ref. 38). Others, reporting larger implants, have used relatively inbred strains of monkeys, potentially inhibiting an immunological response[41]. Immunosuppression is being used with human fetal transplants. This is problematic since use of cyclosporin is not without its own level of morbidity. Studies in non-human primates assessing the need for immunosuppression following fetal allografts are clearly needed, and could directly impact upon the clinical data currently being gathered. Indeed, if grafts function in part by enhancing endogenous dopamine neuronal activity, then perhaps allografts, or even xenografts, could be placed in the striatum of immunosuppressed patients in an attempt to invoke the trophic benefits of the implant, after which, the immunosuppression could potentially be discontinued. This approach currently merits experimental investigation in animals, but the use of xenografts could bypass the problematic question of using aborted fetal cells. Lastly, the efficacy of fetal grafting for Parkinson's disease may be attenuated since all graft recipients receive long-term levodopa therapy. In rats, chronic levodopa treatment impairs fetal graft survival and host dopaminergic innervation[143]. Indeed while multiple and converging lines of experimental evidence would suggest that fetal ventral mesencephalic cells are better than chromaffin cells as a donor tissue, it would appear that both the disease process and conventional pharmacotherapy would be potentially more deleterious to fetal cells than chromaffin cells.

FUTURE CONSIDERATIONS: QUESTIONS FOR THE 1990s

Throughout this review, we have identified problem areas in neural transplantation. As serious scientific inquiry into the concept of functional

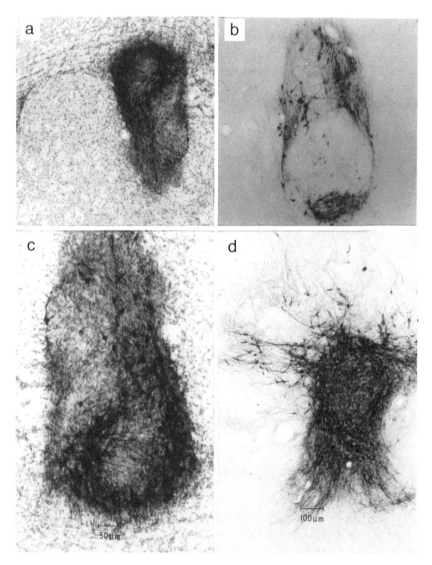

Figure 5 TH-immunostained sections through the striatum of immunosuppressed unilateral nigrostriatal lesioned rats which received implants of human ventral mesence-phalon, maintained in a hibernation medium for 1 day ((a), (b) and (c)) and 4 days (d). Note the robust survival of cells in all panels and the outgrowth of fibers (d) into the host parenchyma. (a) and (b) are the same magnification as (d)

neural implants has been underway for just over a decade, and while exceptional progress has been made, it is not surprising that experimentation to date has raised as many questions as it has provided answers. Perhaps the most fundamental of remaining questions concerns mechanisms of action. Stated more precisely, what are the mechanisms of action underlying the functional recovery in Parkinson's disease and other animal model systems which have been studied? Do these mechanisms vary from model system to model system and which of these model systems will best predict the clinical situation?

Admittedly, this is a complex question with many sub-issues. Among those which need to be addressed are the following:

(1) What are the respective roles of the graft and host brain in functional recovery?

(2) How well are grafted neurons incorporated into the host brain's neural networks, and what is their contribution to functional recovery?

(3) How important are trophic factors in promoting functional recovery? Which trophic factors are involved? Which cell populations are the targets?

(4) Is graft-induced regeneration qualitatively different from normal regenerative processes?

This list, of course, could easily be expanded and various facets of these questions are under active investigation. It does, however, provide a perspective of the challenges facing us over the next decade.

An additional vital challenge that remains is the development of better donor tissues. Most studies in the 1980s used either fetal brain tissue or neural/paraneural cells from the body for transplants. As described earlier, each of these donor tissues has its limitations. In addition, neither fetal dopaminergic grafts nor paraneural grafts of the adrenal medulla have yet proven to be particularly efficacious in the clinical treatment of Parkinson's disease. Cell lines, developed and designed for specific transplant goals such as to deliver a specific neurotransmitter or growth factor to the implant site, may prove to have significant advantages over other types of donor tissues[144-147]. Indeed, many of the practical problems encountered using fetal or peripheral tissues can be avoided by developing cell lines for implantation. Recent studies have demonstrated that implants of cells genetically modified to produce NGF are capable of preventing the death of cholinergic basal forebrain neurons which normally results from fimbria fornix transection[145,146]. Furthermore, fibroblasts can be modified to produce levodopa and attenuate lesion-induced motor dysfunction in a rat model of Parkinson's disease[147]. However, the cells in this study did not produce dopamine. This study points out the difficulty of engineering cells to produce a specific neurotransmitter, since genes for multiple enzymes along the catecholaminergic biosynthetic pathway need to be inserted for the production of the neurotransmitter dopamine to occur. While important progress has been made in this area, and the concept of using modern methods of molecular biology genetically to design cells for specific transplant purposes seems to be especially promising, a number of difficult questions must be answered before engineered cell lines can be considered for any clinical use.

First and foremost are safety issues. Will the implanted cells remain under growth control in the host brain? Do donor cells harbor viruses or any other infectious agents such as prions which can be transmitted to the host? What other factors, in addition to those selected for, are produced by the donor cells and what effect do they have upon the host? What are the long-term effects of the implanted cells on the host and will they produce the desired molecules in a stable fashion over a time of years? How can the implanted cells be removed if this becomes necessary? These and other questions will require much careful thought and experimentation over the coming years.

Finally, there is the challenge of combining neural implantation with other technologies to create new and potentially more effective treatment strategies. The concept of infusing NGF into the striatum along with a chromaffin cell graft is one example of this approach. Another promising approach involves implanting donor cells in thin polymer capsules. This encapsulation procedure allows nutrients from the host brain to infuse into the graft and maintain viability and molecules under $50\,kDa$ to diffuse out into the host brain. Among the advantages of encapsulated cell grafts are:

(1)   Most antigens which could generate an immune response are larger than $50\,kDa$ and would not gain access to the grafted cells. This

could potentially obviate the use of immunosuppression in allograft and xenograft situations. Indeed, viable mouse ventral mesencephalic neurons can survive grafting within the cerebral cortex of non-immunosuppressed rats when placed in polymer capsules prior to implantation[148];

(2) Donor cells are confined to the interior of the capsule and thus cannot overgrow the host brain;

(3) The capsule can be designed for recovery should it be necessary to remove the graft; and

(4) Trophic factors or other drugs can be incorporated into the polymer capsule which are slowly released over time to promote either graft survival or potentiate host recovery.

Of course, encapsulated cell grafts are limited to providing diffusable substances to surrounding parenchyma and will not provide a fiber innervation pattern to the host brain.

CONCLUDING REMARKS

What can we presently expect from clinical transplants? Using present techniques, neural grafting will not cure Parkinson's disease and no data exist to suggest that implants will slow the progression of nigrostriatal degeneration or provide any benefits compared with conventional pharmacological therapy. Indeed, the long-term functional improvements gleaned experimentally following fetal dopaminergic implants may not be a good predictor of graft function in humans, since all animal models of Parkinson's disease are based upon acute lesions of the ventral mesencephalon. The slow progression of cell loss and dopamine insufficiency has yet to be mimicked in non-humans. Neural grafts may improve some of the symptoms of Parkinson's disease for a period of time. However, the natural course of the disease will continue. Unless the magnitude of increased dopaminergic tone greatly exceeds the threshold level below which disability is produced, the benefits derived from the implant will not be sustained over time. This may be why 'responding' adrenal graft recipients generally return to preoperative levels of function within 18 months following implantation[129]. A goal of future research is to find ways of achieving levels of functional dopamine pools well in excess of the levels at which symptoms appear. Thus, the continued decrement of host striatal dopamine induced by the disease process will not quickly lead to dysfunction. This potentially may be achieved through improvements in grafting techniques or supplementation of implants with growth factors. Given enough time, the disease may ultimately 'catch up to and overtake' the transplant. If this time period can be protracted, however, then neural grafting has the potential to be a safe, effective and valuable tool in the treatment of Parkinson's disease.

ACKNOWLEDGEMENTS

The authors thank Drs Massimo S. Fiandaca, John T. Hansen, Mary F.D. Notter, Gouying Bing, Isao Date, Suzanne Y. Felten, and John A. Olschowka for collaborating on some of the experiments described in this paper. We would also like to thank Dr Barry Hoffer for helpful discussions and for sharing his clinical data with us. Supported by NS25655 (JHK), R37 AG06060 (DLF), R2P50 MH40381, NS25778 (DMG) and the Pew Foundation.

REFERENCES

1. Björklund, A. and Stenevi, U. (1985). *Neural Grafting in the Mammalian CNS.* (Amsterdam: Elsevier Science)
2. Sladek Jr., J.R. and Gash, D.M. (1984). *Neural Transplants, Development, Plasticity, and Function.* (New York: Plenum Press)
3. Gash, D.M. and Sladek Jr., J.R. (1988). *Transplantation into the Mammalian CNS. Prog. Brain Res.,* **78**. (Amsterdam: Elsevier Science)
4. Dunnett, S.B. and Richards, S.-J. (1990). *Neural Transplantation. Prog. Brain Res.,* **82**. (Amsterdam: Elsevier Science)
5. Sladek Jr., J.R. and Shoulson, I. (1988). Neural transplantation: a call for patience rather than patients. *Science,* **240**, 1386–8
6. Gash, D.M., Collier, T.C. and Sladek Jr., J.R. (1985). Neural transplantation: A review of recent developments and potential applications to the aged brain. *Neurobiol. Aging,* **6**, 131–50
7. Kordower, J.H., Fiandaca, M.S., Notter, M.F.D. *et al.* (1990). Scientific basis for dopaminergic brain grafting. In Koller, W.C. and Paulson, G.

(eds.) *Therapy of Parkinson's disease*, pp. 443–72. (New York: Marcel Dekker Inc.)

8. Freed, W.J., Poltorak, M. and Becker, J.B. (1990). Intracerebral adrenal medulla grafts: a review. *Exp. Neurol.,* **110**, 139–66

9. Yurek, D. and Sladek Jr., J.R. (1989). Dopamine cell replacement: Parkinson's disease. *Annu. Rev. Neurosci.,* **13**, 415–40

10. Lindvall, O. (1989). Transplantation into the human brain: present status and future possibilities. *J. Neurol. Neurosurg. Psychiatr.,* (Suppl.), 39–54

11. Lindvall, O., Dunnett, S.B., Brundin, P. *et al.* (1987). Transplantation of catecholamine-producing cells to the basal ganglia in Parkinson's disease: experimental and clinical studies. In Rose, F.C. (ed.) *Parkinson's Disease: Clinical and Experimental Advances,* pp. 189–206. (London: John Libby and Co.)

12. Ungerstedt, U. (1971). Post-synaptic supersensitivity after 6-OHDA induced degeneration of the nigrostriatal dopamine system. *Acta Phys. Scand.,* **82** (Suppl. 367), 69–93

13. Dunnett, S.B., Wishaw, I.Q., Rogers, D.C. *et al.* (1987). Dopamine-rich grafts ameliorate whole body motor asymmetry and sensory neglect but not independent limb use in rats with 6-hydroxydopamine lesions. *Brain Res.,* **415**, 63–78

14. Dunnett, S.B., Björklund, A., Schmidt, R.H. *et al.* (1981). Behavioral recovery following transplantation of substantia nigra in rats subjected to 6-OHDA lesions on the nigrostriatal pathway. II. Bilateral lesions. *Brain Res.,* **229**, 457–60

15. Herman, J.P., Chouili, K., Le Moal, M. (1986). Reinnervation of the nucleus accumbens and frontal cortex of the rat by dopaminergic grafts and effects upon hoarding behavior. *Brain Res.,* **372**, 210–16

16. Björklund, A. and Stenevi, U. (1979). Reconstruction of the nigrostriatal dopamine pathway by intracerebral nigral transplants. *Brain Res.,* **177**, 555–60

17. Björklund, A. and Stenevi, U. (1979). Regeneration of monoaminergic and cholinergic neurons in the mammalian central nervous system. *Physiol. Rev.,* **59**, 62–100

18. Perlow, M.J., Freed, W.J., Hoffer, B.J. *et al.* (1979). Brain grafts reduce motor abnormalities produced by destruction of the nigrostriatal pathway. *Science,* **204**, 646–7

19. Freed, W.J., Perlow, M.J., Karoum, F. *et al.* (1980). Restoration of dopamine brain function by grafting fetal substantia nigra to the caudate nucleus: long term behavioral, biochemical, and histological studies. *Ann. Neurol.,* **8**, 510–23

20. Björklund, A., Stenevi, U., Dunnett, S.B. *et al.* (1981). Functional

reactivation of the deafferented neostriatum by nigral transplants. *Nature (London)*, **289**, 497–9

21. Dunnett, S.B., Björklund, A., Stenevi, U. *et al.* (1981). Behavioral recovery following transplantation of substantia nigra in rats subjected to 6-OHDA lesions of the nigrostriatal pathway. I. Unilateral lesions. *Brain Res.*, **215**, 147–61

22. Stenevi, U., Björklund, A. and Svengaard, N.-A. (1976). Transplantation of central and peripheral monoamine neurons to the adult rat brain: techniques and conditions for survival. *Brain Res.*, **114**, 1–31

23. Freed, W.J., Hoffer, B.J., Olson, L. *et al.* (1984). Transplantation of catecholaminergic-containing tissues to restore the functional capacity of the damaged nigrostriatal system. In Sladek Jr., J.R. and Gash, D.M. (eds.) *Neural Transplants, Development, Plasticity and Function*, pp. 373–406. (New York: Plenum Press)

24. Björklund, A., Schmidt, R.H. and Stenevi, U. (1980). Functional reinnervation of the neostriatum in the adult rat by use of intraparenchymal grafting of dissociated cell suspensions from the substantia nigra. *Cell Tissue Res.*, **212**, 39–49

25. Schultzberg, M., Dunnett, S.B., Björklund, A. *et al.* (1984). Dopamine and cholecystokinin immunoreactive neurons in mesencephalic grafts reinnervating the neostriatum: evidence for selective growth regulation. *Neuroscience*, **12**, 17–32

26. Björklund, A., Dunnett, S.B., Stenevi, U. *et al.* (1980). Reinnervation of the denervated striatum by substantia nigra transplants: functional consequences as revealed by pharmacological and sensory-motor testing. *Brain Res.*, **199**, 307–33

27. Mahalick, T.J., Finger, T.E., Stromberg, I. *et al.* (1985). Substantia nigra transplants into denervated striatum of the rat: ultrastructure of graft–host interconnections. *J. Comp. Neurol.*, **240**, 60–70

28. Schmidt, R.H., Ingvar, M., Lindvall, O. *et al.* (1982). Functional activity of substantia nigra grafts reinnervating the striatum: neurotransmitter metabolism and [^{14}C]-2-deoxy-D-glucose autoradiography. *J. Neurochem.*, **38**, 737–48

29. Wuerthele, S.M., Freed, W.J., Olson, L. *et al.* (1981). Effects of dopamine agonists and antagonists on the electrical activity of substantia neurons transplanted into the lateral of the rat. *Exp. Brain Res.*, **44**, 1–10

30. Freed, W.J., Ko, G.N., Niehoff, D. *et al.* (1983). Normalization of spiroperidol binding in the rat striatum by homologous grafts of substantia nigra. *Science*, **222**, 937–9

31. Brundin, P., Strecker, R.E., Clarke, D.J. *et al.* (1988). Can human fetal dopamine neuron grafts provide a therapy for Parkinson's disease? In

Gash, D.M. and Sladek Jr., J.R. (eds.) *Transplantation into the Mammalian CNS. Prog. Brain Res.*, **78**, 441–8. (Amsterdam: Elsevier Science)

32. Björklund, A., Stenevi, U., Dunnett, S.B. *et al.* (1982). Cross-species neural grafting in a rat model of Parkinson's disease. *Nature (London)*, **298**, 652–4

33. van Horne, C.G., Mahalik, T., Hoffer, B. *et al.* (1990). Behavioral and electrophysiological correlates of human mesencephalic dopamine xenograft function in the rat striatum. *Brain Res. Bull.*, **25**, 325–34

34. Stromberg, I., Almqvist, P., Bygdeman, M. *et al.* (1989). Human fetal mesencephalic tissue grafted to dopamine-denervated striatum of athymic rats: light and electron microscopic histochemical and *in vivo* chronoamperometric studies. *J. Neurosci.*, **9**, 614–24

35. Langston, J.W., Ballard, P., Tetrud, J.W. *et al.* (1983). Chronic parkinsonism in humans due to a product of meperidine analogue synthesis. *Science*, **219**, 979–80

36. Burns, S., Chiueh, C.C., Markey, S. *et al.* (1983). Primate model of Parkinson's disease: selective destruction of substantia nigra pars compacta dopaminergic neurons by N-methyl-4-phenyl-1,2,3,6-tetrahydropyridine. *Proc. Natl. Acad. Sci. USA*, **80**, 4546–50

37. Markey, S.P., Johannessen, J.N., Chiueh, C.C. *et al.* (1984). Intraneuronal generation of a pyridium metabolite may cause drug-induced parkinsonism. *Nature (London)*, **311**, 464–7

38. Bakay, R.A.E., Barrow, D.L., Fiandaca, M.S. *et al.* (1987). Biochemical and behavioral correction of MPTP-like syndrome by fetal cell transplantation. *Ann. N.Y. Acad. Sci.*, **495**, 623–40

39. Sladek Jr., J.R., Collier, T.C., Haber, S.N. *et al.* (1986). Survival and growth of fetal catecholamine neurons transplanted into the primate brain. *Brain Res. Bull.*, **17**, 809–18

40. Sladek Jr., J.R., Redmond Jr., D.E., Collier, T.C. *et al.* (1988). Fetal dopamine neural grafts: extended reversal of methylphenyltetrahydropyridine-induced parkinsonism in primates. In Gash, D.M. and Sladek Jr., J.R. (eds.) *Transplantation into the Mammalian CNS. Prog. Brain Res.*, **78**, 497–506. (Amsterdam: Elsevier Science)

41. Fine, A., Hunt, S.B., Oertel, W.H. *et al.* (1988). Transplantation of embryonic dopaminergic neurons to the corpus striatum of marmosets rendered parkinsonian by 1-methyl-4-phenyl-1,2,3,6-tetrahydropyridine. In Gash, D.M. and Sladek Jr., J.R. (eds.) *Transplantation into the Mammalian CNS. Prog. Brain Res.*, **78**, 479–90. (Amsterdam: Elsevier Science)

42. Redmond Jr., D.E., Naftolin, F., Collier, T.J. *et al.* (1988). Cryopreservation, culture, and transplantation of human fetal mesencephalic tissue

into monkeys. *Science,* **242**, 768–71
43. Elsworth, J.D., Deutch, A.Y., Redmond Jr., D.E. *et al.* (1989). Symptomatic and asymptomatic 1-methyl-4-phenyl-1,2,3,6-tetrahydropyridine treated primates: biochemical changes in striatal regions. *Neuroscience,* **33**, 323–31
44. Sladek, J.R., Collier, T.J. and Haber, S.N. (1987). Reversal of parkinsonism by fetal nerve cell transplants in the primate brain. *Ann. N.Y. Acad. Sci.,* **495**, 641–57
45. Sladek Jr., J.R. (1990). Presented at the *Fernstrom Symposium,* Lund, Sweden
46. Itakura, T., Kamei, I., Nakai, K. *et al.* (1988). Autotransplantation of the superior cervical ganglion into the brain: a possible therapy for Parkinson's disease. *J. Neurosurg.,* **68**, 955–9
47. Bing, G., Notter, M.F.D., Hansen, J.T. *et al.* (1988). Comparison of adrenal medullary, carotid body and PC12 cell grafts in 6-OHDA lesioned rats. *Brain Res. Bull.,* **20**, 399–406
48. Jaeger, C.A. (1985). Immunocytochemical study of PC-12 cells grafted into the brain of immature rats. *Exp. Brain Res.,* **59**, 615–24
49. Jaeger, C.B. (1987). Morphological and immunocytochemical characteristics of PC 12 cell grafts in the rat brain. *Ann. N.Y. Acad. Sci.,* **495**, 334–50
50. Hefti, F., Hartikka, J. and Schlumpf, M. (1985). Implantation of PC 12 cells into the corpus striatum of rats with lesions of the dopaminergic system. *Brain Res.,* **348**, 283–8
51. Allen, Y.S., Kershaw, T.R., Prentice, H. *et al.* (1988). The influence of NGF treatment and endogenous trophic factors on the survival of PC 12 cells grafted into the adult rat brain. In Gash, D.M. and Sladek Jr., J.R. (eds.) *Transplantation into the Mammalian CNS. Prog. Brain Res.,* **78**, 637–42. (Amsterdam: Elsevier Science)
52. Freed, W.J., Morihisa, M., Spoor, H.E. *et al.* (1981). Transplanted adrenal chromaffin cells in rat brain reduce lesion-induced rotational behavior. *Nature (London),* **292**, 351–2
53. Freed, W.J., Cannon-Spoor, H., Krauthamer, E. *et al.* (1986). Intrastriatal adrenal medulla grafts in rats. *J. Neurosurg.,* **65**, 664–70
54. Freed, W.J., Cannon-Spoor, H., Krauthamer, E. *et al.* (1985). Factors influencing the efficacy of adrenal medulla and embryonic substantia nigra grafts. In Bjorklund, A. and Stenevi, U. (eds.) *Neural Grafting in Mammalian CNS,* pp. 491–504. (Amsterdam: Elsevier Science)
55. Freed, W.J., Karoum, F., Spoor, H.E. *et al.* (1983). Catecholamine content of intracerebral adrenal medulla grafts. *Brain Res.,* **269**, 184–9
56. Strömberg, I., Herrera-Marschitz, M., Hultgren, L. *et al.* (1984). Adrenal medullary implants in the dopamine-denervated rat striatum. I. Acute

catecholamine levels in grafts and host caudate as determined by HPLC-electrochemistry and fluorescence histochemical image analysis. *Brain Res.*, **297**, 41–51

57. Herrera-Marschitz, M., Stromberg, I., Olsson, D. *et al.* (1984). Adrenal medullary implants in the dopamine-denervated rat striatum. II. Acute behavior as a function of graft amount and location and its modulation by neuroleptics. *Brain Res.*, **297**, 53–61

58. Morihisa, J.M., Nakamura, R.K., Freed, W.J. *et al.* (1984). Adrenal medulla grafts survive and exhibit catecholamine-specific fluorescence in the primate brain. *Exp. Neurol.*, **84**, 643–53

59. Hansen, J.T., Kordower, J.H., Fiandaca, M.S. *et al.* (1988). Adrenal medullary autografts into the basal ganglia of cebus monkeys: graft viability and fine structure. *Exp. Neurol.*, **102**, 65–76

60. Hansen, J.T., Bing, G., Notter, M.F.D. *et al.* (1989). Adrenal chromaffin cells as transplants in animal models of Parkinson's disease. *J. Elec. Microsc. Tech.*, **12**, 308–15

61. Bankiewicz, K.S., Plunket, R.J., Kopin, I.J. *et al.* (1988). Transient behavioral recovery in hemiparkinsonian primates after adrenal medullary allografts. In Gash, D.M. and Sladek Jr., J.R. (eds.) *Transplantation into the Mammalian CNS; Prog. Brain Res.*, **78**, 543–50. (Amsterdam: Elsevier Science)

62. Jankovic, J., Grossman, R., Goodman, C. *et al.* (1989). Clinical, biochemical and neuropathologic findings following transplantation of adrenal medulla to caudate nucleus for the treatment of Parkinson's disease. *Neurology*, **39**, 1227–34

63. Hirsch, E.C., Duyckaerts, C., Javoy-Agid, F. *et al.* (1990). Does adrenal graft enhance recovery of dopaminergic neurons in Parkinson's disease? *Ann. Neurol.*, **27**, 676–82

64. Peterson, D.I., Lynne Price, M. and Small, C.S. (1989). Autopsy findings in a patient who had adrenal to brain transplant for Parkinson's disease. *Neurology*, **39**, 235–8

65. Hurtig, H., Joyce, J., Sladek Jr., J.R. *et al.* (1989). Post-mortem analysis of adrenal medulla-to-caudate autograft in a patient with Parkinson's disease. *Ann. Neurol.*, **25**, 607–14

66. Waters, C., Itabashi, H.H., Apuzzo, M.L.J. *et al.* (1990). Adrenal to caudate transplantation-postmortem study. *Movement Disorders*, **5**, 248–50

67. Frank, F., Sturiale, C., Gaist, G. *et al.* (1988). Adrenal medulla autograft in a human brain for Parkinson's disease. *Acta Neurochir.*, **94**, 39

68. Kordower, J.H., Cochran, E., Penn, R. *et al.* (1991). Putative chromaffin cell survival and enhanced host derived TH-fiber innervation following

a functional adrenal medulla autograft for Parkinson's disease. *Ann. Neurol.*, **29**, 405–12

69. Sagan, J., Pappas, G.D. and Perlow, M.J. (1987). Fine structure of adrenal medullary grafts in the pain modulatory regions of the periaqueductal gray. *Exp. Brain Res.*, **67**, 380–90

70. Jousselin-Hosaja, M. (1988). Ultrastructural evidence for the development of adrenal medullary grafts in the brain. *Exp. Brain Res.*, **73**, 637–43

71. Kordower, J.H., Fiandaca, M.S., Notter, M.F.D. *et al.* (1990). Peripheral nerve provides NGF-like trophic support for grafted Rhesus adrenal chromaffin cells. *J. Neurosurg.*, **73**, 418–28

72. Whitmore, S.R., Ebendal, T., Lärkfort, L. *et al.* (1986). Developmental and regional expression of β nerve growth factor messenger RNA and protein in the rat central nervous system. *Proc. Natl. Acad. Sci. USA*, **83**, 817–21

73. Strömberg, I., Herrera-Marschitz, M., Ungerstedt, U. *et al.* (1985). Chronic implants of chromaffin tissue into the dopamine-denervated striatum: effects of NGF on graft survival, fiber growth and rotational behavior. *Exp. Brain Res.*, **60**, 335–49

74. Pezzoli, G., Fahn, S. and Dwork, A. (1988). Non-chromaffin tissue plus nerve growth factor reduces experimental parkinsonism in aged rats. *Brain Res.*, **459**, 398–403

75. Bing, G., Notter, M.F.D., Hansen, J.T. *et al.* (1990). Cografts of adrenal medulla with C6 glioma cells in rats with 6-hydroxydopamine-induced lesions. *Neuroscience*, **34**, 687–97

76. Unsicker, K., Vey, J., Hoffman, H.-D. *et al.* (1984). C6 glioma cell-condition medium influences neurite outgrowth and survival of rat chromaffin cells in culture *in vitro*. *Proc. Natl. Acad. Sci. USA*, **81**, 2242–6

77. Notter, M.F.D., Hansen, J.T., Okawara, S. *et al.* (1989). Rodent and primate adrenal medullary cells *in vitro*: phenotypic plasticity in response to coculture with C6 glioma cells or NGF. *Exp. Brain Res.*, **76**, 38–46

78. Johnson Jr., E., Taniuchi, M., Clarke, H.B. *et al.* (1988). Regulation of NGF receptors on Schwann cells. In Gash, D.M. and Sladek Jr., J.R. (eds.) *Transplantation into the Mammalian CNS: Prog. Brain Res.*, **78**, 327–32. (Amsterdam: Elsevier Science)

79. Manthorpe, M., Skaper, S.D., Williams, L.R. *et al.* (1986). Purification of adult rat sciatic nerve ciliary neuronotropic factor. *Brain Res.*, **367**, 282–6

80. Murphy, P.R., Myal, Y., Sato, Y. *et al.* (1989). Elevated expression of basic fibroblast growth factor messenger ribonucleic acid in acoustic neuromas. *Mol. Endocrinol.*, **3**, 225–31

81. Barker, P., Acheson, A., Pareek, S. *et al.* (1990). Detection of brain

derived neurotrophic factor-like (BDNF) biological activity and mRNA in sciatic nerve fibroblasts and Schwann cells. *Soc. Neurosci. Abstr.*, **16**, 1136

82. Bing, G., Notter, M.F.D., Hansen, J.T. *et al.* (1987). Adrenal medullary transplants. IV. Cografts with growth factor producing cells. *Soc. Neurosci.*, Abstr., **13**, 161

83. Date, I., Felten, S.Y. and Felton, D.L. (1991). Cografts of adrenal medulla with peripheral nerve enhance the survivability of transplanted adrenal chromaffin cells and recovery of the host nigrostriatal dopaminergic system in MPTP-treated young mice. *Brain Res.*, **537**, 33–9

84. Dinarello, C.A. (1984). Interleukin-1. *Rev. Infec. Dis.*, **6**, 51–95

85. Fontano, A., Kristensen, F., Dubs, R. *et al.* (1982). Production of prostaglandin E and interleukin-1-like factor by cultured astrocytes and C6 cells. *J. Immunol.*, **129**, 2413–9

86. Nathan, C.F., Murray, H.W. and Cohn, Z.A. (1980). The macrophage as an effector cell. *N. Engl. J. Med.*, **303**, 622–6

87. Giulian, D. and Lachman, L.B. (1985). Interleukin-1 stimulation of astroglial proliferation after brain injury. *Science*, **228**, 497–9

88. Giulian, D., Young, D.G., Woodward, J. *et al.* (1988). Interleukin-1 is an astroglial growth factor in the developing brain. *J. Neurosci.*, **8**, 709–14

89. Lindholm, D., Heumann, R., Meyer, M. *et al.* (1987). Interleukin-1 regulates synthesis of NGF in non-neuronal cells of rat sciatic nerve. *Nature (London)*, **330**, 658–9

90. Bakay, R.A.E., Herring, C., Watts, R. *et al.* (1990). Delayed and acute stereotaxic cografting in the treatment of hemiparkinsonian monkeys. *Soc. Neurosci. Abstr.*, **16**, 809

91. Nieto-Sampedro, M., Kesslak, J.P., Gibbs, R. *et al.* (1987). Effects of conditioning lesions on transplant survival, connectivity, and function. *Ann. N.Y. Acad. Sci.*, **495**, 108–19

92. Kromer, L.F. and Cornbrooks, C.J. (1987). Identification of trophic factors and transplanted cellular environments that promote CNS axonal regeneration. *Ann. N.Y. Acad. Sci.*, **495**, 207–24

93. Bregman, B.S. and Reier, P.J. (1986). Neural tissue implants rescue axotomized rubrospinal cells from retrograde death. *J. Comp. Neurol.*, **244**, 86–95

94. Marciano, F.F., Weigand, S.J., Sladek Jr., J.R. *et al.* (1989). Fetal hypothalamic transplants promote survival and functional regeneration of axotomized adult supraoptic magnocellular neurons. *Brain Res.*, **483**, 135–43

95. Sofrieniew, M.V., Isaacson, O. and Björklund, A. (1986). Cortical grafts prevent atrophy of basal forebrain neurons induced by excitotoxic cortical

damage. *Brain Res.,* **378**, 409–15

96. Labbé, R., Firl, J.R., Mufson, E.J. *et al.* (1983). Fetal brain transplants: reduction of cognitive deficits in rats with frontal cortex lesions. *Science,* **221**, 470–2

97. Kesslak, J.P., Nieto-Sampedo, M., Globus, J. *et al.* (1986). Transplants of purified astrocytes promote behavioral recovery after frontal cortex ablation. *Exp. Neurol.,* **92**, 377–90

98. Bohn, M.C., Cupit, L., Marciano, F. *et al.* (1987). Adrenal medulla grafts enhance recovery of striatal dopaminergic fibers. *Science,* **237**, 913–15

99. Date, I., Felten, S.Y. and Felton, D.L. (1991). The nigrostriatal dopaminergic system in MPTP-treated mice shows more prominent recovery by syngeneic adrenal medullary graft than by allogeneic or xenogeneic graft. *Brain Res.,* **545**, 191–8

100. Fiandaca, M.S., Kordower, J.H., Jiao, S.-S. *et al.* (1988). Adrenal medullary autografts into the basal ganglia of Cebus monkeys: injury-induced regeneration. *Exp. Neurol.,* **102**, 76–91

101. Bankiewicz, K.S., Plunkett, R.J., Jacobowitz, D.M. *et al.* (1990). Fetal nondopaminergic neural implants in parkinsonian primates: histochemical and behavioral studies. *J. Neurosurg.,* **72**, 231–44

102. Plunkett, R.J., Bankiewicz, K.S., Cummings, A.C. *et al.* (1990). Evaluation of hemiparkinsonian monkeys after adrenal autografting or cavitation alone. *J. Neurosurg.,* **73**, 918–26

103. Finklestein, S.P., Apostolides, P.J., Caday, C.G. *et al.* (1988). Increased basic fibroblast growth factor (bFGF) immunoreactivity at the site of focal brain wounds. *Brain Res.,* **460**, 253–9

104. Date, I., Notter, M.F.D., Felten, S.Y. *et al.* (1991). MPTP-treated young mice, but not aging mice show partial recovery of the nigrostriatal dopaminergic system by stereotaxic injection of acidic fibroblast growth factor (aFGF). *Brain Res.,* **526**, 156–60

105. Otto, D. and Unsicker, K. (1990). Basic FGF reverses chemical and morphological deficits in the nigrostriatal system of MPTP-treated mice. *J. Neurosci.,* **10**, 1912–21

106. Date, I., Felten, S.Y., Olschowka, J.A. and Felten, D.L. (1990). Limited recovery of striatal dopaminergic fibers by adrenal medullary grafts in MPTP-treated aging mice. *Exp. Neurol.,* **107**, 197–207

107. Murphy, M., Drago, J. and Bartlett, P.F. (1990). Fibroblast growth factor stimulates the proliferation and differentiation of neural precursor cells *in vitro. J. Neurosci. Res.,* **25**, 463–75

108. Pettmann, B., Weibel, M., Sensenbrenner, M. *et al.* (1985). Purification of two astroglial growth factors from bovine brain. *FEBS Lett.,* **189**, 102–8

109. Morrison, R.S. and De Vellis, J. (1981). Growth of purified astrocytes in

a chemically defined medium. *Proc. Natl. Acad. Sci. USA,* **78**, 7205–9

110. Lavoie, B., Smith, Y. and Parent, A. (1989). Dopaminergic innervation of the basal ganglia in Squirrel monkey as revealed by tyrosine hydroxylase immunohistochemistry. *J. Comp. Neurol.,* **289**, 36–52

111. Felten, D.L. and Sladek Jr., J.R. (1983). Monoamine distribution in the primate brain. V. Monoaminergic nuclei: anatomy, pathways, and local organization. *Brain Res. Bull.,* **10**, 171–284

112. Gupta, M., Gupta, B.K., Thomas, R. *et al.* (1986). Aged mice are more sensitive to 1-methyl-4-phenyl-1,2,3,6,tetrahydropyridine treatment than young adults. *Neurosci. Lett.,* **70**, 326–31

113. Bernheimer, H., Birkmayer, W., Hornykiewicz, O. *et al.* (1973). Brain dopamine and the syndromes of Parkinson and Huntington's disease. *J. Neurol. Sci.,* **20**, 415–55

114. Riederer, P. and Wuketich, S. (1976). Time course of nigrostriatal degeneration in Parkinson's disease. *J. Neural Transmission,* **38**, 277–301

115. Lindvall, O., Backlund, E.-O., Farde, L. *et al.* (1987). Transplantation in Parkinson's disease: two cases of adrenal medullary grafts to the putamen. *Ann. Neurol.,* **22**, 457–68

116. Olanow, C.W. (1990). Oxidation reactions in Parkinson's disease. *Neurology,* **40**, 32–7

117. Spina, M.B. and Cohen, G. (1989). Dopamine turnover and glutathione oxidation: implications for Parkinson's disease. *Proc. Natl. Acad. Sci. USA,* **86**, 1398–400

118. Backlund, E.-O., Granberg, P.O., Hamberger, B. *et al.* (1985). Transplantation of adrenal medullary tissue to striatum in parkinsonism. First clinical trials. *J. Neurosurg.,* **62**, 169–73

119. De Long, M. (1990). Primate models of movement disorders of basal ganglia origin. *Trends Neurosci.,* **13**, 281–5

120. Madrazo, I., Drucker-Colín, R., Daíz, V. *et al.* (1987). Open microsurgical autograft of adrenal medulla to the right caudate nucleus in two patients with intractable Parkinson's disease. *N. Engl. J. Med.,* **316**, 831–4

121. Madrazo, I., Drucker-Colín, R., Leon, V. *et al.* (1987). Adrenal medulla transplanted to caudate nucleus for treatment of Parkinson's disease: report of 10 cases. *Surg. Forum,* **38**, 510–11

122. Jiao, S., Zhang, W., Cao, J. *et al.* (1988). Study of adrenal medullary tissue transplantation to striatum in parkinsonism. In Gash, D.M. and Sladek Jr., J.R. (eds.) *Transplantation into the Mammalian CNS. Prog. Brain Res.,* **78**, 575–82. (Amsterdam: Elsevier Science)

123. Penn, R.D., Goetz, C.G., Tanner, C.M. *et al.* (1988). The adrenal medullary transplant operation for Parkinson's disease: clinical observations in 5 patients. *Neurosurgery,* **22**, 999–1004

124. Goetz, C.G., Olanow, C.W., Koller, W.C. *et al.* (1989). Adrenal medullary transplant to the striatum of patients with advanced Parkinson's disease: multicenter study. *N. Engl. J. Med.,* **320**, 337–40

125. Ahlskog, J.E., Kelly, P.J., Stoddard, S. *et al.* (1990). Adrenal medullary transplantation into the brain for the treatment of Parkinson's disease: clinical outcome and neurochemical studies. *Mayo Clin. Proc.,* **65**, 305–28

126. Kelly, P.J., Ahlskog, J.E., van Heerden, J.A. *et al.* (1989). Adrenal medullary transplantation into the brain for the treatment of Parkinson's disease. *Mayo Clin. Proc.,* **64**, 282–90

127. Allen, G.S., Burns, R.S., Tulipan, N.B. *et al.* (1989). Adrenal medullary transplantation into the caudate nucleus in Parkinson's disease: initial clinical results in 18 patients. *Arch. Neurol.,* **46**, 487–91

128. Apuzzo, M.L.J., Neal, J.H., Waters, C.H. *et al.* (1990). Utilization of unilateral and bilateral stereotactically placed adrenomedullary–striatal autografts in Parkinsonian humans: rationale, techniques, and observations. *Neurosurgery,* **26**, 746–57

129. Olanow, C.W., Koller, W., Goetz, C.G. *et al.* (1990). Autologous transplantation of adrenal medulla in Parkinson's disease: 18 month results. *Arch. Neurol.,* **47**, 1286–9

130. Lopez-Lozano, J.J., Bravo, G. and Abascal, T. (1990). A long-term study of Parkinson's patients subjected to autoimplants of perfused adrenal medulla into the caudate nucleus. *Transplant. Proc.,* **22**, 2243–6

131. Molina, H. (1990). Neural transplantation in Parkinson's disease – the Cuban experience. Presented at the *IIIrd International Symposium on Neural Transplantation,* Cambridge, England, June 20–22

132. Olson, L., Backlund, E.-O., Ebendal, T. *et al.* (1991). Intraputaminal infusion of nerve growth factor to support adrenal medullary autografts in Parkinson's disease: one year follow-up of first clinical trial. *Arch. Neurol.,* **48**, 373–81

133. Stoddard, S.L., Ahlskog, J.E., Kelly, P.J. *et al.* (1989). Decreased adrenal medullary catecholamines in adrenal transplanted parkinsonian patients compared to nephrectomy patients. *Exp. Neurol.,* **104**, 218–22

134. Lindvall, O., Rehncrona, S., Gustaavii, N. *et al.* (1988). Fetal dopamine-rich mesencephalic grafts in Parkinson's disease. *Lancet,* **1**, 1483–4

135. Lindvall, O., Rehncrona, S., Brundin, P. *et al.* (1989). Human fetal dopamine neurons grafted into the striatum in two patients with Parkinson's disease: a detailed account of methodology and 6 month follow-up. *Arch. Neurol.,* **46**, 615–31

136. Lindvall, O., Brundin, P., Widner, H. *et al.* (1990). Grafts of fetal dopamine neurons survive and improve motor function in Parkinson's disease. *Science,* **247**, 575–7

137. Freed, W.J. (1990). Fetal brain grafts and Parkinson's disease. *Science*, **250**, 1434

138. Miletich, R.S., Bankiewicz, K.S. and Plunkett, R.J. (1990). Fetal brain grafts and Parkinson's disease. *Science*, **250**, 1434–5

139. Freed, C.R., Breeze, R.E., Rodenberg, N.L. *et al.* (1990). Transplantation of human fetal dopamine cells for Parkinson's disease. Results at 1 year. *Arch. Neurol.*, **47**, 505–12

140. Lindvall, O. and Björklund, A. (1989). Transplantation strategies in the treatment of Parkinson's disease: experimental basis and clinical trials. *Acta Neurol. Scand.*, **126**, 197–210

141. Collier, T.C., Sladek, C.D., Gallagher, M.J. *et al.* (1988). Cryopreservation of fetal rat and nonhuman primate mesencephalic neurons: viability in culture and neural transplantation. In Gash, D.M. and Sladek Jr., J.R. (eds.) *Transplantation into the Mammalian CNS. Prog. Brain Res.*, **78**, 631–6. (Amsterdam: Elsevier Science)

142. Freemant, T.B. and Kordower, J.H. (1991). Human cadaver embryonic substantia nigra grafts: ontogeny, preoperative graft preparation and tissue storage. *Eric K. Fernström Symposium: Intracerebral Transplantation in Movement Disorders: Experimental Basis and Clinical Experience*, in press

143. Steece-Collier, K., Yurek, D. and Collier, T.J. (1991). Neuropharmacological interactions of L-dopa and dopamine grafts: possible impaired development of grafted embryonic neurons. *Erik K. Fernström Symposium: Intracerebral Transplantation in Movement Disorders: Experimental Basis and Clinical Experience*, in press

144. Gage, F.H., Wolff, J.A., Rosenberg, M.B. *et al.* (1987). Grafting genetically modified cells into the brain: possibilities for the future. *Neuroscience*, **23**, 795–807

145. Rosenberg, M.B., Friedmann, T., Robertson, R.C. *et al.* (1988). Grafting genetically modified cells to the damaged brain: restorative effects of NGF expression. *Science*, **242**, 1575–8

146. Stromberg, I., Wetmore, C.J., Ebendal, T. *et al.* (1990). Rescue of basal forebrain cholinergic neurons after implantation of genetically modified cells producing recombinant NGF. *J. Neurosci. Res.*, **25**, 405–11

147. Wolff, J.A., Fisher, L.J., Xu, L. *et al.* (1989). Grafting fibroblasts genetically modified to produce L-dopa in a rat model of Parkinson's disease. *Proc. Natl. Acad. Sci. USA*, **86**, 9011–14

148. Aebischer, P., Winn, S.R. and Galletti, P.M. (1988). Transplantation of neural tissue in polymer capsules. *Brain Res.*, **448**, 36–48

11

Protective therapy for Parkinson's disease

C. W. Olanow

Protective therapy for Parkinson's disease can be defined as an intervention which slows or stops the progression of neuronal degeneration. In the absence of a specific marker of dopamine neuronal activity, such a protective therapy may be difficult to evaluate, particularly if beneficial effects are subtle. However, identification of a protective therapy might not only alter the natural progression of Parkinson's disease, it might also provide important clues regarding etiological and pathogenetic mechanisms.

Removal or treatment of a specific causative factor is the preferred treatment for Parkinson's disease but, at present, the etiology remains unknown. Interest has, therefore, been directed towards attempts to define and treat the pathogenetic mechanism responsible for cell death. Possibilities that are currently being explored include mitochondrial disorders, excitatory transmitter-induced neurotoxicity, intracellular accumulation of free calcium with activation of destructive protease, lipase and endonuclease enzymes, and a deficiency of cell-sustaining trophic factors. Most attention, however, has focused on the possibility that oxidative stress contributes to the pathogenesis of Parkinson's disease[1-3] (Chapter 4).

Oxidation reactions are essential biological reactions which are necessary for the formation of high energy compounds used to fuel cellular metabolic processes. These reactions can generate highly reactive oxidant species, which include peroxides and the superoxide and hydroxyl free radicals. Free radicals have the potential to react with and damage most biological molecules including DNA[4], essential proteins[5] and membrane lipids[6]. Naturally occurring antioxidant defense mechanisms protect against free radical-induced tissue damage. These defenses can be divided into the preventative and chain-breaking systems. The *preventative system* consists of enzymes such as superoxide dismutase, catalase and glutathione peroxidase, which clear oxidant species and limit the formation of the highly reactive hydroxyl radical. *Chain-breaking agents* or free radical scavengers react directly with other free radicals and prevent their reaction with other, more critical biological molecules. They also react with other radicals to inhibit chain reactions such as lipid peroxidation. The major free radical scavengers are α-tocopherol (vitamin E), ascorbate (vitamin C), uric acid (urate) and β-carotene. These have potential therapeutic importance because they can be augmented by dietary administration. Other important defense mechanisms are *proteins which bind transition metals*, such as iron, copper and manganese, and maintain them in a relatively unreactive form so that they cannot promote redox reactions. These proteins include ferritin, transferrin, hemoglobin, hemosiderin, bilirubin, ceruloplasmin, etc. Under physiological conditions, there is a balance between pro-oxidant and antioxidant forces. A dominance of pro-oxidant activities or a deficiency of antioxidant defense mechanisms could lead to a state of oxidant stress and resultant tissue damage. Oxidant stress with free radical formation has been implicated in the pathogenesis of a variety of clinical disorders including stroke, myocardial infarction, arthritis, cataracts, cancer and, more recently, Parkinson's disease. In the case of Parkinson's disease, the hypothesis that oxidation reactions may contribute to cell death is based on the following considerations:

(1)   The brain appears to be vulnerable to oxidant stress[3]. It consumes approximately 20% of total body oxygen but comprises only 2% of total body weight. Selective brain areas are rich in iron which promotes oxidation but relatively deficient in protective mechanisms which defend against oxidant stress. The brain contains an abundance of membrane lipids which are a substrate for free radicals but has only a limited capacity for tissue repair.

(2)   MPTP-parkinsonism in humans and experimental animals is dependent upon an oxidation reaction in which the protoxin MPTP is

oxidized to MPP^+ by monoamine oxidase B $(MAO-B)^7$.

Current evidence suggests that MPP^+ exerts its toxic effects at the rotenone binding site on complex I of the mitochondrial respiratory enzyme chain[8]. It is noteworthy that a reduction in complex I has also been identified in Parkinson's disease[9,10]. A deficiency of mitochondrial complex I could lead to a depletion in the synthesis of ATP and a reduction in the capacity to trap electrons and oxidant species as they pass along the electron transport chain. There are conflicting reports as to whether oxidative stresss contributes to MPTP toxicity[11-14]. The importance of MAO-B oxidation, however, is clearly established by studies which demonstrate that MPTP toxicity in animals can be completely prevented by selective inhibitors of MAO-B, such as deprenyl or pargyline[15,16]

(3) Dopamine (DA) neurons may be particularly vulnerable to oxidative stress. Dopamine is metabolized by either monoamine oxidase (MAO) or by auto-oxidation to form a pool of hydrogen peroxide.

Enzymatic oxidation of dopamine

$$DA + O_2 + H_2O \xrightarrow{MAO} \text{3,4 Dihydroxyphenylacetaldehyde} + NH_3 + H_2O_2$$

Auto-oxidation of dopamine

$$DA + O_2 \longrightarrow \cdot SQ + O_2^- + H^+$$
$$DA + O_2 + 2H^+ \longrightarrow \cdot SQ + H_2O_2$$

For each mole of dopamine that is metabolized, a mole of hydrogen peroxide (H_2O_2) is formed. Hydrogen peroxide is normally disposed of by glutathione in a reaction catalyzed by glutathione peroxidase.

$$H_2O_2 + 2GSH \longrightarrow GSSG + 2H_2O$$

However, H_2O_2 which is not cleared by glutathione can interact with iron and be reduced to form the highly reactive cytotoxic hydroxyl radical $(OH^\cdot)$.

Fenton reaction

$$H_2O_2 + Fe^{2+} \longrightarrow \cdot OH + OH^- + Fe^{3+}$$

Iron-catalyzed Haber–Weiss reaction

$$H_2O_2 + O_2^- \xrightarrow{Fe} O_2 + OH \cdot + OH^-$$

The formation of hydroxyl radicals due to the metabolism of dopamine might be promoted by:

(a) An increase in dopamine turnover resulting in an accumulation of peroxides;

(b) A deficiency in glutathione, thereby reducing the capacity to clear peroxides;

(c) An increased concentration of iron, thus increasing the likelihood of a reaction with available peroxide molecules.

The oxidative metabolism of dopamine thus has the potential to create a state of oxidant stress with increased levels of peroxides and cytotoxic radicals, and thereby endanger neighbouring dopamine neurons.

Neuromelanin may also contribute to the vulnerability of dopamine neurons. Neuromelanin is a by-product of the auto-oxidation of dopamine and accumulates with age[17,18]. It has an affinity to bind transition metals and can provide electrons to convert iron from its Fe^{3+} to its Fe^{2+} state so that it can participate in reactions which generate toxic oxidant species. Neuromelanin can thus endanger dopamine neurons by promoting the site-specific binding and reduction of iron (and copper) and the formation of cytotoxic hydroxyl radicals. It is noteworthy that the decline in dopamine neurons that occurs with aging and Parkinson's disease appears preferentially to affect melanized neurons[18,19].

(4) There is evidence that, in patients with Parkinson's disease, a state of oxidative stress exists within the substantia nigra. This is based on reports of increased iron[20,21], decreased ferritin[22], decreased glutathione[23,24], and increased lipid peroxidation[25]. Iron, when it is in a reactive form, can promote oxidation reactions and the formation of free radicals[26]. When iron is bound to proteins such as ferritin, it is relatively unreactive[27]. The findings of increased iron and decreased ferritin in the nigra of patients with Parkinson's disease suggest that iron is present as a reactive low molecular weight complex capable of enhancing free radical formation. As glutathione is the primary mechanism for clearing peroxide, a deficiency in glutathione could increase the steady-state concen-

tration of peroxide and increase the chance that it will react with iron to form the hydroxyl radical. The finding of increased lipid peroxidation in the nigra of patients with Parkinson's disease supports the notion that this is in fact occurring. Taken together, these findings indicate that a state of oxidant stress exists in the nigra of patients with Parkinson's disease.

These observations provide a theoretical rationale for considering the possibility that oxidant stress contributes to neuronal damage in Parkinson's disease. While oxidant stress could be the primary cause of tissue injury, it might also develop as a consequence of tissue injury from an alternate cause. In either case, the existence of a state of oxidant stress suggests that an antioxidant therapy might protect residual dopamine neurons and slow the progression of neuronal damage in Parkinson's disease. The ideal antioxidant would be one that can cross the blood–brain barrier, prevent the formation of reactive oxidant species, preserve free radicals that serve physiological functions, and is safe and inexpensive. Some candidate antioxidant strategies for consideration as possible neuroprotective agents in Parkinson's disease are summarized in Table 1.

MAO INHIBITORS

Much of the current interest in protective therapy for Parkinson's disease has centered on the selective MAO-B inhibitor deprenyl (Selegiline). This is based on two recent clinical trials which demonstrated clearly and unequivocally that deprenyl delays the time until a predetermined level of disability develops in patients with early, otherwise untreated, Parkinson's disease[28,29]. These studies were initiated based on the hypothesis that an MAO-B inhibitor such as deprenyl might prevent the oxidation of an MPTP-like protoxin and/or diminish the formation of peroxides and free radicals generated by the oxidation of dopamine. These hypotheses are supported by experiments which demonstrate that deprenyl prevents the development of MPTP-parkinsonism[15,16] and diminishes oxidant stress due to increased dopamine turnover[30].

Deprenyl was initially developed as a possible antidepressant agent without the 'cheese effect' associated with inhibition of MAO-A[31,32]. However, in doses which selectively inhibit MAO-B, deprenyl provides

Table 1 Possible antioxidant strategies for Parkinson's disease

(1) Prevent hydroxyl radical formation
    (a) MAO inhibitors
        (i) MAO-B inhibitors
        (ii) MAO-A $\pm$ MAO-B inhibitors
    (b) Enhance glutathione or glutathione peroxidase activity

(2) Free radical scavengers
    (a) α-tocopherol (vitamin E)
    (b) Ascorbate (vitamin C)
    (c) β-carotene
    (d) Spin traps

(3) Iron chelators which maintain iron in an unreactive form

(4) Reduce dopamine turnover
    (a) Minimize cumulative levodopa dose (decrease substrate)
    (b) Dopamine agonists

(5) Miscellaneous
    (a) N-acetyl-carnitine
    (b) 21 amino steroids (lazaroids)

little if any antidepressant effect[33–35]. In Parkinson's disease, deprenyl was first tested in combination with levodopa based on the idea that inhibition of MAO-B might increase the availability of striatal dopamine[36]. These studies indicated that, as an adjunct to levodopa in patients with advanced Parkinson's disease, deprenyl provided mild antiparkinsonian effects and a slight reduction in motor fluctuations. These observations have been confirmed in prospective double-blind controlled studies[37] and it is for this indication that deprenyl is currently approved for use in the United States. Interest in the possibility that deprenyl might provide more than symptomatic benefits was suggested by Knoll who reported an extension of life span in deprenyl-fed rats[38]. A retrospective analysis of Parkinson patients who had taken deprenyl with levodopa demonstrated that they had prolonged survival in comparison to patients taking levodopa alone[39]. While this study was retrospective and uncontrolled, it pointed to the need for a more critical evaluation of deprenyl as possible protective therapy for Parkinson's disease.

Two prospective, double-blind, placebo-controlled trials of deprenyl as monotherapy for patients with early Parkinson's disease have now been performed. The Tetrud–Langston Study compared 54 patients randomized to deprenyl 10 mg, or placebo[29]. The 'Deprenyl and Tocopherol Antioxidative Therapy of Parkinsonism (DATATOP) Study' evaluated 800 patients as part of a multicenter study[28]. It was performed according to a 2 × 2 factorial design in which patients with early, untreated Parkinson's disease were randomized to one of four treatment groups: deprenyl 10 mg, α-tocopherol 2000 IU, the combination of deprenyl and α-tocopherol, or placebo. Following randomization to study group, patients were monitored until they reached a predetermined end-point defined as disability necessitating the introduction of symptomatic therapy in the form of Sinemet. As part of the study, a wash-out examination was performed 1 month after patients reached end-point and the study drug was discontinued. Secondary variables that were monitored included the activities of daily living (ADL) and motor subsets of the Unified Parkinson's Disease Rating Scale (UPDRS), Hoehn and Yahr stage and Schwab–England ADL Score.

Both studies demonstrated that patients who received deprenyl had a highly significant delay in reaching end-point. In the Tetrud–Langston study, patients randomized to placebo reached end-point after an average of 312.1 days, whereas deprenyl-treated patients did not reach end-point for an average of 548.9 days ($p < 0.002$). Similar results were observed in an interim analysis of the DATATOP study. After a mean follow-up of 12 months, 176 placebo-treated subjects but only 97 deprenyl-treated subjects had reached end-point ($p < 10^{-8}$). The risk of reaching end-point for patients receiving deprenyl ($\pm$ tocopherol) was decreased by 57% in comparison to those who did not receive deprenyl ($\pm$ tocopherol) (hazard ratio 0.43, $p < 10^{-10}$). The Kaplan–Meier plots showing the probability of reaching end-point for patients randomized to deprenyl and placebo in the DATATOP studies are shown in Figure 1. Based on these findings, the deprenyl arms of the DATATOP study were prematurely terminated according to the predetermined early stopping rules.

A reduction in the rate of progression of secondary variables was also observed in deprenyl-treated patients. In the Tetrud–Langston study, total UPDRS score deteriorated by 17.85 points per year in placebo-treated patients compared to 9.44 points in those treated with deprenyl

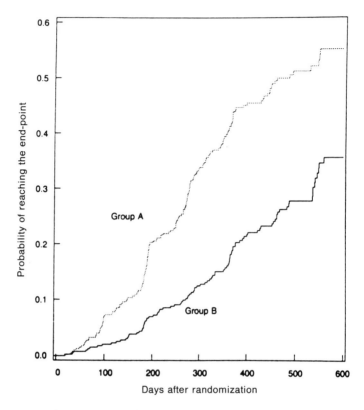

Figure 1   Kaplan-Meier curve demonstrating the cumulative probability of reaching end-point for patients randomized to Group A (placebo) and Group B (deprenyl) in the DATATOP study. Note that the hazard ratio comparing deprenyl to placebo-treated patients with respect to the risk of reaching end-point per unit of time is 0.43 ($p < 10^{-10}$). Reproduced with permission of *New England Journal of Medicine*

($p < 0.01$). Similarly, in the DATATOP study, total UPDRS score deteriorated by 13.11 points per year in placebo-treated patients but by only 5.50 points per year in those on deprenyl. A statistically significant slowing in the rate of deterioration of the Hoehn–Yahr and Schwab–England scores was also observed in deprenyl-treated patients in both studies. Interim analysis comparing tocopherol to placebo did not show a significant difference in reaching end-point and this component of the study was not prematurely terminated.

Conclusive evidence is thus provided indicating that deprenyl delays the development of disability in patients with early Parkinson's disease. These results are consistent with the hypothesis that deprenyl protects against neuronal degeneration by preventing the oxidation of a protoxin or by diminishing the accumulation of peroxides and free radicals due to the oxidative metabolism of dopamine. However, while the observations appear to be incontrovertible, the responsible mechanism is far from established. The possibility must be considered that deprenyl delays the development of disability by a symptomatic mechanism which masks rather than slows underlying disability[40].

There are several mechanisms by which deprenyl might reduce symptomatic effects capable of influencing the emergence of end-point and the detection of disability. These include:

(1) *Increased striatal dopamine* Deprenyl inhibits MAO-B oxidation and re-uptake of dopamine in the striatum and thus might be expected to increase striatal dopamine and provide symptomatic effects in patients with Parkinson's disease. However, acute injections of deprenyl do not increase the content, turnover, or release of dopamine in the striatum of rats[41], and trials of deprenyl as monotherapy in Parkinson's disease patients have shown little detectable clinical antiparkinsonian benefit[28,29,42]. Further, deprenyl does not induce increased locomotion or stereotypy in rats[43]. But, deprenyl does appear to have a cumulative effect[44] and chronic administration of deprenyl does induce an increase in striatal dopamine content in rodents[45]. Information on the effect of deprenyl on dopamine metabolism in primates is needed.

(2) *Increased striatal phenylethylamine* Recently, it has been suggested that an accumulation of phenylethylamine (PE) in the striatum may contribute to the clinical effects of deprenyl[46]. PE is a biogenic amine which is generated from phenylalanine by aromatic amino acid decarboxylase and is a relatively specific substrate for MAO-B. It is synthesized at the same rate as dopamine but has a rapid turnover to account for its low endogenous concentration under physiological conditions. Inhibition of MAO-B results in a rapid and marked accumulation of striatal PE. In high, but not low concentrations, PE can stimulate the release and inhibit the re-uptake of dopamine and may directly stimulate dopamine receptors[47]. In the rat striatum, deprenyl potentiates

dopaminergic responses and is associated with a marked increase in PE but not dopamine[48]. Inhibition of MAO-B by deprenyl thus appears to enhance dopaminergic effects through a mechanism which does not depend on an increase in dopamine. It has been proposed that PE acts as a neuromodulator which amplifies the dopaminergic response[47]. An increase in PE might account for deprenyl providing symptomatic effects in parkinsonian patients in the absence of an increase in striatal dopamine.

(3) *Amphetamine metabolites* Deprenyl is virtually entirely metabolized to methamphetamine and to a lesser extent amphetamine[49]. Amphetamine promotes the release and inhibits the re-uptake of dopamine and therefore could be associated with dopaminergic effects. However, L-deprenyl is used exclusively in clinical practice as it is a more potent inhibitor of MAO-B than its D-isomer[50]. Accordingly, L-deprenyl is metabolized to L-methamphetamine and L-amphetamine which have much less potency than D-methamphetamine or D-amphetamine and accumulate in only small quantities[51]. It is thus unlikely that anitparkinsonian benefits associated with L-deprenyl monotherapy result from a central amphetamine-like effect. Further, deprenyl has not been demonstrated to have amphetamine-like effects in human controls or in patients with narcolepsy[52]. Studies of selective MAO-B inhibitors which do not have amphetamine metabolites should help to resolve this issue.

(4) *Antidepressant effects* Deprenyl was originally developed as a possible antidepressant agent. Controlled clinical trials demonstrate that, in the dose ranges which selectively inhibit MAO-B, little, if any, antidepressant effects have been documented[33-35]. In the Tetrud–Langston and DATATOP studies, patients were excluded from participation if they had evidence of clinical depression, and no significant antidepressant effects were observed in deprenyl-treated patients. Still, reports of 'a feeling of well-being' have been described in patients on deprenyl[53] and there exists the possibility that a subclinical antidepressant or mood effect may have influenced the interpretation of end-point.

(5) *Sensitization of dopamine neurons* Chronic amphetamine treat-

ment has been demonstrated to sensitize dopamine neurons, resulting in an increase in firing rate and release of dopamine[54]. It is possible that deprenyl, either directly, or by way of its amphetamine metabolites, could similarly sensitize dopamine neurons. This mechanism might account for dopaminergic effects that are seen with chronic but not acute deprenyl administration.

To try and differentiate protective versus symptomatic effects, wash-in and wash-out analyses were performed as part of the Tetrud–Langston and DATATOP studies. The wash-in analysis compared clinical score at baseline to that obtained 1 and 3 months after initiation of study drug. The wash-out analysis compared clinical score at end-point with clinical score 1 month after end-point had been reached and the study drug discontinued. Clinical improvement with drug wash-in or deterioration with drug wash-out would be indications of a symptomatic effect.

In the Tetrud–Langston study, there was no significant clinical change following wash-in or wash-out and no evidence for a symptomatic mechanism was detected.

In the larger DATATOP study, a statistically significant improvement was detected 1 and 3 months after initiation of deprenyl. Similar improvement was not detected in placebo-treated patients. This improvement, while deemed clinically trivial by the authors, nonetheless was highly significant for a variety of clinical parameters including motor and ADL subsets of the UPDRS. While the magnitude of this symptomatic improvement was only 1.7 points in total UPDRS score and its clinical relevance uncertain, a symptomatic effect was clearly identified. Failure to identify this effect in the Tetrud–Langston study and in other clinical trials probably reflects the large number of patients employed in the DATATOP study and its power to detect subtle clinical change. The question is whether a symptomatic effect of such a slight magnitude could account for the robust difference in reaching end-point in deprenyl- versus placebo-treated patients? To address this issue further, placebo and deprenyl patients were subdivided into those who demonstrated clinical improvement at 1 month and those who had not. A Kaplan–Meier analysis of these four groups continued to show a significant difference in the risk of reaching end-point favoring patients randomized to deprenyl, even when symptomatic benefits had not been detected. Indeed, a comparison of patients randomized to deprenyl who *had not* improved, with patients randomized to placebo who *had* improved, continues to show a decreased rate in reaching end-point in favor of deprenyl-treated patients ($p < 0.01$)[55]. Nonetheless, it is clear that deprenyl monotherapy does exert a small symptomatic effect in patients with early Parkinson's disease.

Wash-out examinations did not show a significant deterioration in UPDRS score in either deprenyl or placebo patients. This would support the hypothesis that deprenyl acts by a protective mechanism. However, it is uncertain if a 1-month follow-up is sufficiently long to permit adequate recovery of MAO-B. Deprenyl is an irreversible, suicide inhibitor of MAO-B and doses of 10 mg per day result in 100% inhibition of platelet and approximately 80% inhibition of brain MAO-B activity[56,57]. The plasma half-life of deprenyl is approximately 40 h, but restoration of MAO-B activity is a function of regeneration of the enzyme. It is estimated that 50% normalization of brain MAO-B activity in the rat occurs in approximately 10 days[58] but the half-life for turnover of MAO-B in the baboon is estimated to be 30 days using position emission tomography[59]. It is possible that MAO-B activity has not sufficiently regenerated at 1 month to permit detection of symptomatic deterioration. Further, clinical deterioration leading to a determination of end-point occurred abruptly rather than in a gradual or linear fashion. End-point thus might represent a loss of compensatory mechanisms which, in the case of deprenyl-treated patients, may be drug-related. Evaluation of wash-out performed at end-point might thus prejudice against the detection of a symptomatic deterioration which might otherwise have been observed if performed at an earlier time point, when patients were enjoying the benefit associated with deprenyl therapy. It is thus possible that a longer duration wash-out, performed at a time in the study when patients had not yet reached end-point, might have permitted detection of symptomatic deterioration that was not appreciated under the study conditions. Such an evaluation is now being performed as part of the modification of the DATATOP protocol and this information should soon be forthcoming.

In summary, wash-in evaluation shows evidence of a small but definite symptomatic effect but it is unclear whether this accounts for the delay in end-point. Wash-out evaluation shows no evidence of a symptomatic effect but may not have been performed under ideal conditions. In evaluating these data, it is important to recognize that currently employed scoring systems may be relatively insensitive and fail to detect clinically significant changes which might influence the determination of end-point.

For the present, it remains unclear as to whether the symptomatic effect is entirely responsible for the delay in development of disability observed or whether a protective component contributes in some part. If deprenyl acts through a 'symptomatic' mechanism, its importance in the management of Parkinson's disease and in understanding the basis of cell death in Parkinson's disease would be greatly diminished. To date, no MPTP-like protoxin has been identified despite extensive epidemiological studies, and there exists no conclusive proof linking oxidant stress and free radical mechanisms to the pathogenesis of Parkinson's disease. It is not likely that further analyses of the DATATOP and Tetrud–Langston studies will resolve these issues. Additional clinical and/or laboratory studies will probably be necessary to clarify the role of deprenyl in Parkinson's disease. New clinical trials in which parkinsonian patients are assessed before and after randomization to treatment with deprenyl or placebo for *a fixed period of time* might permit detection of a protective effect without confounding symptomatic effects if a long enough wash-out period is employed. Evidence that deprenyl interferes with the natural progression of other neurodegenerative disorders, such as parkinsonism, ALS or Alzheimer's disease, in which no known symptomatic therapy is presently available, would provide strong evidence for a neuroprotective effect. Trials of other MAO-B inhibitors, which lack amphetamine metabolites and induce short-lasting reversible inhibition of MAO-B, might help to resolve questions regarding symptomatic effects. It may also be important to consider whether inhibition of MAO-A might be necessary to achieve a protective effect. Dopamine neuronal damage can occur with MPTP analogs which are oxidized by MAO-A[60]. Also, it is assumed that dopamine is primarily metabolized in the human brain by MAO-B because 80% of MAO is in the B form[61]. However, MAO within dopamine neurons is in the A form[62,63] and dopamine metabolism is primarily terminated by re-uptake under normal circumstances. It may be that MAO-A plays a more important role in the enzymatic deamination of dopamine than is currently appreciated. Inhibition of MAO-A, either alone or in combination with MAO-B, may thus be necessary to prevent oxidation of a protoxin or significantly to diminish peroxide formation from the metabolism of dopamine and so provide protective effects for patients with Parkinson's disease.

It has also been suggested that deprenyl may provide protective effects by a mechanism which does not depend on MAO-B inhibition[64]. Tatton and Greenwood report that deprenyl protects nigral neurons of MPTP-treated mice even when administered 72 h after MPTP damage has occurred. The authors propose that deprenyl may act as a trophic factor.

The door may now be open for a 'neuroprotective era' in the treatment of Parkinson's disease. A theoretical basis exists for considering the possibility that oxidative stress contributes to the pathogenesis of Parkinson's disease, and clinical trials of antioxidative agents as protective therapy have been initiated. Deprenyl has been demonstrated to delay the emergence of disability in patients with early Parkinson's disease, although the responsible mechanism has not yet been defined. If it can be established with certainty that deprenyl does have a protective effect on residual dopamine neurons, it will have profound clinical and biological implications which include:

(1) Support for the hypothesis that oxidant stress and free radical formation contribute to the pathogenesis of Parkinson's disease.

(2) A recommendation that deprenyl and/or other antioxidant agents be used in the treatment of patients with Parkinson's disease.

(3) A re-evaluation of the manner in which we use levodopa. The possibility that levodopa, by way of its oxidation to dopamine, might promote oxidant stress by favoring the formation of peroxides and free radicals would have to be considered and some urgency would be attached to the development of other antiparkinsonian drugs which do not undergo oxidative metabolism.

(4) A search for a preclinical marker of Parkinson's disease that would enable the detection of at-risk individuals prior to the development of clinical features and permit the introduction of antioxidant therapy at this early time point.

(5) Research into the development of new and more effective antioxidant agents that can stop or reverse the progression of Parkinson's disease.

OTHER ANTIOXIDANTS

Free radical scavengers

α-tocopherol (vitamin E) is the only antioxidant agent other than deprenyl that has been rigorously tested for its potential role as a protective agent in Parkinson's disease. Tocopherols of which α-tocopherol is the most abundant isomer, are present in plant oils and are an essential dietary component. Vitamin E is the major lipid soluble free radical scavenger in biological systems. It inhibits the chain reaction of lipid peroxidation in membranes and protects them from oxidative damage[65,66]. Tocopherol acts to inhibit lipid peroxidation by binding directly with peroxyl radicals to form the stable tocopheroxyl radical. The tocopheroxyl radical is unreactive due to resonance stabilization, and tends spontaneously to degrade, by accepting another electron from a second peroxyl radical, to become a non-radical. Alternatively, tocopheroxyl radicals can also be recycled back to tocopherol through reduction reactions with ascorbate or glutathione and as well by electrons provided by the mitochondrial electron transport chain[67,68]. Dietary supplement can increase tissue and brain concentrations of vitamin E[69] and protect against lipid peroxidation. In high doses, vitamin E diminishes the age-related accumulation of lipofuscin which is thought to be a product of lipid peroxidation[70]. By contrast, hypovitaminosis E is associated with massive lipofuscin accumulation[71]. Vitamin E supplementation is reported to be beneficial for a variety of disorders thought to be associated with excess free radicals, including cancer, arthritis, cataracts and pulmonary abnormalities due to air pollutants such as cigarette smoke[66]. Vitamin E deficiency is associated with a neurological syndrome which includes cerebellar dysfunction and peripheral neuropathy but not basal ganglia dysfunction or parkinsonian syndromes[72]. Nonetheless, vitamin E was selected to be evaluated as part of the DATATOP study because it is a potent lipophilic antioxidant which has the capacity to penetrate the central nervous system. Further, it is thought to have relatively less pro-oxidant potential in comparison to other antioxidants such as ascorbate and β-carotene (see below). An open-label trial of vitamin E in patients with early, untreated Parkinson's disease suggested that it delayed the time until symptomatic therapy was required[73]. A prospective, double-blind, placebo-controlled study of vitamin E is now being carried out as part of the DATATOP study[28].

Patients with early untreated Parkinson's disease were randomized to treatment with either 2000 units of α-tocopherol (± deprenyl) or placebo (± deprenyl). Patients were followed until they developed disability necessitating levodopa therapy (end-point). Survival analysis will be performed to determine if α-tocopherol delays the development of disability in comparison to placebo. A demonstration that vitamin E delays the development of disability would be a strong argument that antioxidants have protective effects in patients with Parkinson's disease, as vitamin E is not suspected on clinical or theoretical grounds of providing a symptomatic effect. On the other hand, there is no certainty that such an observation will be found, and it remains questionable whether vitamin E can accumulate within the central nervous system in sufficient quantity to provide a satisfactory antioxidant effect.

Ascorbic acid (vitamin C) is an outstanding antioxidant in human plasma[74]. Ascorbate is thought to act by trapping peroxyl radicals in the aqueous phase and preventing their diffusion into lipids. Ascorbate can completely protect plasma lipids from oxidative damage by blocking the initiation of lipid peroxidation. By contrast, α-tocopherol acts within plasma membrane to slow the rate at which lipid peroxidation occurs, but does not prevent its initiation. In plasma, ascorbate provides greater protection against lipid peroxidation than other endogenous antioxidants, including tocopherols, thioles, bilirubin and urate[74]. It would thus appear that ascorbate might be an antioxidant worthy of trial in Parkinson's disease. However, it acts primarily in the aqueous phase and is much less effective once lipid peroxidation in membranes has begun, as it likely has in Parkinson's disease where 60–80% of dopamine neurons have undergone degeneration by the time clinical features are evident. There is also concern as to the potential of ascorbate to act as a pro-oxidant. Ascorbate promotes the conversion of Fe^{3+} to Fe^{2+} in which form iron can provide an electron to foster the reduction of oxygen and promote the formation of cytotoxic radicals[75]. Pro-oxidant effects of vitamin C are unlikely to be a problem in plasma, where there is an abundance of the iron-binding protein transferrin, so that virtually all iron is maintained in an unreactive state. In plasma, no pro-oxidant effects of ascorbate are detected. However, this may not be the case within the brain which is rich in iron and where iron-binding capacity may be limited, as evidenced by the lack of iron-binding capacity within the cerebrospinal fluid[76].

The potential of ascorbate to induce pro-oxidant effects may be a particular concern in Parkinson's disease where excess iron accumulates within the substantia nigra. Thus, while ascorbate has been demonstrated to be an outstanding antioxidant in plasma, concerns about its potential to augment oxidant stress in parkinsonian brain have restricted clinical trials of ascorbate in Parkinson's disease.

β-carotene and other carotenoids are unusual lipid antioxidants that quench singlet oxygen[77]. Epidemiological studies suggest that there is a slightly reduced incidence of cancer in patients taking a diet rich in β-carotene[78]. However, β-carotene, like ascorbate, is known to induce pro-oxidant effects that to date have limited its usefulness as a clinical antioxidant. It now appears that the pro-oxidant effects of β-carotene occur only under conditions of a high partial pressure of oxygen[77]. In circumstances where the partial pressure of oxygen is low, as is found in most tissues under physiological conditions, β-carotene is an effective radical-trapping antioxidant. Thus β-carotene would probably be an inappropriate agent to use in disorders associated with high oxygen tension such as retrolental fibroplasia or intraventricular hemorrhage in infants. This may not be the case in Parkinson's disease where degeneration occurs deep within the basal ganglia, where the partial pressure of oxygen is low and where β-carotene is highly reactive towards peroxyl radicals. It may be that a combination of vitamin E (which is most effective in a high concentration of oxygen) and β-carotene (which is most effective at a low concentration of oxygen) might provide synergistic antioxidant effects for patients with Parkinson's disease.

Spin traps may be another mechanism for providing protection against lipid peroxidation. Exogenous traps have been used to detect and measure free radicals through a process known as spin-trapping[79]. Spin traps such as phenyl-butyl-nitrone (PBN) react with free radicals to form stable nitroxide radicals that can be measured by electron paramagnetic resonance (EPR) techniques. Similarly, salicylates have been used to trap hydroxyl free radicals. Recent studies of stroke in gerbils have demonstrated that spin-traps such as PBN cannot only be used to quantify free radical formation but also to provide protection against cerebral ischemia[80]. These observations not only suggest that free radicals may play a primary role in the development of pathological processes such as stroke but that spin-trapping agents such as PBN may be of value in preventing tissue injury due to free radical formation, such as may occur in Parkinson's disease.

Iron chelators

Chelation of iron, so that it is in an unreactive form, inhibits lipid peroxidation and may be a viable approach to protective therapy for patients with Parkinson's disease[81-83]. Iron is a transition metal which is capable of either accepting or donating an electron to promote redox reactions. More specifically, iron catalyzes the formation of the highly reactive hydroxyl radical from both the Fenton and Haber–Weiss reactions. Iron thus serves to convert poorly reactive species such as O_2^- and H_2O_2 into highly reactive species such as .OH. Iron is known to be incorporated into the structure of the D_2 dopamine receptor and is critical for numerous physiological functions within the brain, including catecholamine synthesis and degradation and myelin formation. However, brain iron is present in concentrations which far exceed its known physiological functions. Further, the capacity of proteins, such as ferritin and transferrin, to maintain iron in an unreactive form appears to be limited in the brain in comparison to plasma. The high iron concentration in the brain may serve some as yet unknown function, but there is the obvious concern that if iron is present in a reactive form it will stimulate radical production. Findings of increased iron and decreased ferritin in the substantia nigra of patients with Parkinson's disease suggest that iron-mediated oxidant stress may contribute to cell death in Parkinson's disease. If so, then iron chelators which maintain iron in a non-reactive form and limit its participation in redox reactions might protect surviving dopamine neurons in parkinsonian patients from damage due to oxidant stress. Desferrioxamine (desferal) is a potent iron chelator which can inhibit most iron-dependent oxidation reactions and protect tissue from lipid peroxidation[82,83]. Co-administration of the iron chelator desferal attenuates the damage associated with the neurotoxin 6-hydroxy-dopamine, suggesting that iron plays a crucial role in the mechanism of dopamine neuronal injury which occurs in this model of parkinsonism[84]. More recently, it has been shown that direct infusion of low molecular weight iron into the pars compacta of the substantia nigra of rodents induces neuronal degeneration and a dose-related decline in ipsilateral striatal markers of dopamine[85]. These effects can be attenuated by combining iron with transferrin, which binds iron and prevents it from participating in oxidation reactions.

A rationale can thus be made for testing iron chelators as possible protective therapy for Parkinson's disease. Iron chelators provide clinical benefit in patients with peripheral iron overload syndromes such as hemochromatosis and transfusional iron excess. However, iron chelators such as desferal do not cross the blood–brain barrier and have not yet been demonstrated to be able to chelate brain iron. An initial report suggested that systemic administration of desferal delayed the rate of progression of Alzheimer's disease[86], which has also been proposed to be associated with oxidant stress. This study was not blinded, and did not employ a comparable control group and therefore must be taken with some reservation. There are also safety issues to consider. Desferal has been reported to cause cerebral and ocular toxicity[87] and to induce coma in iron-deficient rats as well as in two patients with rheumatoid arthritis when administered in conjunction with prochlorperazine[2].

The 21 amino steroids or lazaroids form a class of drugs that interfere with lipid peroxidation as well as other iron-dependent radical reactions. They were initially thought to act by way of iron chelation[88], but this has not been confirmed. Lazaroids have been demonstrated to provide protective effects in experimental models of spinal cord, head trauma, ischemia–reperfusion injury and hemorrhagic shock[89–92]. Some of these drugs are lipid soluble and have a relatively long half-life, making them candidates for study in Parkinson's disease.

There exists considerable interest in determining whether iron chelators can be developed which can penetrate the central nervous system, bind pathological accumulations of iron and provide protective effects by way of antioxidant mechanisms. Further laboratory studies and clinical trials are anticipated.

Antioxidant enzymes

Antioxidant enzymes act to clear oxidant species and prevent the formation of hydroxyl radical. To this extent they are theoretically preferable to chain-breaking antioxidants or free radical scavengers which act only after highly reactive oxidant species, such as hydroxyl radicals, have already been formed and/or the chain reaction of lipid peroxidation begun. There is interest in superoxide dismutase because it is reported to protect against ischemia–reperfusion injury and head trauma, and recombinant forms are now availabe[93–95]. Whether superoxide dismutase will be of value in Parkinson's disease is less clear. Superoxide dismutase converts superoxide radical to peroxide, thus preventing tissue damage from these radicals. This mechanism is likely to be more important in the periphery where there is little free iron, and superoxide may be an important source of tissue injury. However, in the brain, hydroxyl radicals are thought to be the primary mediator of tissue damage due to oxidant stress. Superoxide dismutase, by promoting the conversion of superoxide to peroxide, might actually increase oxidant stress in the parkinsonian brain and *increase* the likelihood that hydroxyl radical will be formed. It is thus highly questionable whether supplementation with superoxide dismutase will provide clinical benefit in parkinsonian patients.

Perhaps a better theoretical approach would be an increase in glutathione or glutathione peroxidase activity which would clear hydrogen peroxide and thereby defend against hydroxyl radical production. Ebselen, which has glutathione peroxidase-like activity, has been demonstrated to inhibit lipid peroxidation in rat liver microsomes[96]. Increased levels of glutathione or glutathione peroxidase might also be achieved by genetic engineering techniques.

Decreased dopamine turnover

The enzymatic or auto-oxidation of dopamine generates a pool of hydrogen peroxide and creates a potential oxidant stress. The more dopamine that is metabolized, the more hydrogen peroxide that is produced and the greater the likelihood that peroxide will interact with iron and generate hydroxyl radical. As levodopa is metabolized to dopamine, it is reasonable to question whether levodopa administration might promote the formation of peroxides and free radicals by way of the following equations[97].

$$\text{Levodopa} \xrightarrow{\text{Dopa-decarboxylase}} DA + CO_2 \tag{1}$$

$$DA + O_2 + H_2O \xrightarrow{\text{MAO}} 3{,}4 \text{ Dihydroxyphenylacetaldehyde} + NH_3 + H_2O_2 \tag{2}$$

$$H_2O_2 + Fe^{2+} \longrightarrow Fe^{3+} + \cdot OH + OH^- \tag{3}$$

$$\Big\downarrow \text{Glutathione peroxidase}$$

$$H_2O$$

High doses of levodopa have not been shown adversely to affect dopamine neurons in mice, rats or non-parkinsonian humans[98-100]. However, this may not be comparable to administering levodopa to patients with Parkinson's disease in whom a state of oxidant stress and compromised defense mechanisms may exist. It is noteworthy that, as primary therapy, levodopa is associated with a higher incidence of adverse reactions (dyskinesia and motor fluctuations) than dopamine agonists which are not oxidatively metabolized[101]. It is currently thought that adverse effects are a function of the capacity of surviving dopamine neurons to store dopamine[102]. A reduced number of dopamine neurons permits less central storage of dopamine and results in motor responses which fluctuate with the plasma availability of levodopa. It can be postulated that the increased incidence of adverse effects in levodopa-treated patients reflects an accelerated loss of dopamine neurons, due to oxidant stress promoted by exogenously administered levodopa. That dopamine agonists may have a protective effect, by decreasing dopamine turnover, is suggested by studies demonstrating that rats fed a diet enriched with the dopamine agonist pergolide have a dramatic reduction in the age-related loss of nigral dopamine neurons and striatal dopamine terminals, in comparison to pair-fed rats[103]. The authors propose that pergolide acts by stimulating dopamine autoreceptors, decreasing dopamine turnover and thereby reducing free radical generation. Dopamine has also been shown to damage dopamine neurons in tissue culture[104] and to contribute to ischemic damage, presumably through free radical mechanisms[105]. These considerations have led to speculation that a strategy designed to minimize the levodopa dose might reduce free radical formation and protect residual dopamine neurons[97].

SUMMARY

A better understanding of the role that oxidative stressplays in the neuronal damage that occurs in Parkinson's disease might permit the development of specific antioxidant agents that interfere with this mechanism. In the search for an antioxidant therapy for Parkinson's disease, it is important to recall that antioxidants may be fraught with problems. Some antioxidants can have undesired pro-oxidant effects, and the consequences of removing iron from the brain remain to be established. Free radicals may also play an important role in physiological functions. White cells destroy invading pathogens and the proliferation of neoplastic cells may be held in check by free radical mechanisms[106,107]. Non-specific inhibition of free radical formation may have adverse consequences on these defense systems. It seems reasonable for the present to limit the use of antioxidants to clinical trials in conditions in which excess formation of free radicals is implicated in the pathogenesis, and to avoid the widespread 'prophylatic' use of antioxidants in otherwise normal individuals until the clinical consequences of these drugs have been more clearly defined.

OTHER APPROACHES TO PROTECTIVE THERAPY

While much interest has centered on oxidant stress as a possible cause of cell death in Parkinson's disease, other mechanisms, acting alone or in combination with oxidant stress, might also play a role.

Acetyl-levo-carnitine (ALC), which does not inhibit MAO-B, has been reported to protect against MPTP-induced toxicity in the non-human primate[108]. It has been proposed that ALC may protect against the consequences of MPP^+ damage to complex I by promoting the formation of high energy compounds or by shunting oxidative metabolism of acylated compounds downstream from complex I[109]. ALC therapy is currently being tested in Alzheimer's disease and may have even more relevance in Parkinson's disease in which a deficiency of complex I in the nigra has been reported.

Excitatory neurotransmitters which stimulate glutamate receptors have been implicated in a number of neurological disorders, including Huntington's chorea and ischemia–reperfusion injury[110,111]. Experimentally, glutamate neurotoxicity can be prevented by glutamate receptor antagonists such as MK-801[112]. In the basal ganglia, fibers from the cortex to the striatum and from the subthalamic nucleus to the internal portion of the globus pallidus utilize glutamate as a neurotransmitter[113]. Dopamine deficiency secondary to nigral lesions results in a disinhibition of these glutaminergic neurons and, likely, a state of glutaminergic over-activity. Interest to date has focused on the symptomatic consequences of excess glutamate activity, and lesions of the subthalamic nucleus and glutamate receptor antagonists have been demonstrated to provide antiparkinsonian benefits[114,115]. It is also possible that excess glutaminergic activity could lead to neurotoxicity and contribute to the continued progression of parkinsonian disability. Support for this hypothesis is provided by studies demonstrating that antagonists of the NMDA receptor protect against damage induced by MPP+ and methamphetamine[116,117]. While these studies have not been confirmed, they raise the possibility that glutamine antagonists, perhaps in combination with antioxidants, may have a protective role in Parkinson's disease. In this regard, it is perhaps noteworthy that excitatory neurotransmitters are released by oxidant stress[118].

Many neurotoxins, including excitatory neurotransmitters, are thought to act on voltage-dependent calcium channels, to permit a rise in free intracellular calcium^{2+} with activation of protease, lipase and endonuclease enzymes[119]. Calcium channel blockers might interfere with this mechanism. Preliminary studies in stroke indicate that central calcium channel blockers, if administered early enough, attenuate the size of the infarction and functional deficit[120]. Whether such an approach would have value in Parkinson's disease remains to be determined. However, preliminary reports indicate that remaining nigral neurons in parkinsonian patients have a high content of the calcium–binding protein calbindin, which may protect against intracellular calcium accumulation and account for their survival[121].

Trophic factors that act on the dopaminergic system are only now beginning to be identified. Low concentrations of a brain-derived neurotrophic factor (BDNF) have been detected in the striatum of normal individuals. BDNF has been demonstrated to augment growth of dopamine neurons in tissue culture and to provide protection against the toxic effects of MPP+ [122]. It is conceivable that a deficiency of a neurotrophic factor(s) contributes to the degeneration of cells in Parkinson's disease and that replacement of such neurotrophic factors may have protective or restorative benefits.

A more precise understanding of the mechanism responsible for cell death in Parkinson's disease could provide the opportunity to introduce protective therapy. Currently, attention has largely focused on the possibility that oxidant stress plays the key role in degeneration of dopamine neurons. Clinical trials of MAO-B inhibitors and α-tocopherol have already been initiated and it is likely that studies of other antioxidants will be forthcoming. There is also the possibility that protective therapy aimed at a mitochondrial lesion, excitotoxic lesion, increased intracellular calcium, or a trophic factor deficiency may be of value. Parkinson's disease may be a heterogeneous condition with different etiologies and multiple pathogenetic mechanisms that operate in varying degrees in different individuals. All of this renders the delineation of a specific protective therapy for patients with Parkinson's disease difficult. Nonetheless, the search for a protective therapy which will interfere with the degenerative process has begun, and hopefully will soon enable us to slow or stop progression of Parkinson's disease.

REFERENCES

1. Cohen, G. (1988). Oxygen radicals and Parkinson's disease. In Halliwell, B. (ed.) *Oxygen Radicals and Tissue Injury*, pp. 130–5. (FASEB)
2. Halliwell, B. and Gutteridge, J.M.C. (1985). Oxygen radicals and the nervous system. *Trends Neurosci.*, **8**, 22–9
3. Olanow, C.W. (1990). Oxidation reactions in Parkinson's disease. *Neurology*, **40**, 32–7
4. Floyd, R.A. and Schneider, J.E. (1990). Hydroxyl free radical damage to DNA. In Vigo-Pelfrey, C. (ed.) *Membrane Lipid Oxidation*, Vol. I. (Boca Raton, Florida: CRC Press)
5. Wolff, S.P., Garner, A. and Dean, R.T. (1986). Free radicals, lipids and protein degradation. *Trends Biol. Sci.*, **11**, 27–31
6. Minotti, G. and Aust, S.D. (1987). The role of iron in the initiation of lipid peroxidation. *Chem. Phys. Lipids*, **44**, 191–208
7. Chiba, K., Trevor, A. and Castagnoli, N. Jr. (1984). Metabolism of the neurotoxic tertiary amine, MPTP, by brain monoamine oxidase. *Biochem. Biophys. Res. Commun.*, **120**, 447–8
8. Heikkila, R.E., Nicklas, W.J., Vyas, I. and Duvoisin, R.C. (1985). Dopaminergic toxicity of rotenone and the MPP ion after their stereotaxic administration to rats: implications for the mechanism of MPTP toxicity. *Neurosci. Lett.*, **682**, 389–94
9. Schapira, A.H.V., Cooper, J.M. *et al.* (1989). Mitochondrial complex I deficiency in Parkinson's disease. *Lancet*, **1**, 1269
10. Mizuno, Y., Ohta, S., Tanaka, M. *et al.* (1989). Deficiencies in complex I subunits of the respiratory chain in Parkinson's disease. *Biochem. Biophys. Res. Commun.*, **163**, 1450–5
11. Wegner, G.C., Jarvis, M.F. and Carelli, R.M. (1985). Ascorbic acid reduces the dopamine depletion induced by MPTP. *Neuropharmacology*,

24, 1261–2

12. Odunze, I.N., Klaidman, L.K. and Adams, J.D. (1990). MPTP toxicity in the mouse brain and vitamin E. *Neurosci. Lett.*, **108**, 346–9

13. Frank, D.M., Arora, P.K., Blumer, J.L. and Sayre, L.M. (1987). Model study on the bioreduction of paraquat, MPP^+ and analogs. Evidence against a 'redox cycling' mechanism in MPTP neurotoxicity. *Biochem. Biophys. Res. Commun.*, **147**, 1095–104

14. Martinovits, G., Melamed, E., Cohen, O., Rosenthal, J. and Uzzan, A. (1986). Systemic administration of antioxidants does not protect mice against the dopaminergic neurotoxicity of 1-methyl-4-phenyl-1,2,5,6-tetrahydropyridine (MPTP). *Neurosci. Lett.*, **69**, 192–7

15. Langston, J.W., Irwin, I., Langston, E.B. and Forno, L.S. (1984). Pargyline prevents MPTP-induced parkinsonian in primates. *Science*, **225**, 1480–2

16. Cohen, G., Pasik, P., Cohen, B. *et al.* (1985). Pargyline and deprenyl prevent the neurotoxicity of 1-methyl-4-phenyl-1,2,3,6-tetrahydropyridine (MPTP) in monkeys. *Eur. J. Pharmacol.*, **106**, 209–10

17. Graham, D.G. (1979). On the origin and significance of neuromelanin. *Arch. Pathol. Lab. Med.*, **103**, 359–62

18. Mann, D.M.A. and Yates, P.O. (1974). Lipoprotein pigments – their relationship to aging in the human nervous system. II. The melanin content of pigmented nerve cells. *Brain*, **97**, 489–98

19. Hirsch, E., Graybiel, A.M. and Agid, Y.A. (1988). Melanized dopaminergic neurons are differentially susceptible to degeneration in Parkinson's disease. *Nature (London)*, **334**, 345–8

20. Sofic, E., Paulus, W., Jellinger, K. *et al.* (1991). Selective increase of iron in the substantia nigra zona compacta of parkinsonian brains. *J. Neurochem.*, **56**, 978–82

21. Dexter, D.T., Wells, F.R., Lees, A.J. *et al.* (1989). Increased nigral iron content and alterations in other metal irons occurring in brain in Parkinson's disease. *J. Neurochem.*, **52**, 1830–6

22. Dexter, D.T., Carayon, A., Vidailhet, M. *et al.* (1990). Decreased ferritin levels in brain in Parkinson's disease. *J. Neurochem.*, **55**, 16–20

23. Perry, T.L. and Young, V.W. (1986). Idiopathic Parkinson's disease, progressive supranuclear palsy and glutathione metabolism in the substantia nigra of patients. *Neurosci. Lett.*, **67**, 269–74

24. Riederer, P., Sofic, E., Rausch, W.D. *et al.* (1989). Transition metals, ferritin, glutathione and ascorbic acid in parkinsonian brains. *J. Neurochem.*, **52**, 515–20

25. Dexter, D.T., Carter, C.J., Wells, F.R. *et al.* (1989). Basal lipid peroxidation in substantia nigra is increased in Parkinson's disease. *J. Neurochem.*, **52**, 381–9

26. Halliwell, B. and Gutteridge, J.M.C. (1988). Iron as a biological pro-oxidant. *ISI Atlas Sci. Biochem.*, **1**, 48–52

27. Halliwell, B., Aruoma, O.I., Wasil, M. and Gutteridge, J.M.C. (1988). The resistance of transferrin, lactoferrin and caeruloplasmin to oxidative damage. *Biochem. J.*, **256**, 311–12

28. The Parkinson's Study Group (1989). Effect of deprenyl on the progression of disability in early Parkinson's disease. *N. Engl. J. Med.*, **321**, 1364–71

29. Tetrud, J.W. and Langston, J.W. (1989). The effect of Deprenyl (Seleghine) on the natural history of Parkinson's disease. *Science*, **245**, 519–22

30. Cohen, G. and Spina, M.B. (1989). Deprenyl suppresses the oxidant stress associated with increased dopamine turnover. *Ann. Neurol.*, **26**, 689–90

31. Knoll, J., Ecseri, Z., Kelemen, K. *et al.* (1965). Phenylisopropylmethylpropinylamine (E-250), a new spectrum psychic energizer. *Arch. Int. Pharmacodyn. Ther.*, **155**, 154–64

32. Elsworth, J.D., Glover, V., Reynolds, G.P. *et al.* (1978). Deprenyl administration in man: a selective monoamine oxidase B inhibitor without the 'cheese effect'. *Psychopharmacology*, **57**, 33–8

33. Mendis, N., Paire, C.M.B., Sandler, M. *et al.* (1981). Is the failure of (−) Deprenyl, a selective monoamine oxidase B inhibitor, to elevate depression related to freedom from the cheese effect? *Psychopharmacology (Berlin)*, **73**, 87–90

34. Fischer, P.A. and Bass, J. (1987). Therapeutic efficacy of (−) Deprenyl as an adjunct therapy in advanced parkinsonism. *J. Neural Transm.*, **25**(Suppl.), 137–47

35. Mann, J.J., Aarons, S.F., Wilner, P.J. *et al.* (1989). A controlled study of the antidepressant efficacy and side-effects of (−) Deprenyl: a selective monoamine oxidase inhibitor. *Arch. Gen. Psychiatr.*, **46**, 45–50

36. Birkmayer, W., Riederer, P., Youdim, M.B.H. and Linauer, W. (1975). The potentiation of the antiakinetic effect after L-dopa treatment by an inhibitor of MAO-B, deprenyl. *J. Neural Transm.*, **36**, 303–26

37. Golbe, L.I., Lieberman, A.N., Muenter, M.D. *et al.* (1988). Deprenyl in the treatment of symptom fluctuations in advanced Parkinson's disease. *Clin. Neuropharmacol.*, **11**, 45–55

38. Knoll, J. (1988). Extension of life span of rats by long-term (−) Deprenyl treatment. *Mt. Sinai J. Med.*, **55**, 67–74

39. Birkmayer, W., Knoll, J., Riederer, P. *et al.* (1985). Improvement of life expectancy due to L-Deprenyl addition to madopar treatment in Parkinson's disease: a long-term study. *J. Neural Transm.*, **64**, 113–27

40. Olanow, C.W. and Calne, D. (1992). Does deprenyl monotherapy in Parkinson's disease act by symptomatic or protective mechanisms? *Neurology*, in press

41. Knoll, J. (1978). The possible mechanism of action (−) Deprenyl in Parkinson's disease. *J. Neural Transm.*, **43**, 117

42. Csanda, E. and Tarczy, M. (1987). Selegiline in the early and late phases of Parkinson's disease. *J. Neural Transm.*, Suppl. 25, 105–13

43. Mantegazza, P. and Riva, M.J. (1963). Amphetamine-like activity of β-phenethylamine after a monoamine oxidase inhibitor *in vivo*. *Pharm. Pharmacol.*, **15**, 472–8

44. Felner, A.E. and Waldmeier, P.C. (1979). Cumulative effect of irreversible MAO inhibitors *in vivo*. *Biochem. Pharmacol.*, **28**, 995–1002

45. Zsilla, G., Foldi, P., Held, G. *et al.* (1986). The effect of repeated doses of (−) Deprenyl on the dynamics of monoaminergic transmission. Comparison with Clorgyline. *J. Pol. J. Pharmacol. Pharm.*, **86**, 211–17

46. Paterson, I.A., Juorio, A.V. and Boulton, A.A. (1990). Possible mechanism of action of deprenyl in parkinsonism. *Lancet*, **336**, 183

47. Paterson, I.A., Juorio, A.V. and Boulton, A.A. (1990). 2-phenyl-ethyl-amine: a modulator of catecholamine transmission in the melanin central nervous system? *J. Neurochem.*, **55**, 1827–37

48. Paterson, I.A., Juorio, A.V., Berry, M.D. and Zhu, M.Y. (1991). Inhibition of monoamine oxidase-B by (−) deprenyl potentiates neuronal responses to dopamine agonists but does not inhibit dopamine metabolism in the rat striatum. *J. Pharmacol. Exp. Ther.*, **258**, 1019–26

49. Reynolds, G.P., Elsworth, J.D., Blau, K. *et al.* (1978). Deprenyl is metabolized to methamphetamine and amphetamine in man. *Br. J. Clin. Pharmacol.*, **6**, 542–4

50. Knoll, J. (1976). Analysis of the pharmacological effects of selective monoamine oxidase inhibitors. In Wolstenholme, G.E.W. and Knight, J. (eds.) *Monoamine Oxidase and Its Inhibition*, pp. 135–61. (Amsterdam: Elsevier)

51. Innes, I.R. and Nickerson, M. (1977). Neuroepinephrine, epinephrine and the sympathomimetic amines. In Goodman, L.S. and Gilman, A. (eds.) *The Pharmacological Basis of Therapeutics*. pp. 477–513. (New York: MacMillan)

52. Schachter, M., Price, P.A. and Parkes, J.D. (1979). Deprenyl in narcolepsy. *Lancet*, **1**, 831–2

53. Tariot, P.N., Cohen, R.M., Sunderland, T. *et al.* (1987). L-deprenyl in Alzheimer's disease: preliminary evidence for behavioral change with monoamine oxidase B inhibition. *Arch. Gen. Psychiatr.*, **44**, 27–33

54. Robinson, T.E. and Becker, J.B. (1986). Enduring changes in brain and behavior produced by chronic amphetamine administration: a review and evaluation of animal models of amphetamine psychosis. *Brain Res. Rev.*, **11**, 157–98

55. Shoulson, I. and Parkinson Study Group (1990). Deprenyl and early Parkinson's disease: symptomatic versus protective efficacy. *Neurology*, **40**(Suppl. 1), 153

56. Maitre, L., Delini-Stula, A. and Waldmeier, P.C. (1987). Relations between the degree of monoamine oxidase inhibition and some psychopharmacological responses to monoamine oxidase inhibitors in rats. In *Monoamine Oxidase and Its Inhibition* (CIBA Foundation Symposium), Vol. 6, pp. 247–70. (New York: Elsevier)

57. Riederer, P. and Youdim, M.B.H. (1986) Monoamine oxidase activity in monoamine metabolism in brains of parkinsonian patients treated with L-Deprenyl. *J. Neurochem.*, **46**, 1359–65

58. Turkish, S., Tu, P.H. and Grenshaw, A.J. (1988). Monoamine oxidase-B inhibition: a comparison of *in vivo* and *ex vivo* measures of reversible effects. *J. Neural Trans.*, **74**, 141–8

59. Arnett, C.D., Fowler, J.S., MacGregor, R.R. *et al.* (1987). Turnover of brain monoamine oxidase measured *in vivo* by position emission tomography using L(11C) Deprenyl. *J. Neurochem.*, **49**, 522–7

60. Kindt, M.V., Youngster, S.K., Sonsalla, P.K. *et al.* (1988). Role for the monoamine oxidase A (MAO-A) in the bioactivation and nigral striatal dopaminergic neurotoxicity of the MPTP analog 2'ME-MPTP. *Eur. J. Pharmacol.*, **146**, 313–18

61. Glover, V., Sandler, M., Owen, F. and Riley, G.J. (1977). Dopamine is a monoamine B substrate in man. *Nature (London)*, **265**, 80–1

62. Westlund, K.N., Denney, R.M., Kochersperger, L.M., Rose, R.M. and Bell, C.W. (1985). Distinct monoamine oxidase A and B populations in primate brain. *Science*, **230**, 181–3

63. Kato, T., Dong, E., Iskii, K. and Kinemuchi, H. (1986). Brain dialysis: *in vivo* metabolism of dopamine and serotonin by monoamine oxidase A but not B in the striatum of unrestrained rats. *J. Neurochem.*, **48**, 1277–82

64. Tatton, W.G. and Greenwood, C.E. (1992). Rescue of dying neurons: a new action for deprenyl and MPTP-parkinsonism. *J. Neurosci. Res.*, in press

65. Ingold, K.U., Webb, A.C., Witter, D. *et al.* (1987). Vitamin E remains the major lipid-soluble, chain-breaking antioxidant in human plasma even in individuals suffering severe vitamin E deficiency. *Arch. Biochem. Biophys.*, **259**, 224–5

66. Packer, L. and Landvik, S. (1990). Vitamin E in biological systems. In Emerit, I., Packer, L. and Auclair, C. (eds.) *Antioxidants in Therapy and Preventive Medicine*, pp. 93–103. (New York: Plenum Press)

67. Packer, J.E., Slater, T.F. and Willson, R.L. (1979). Direct observation of

a free radical interaction between vitamin E and vitamin C. *Nature (London)*, **278**, 737–8

68. Maguire, J.J., Wilson, D.S. and Packer, L. (1989). Mitochondrial electron transport-linked tocopheroxyl radical reduction. *J. Biol. Chem.*, **264**, 21462–5

69. Vatassery, G.T., Brin, M.F., Fahn, S. *et al.* (1988). Effect of high doses of dietary vitamin E on the concentrations of Vitamin E in several brain regions, plasma, liver and adipose tissue of rats. *J. Neurochem.*, **51**, 621–3

70. Constantinides, P., Harkey, M. and McLaury, D. (1986). Prevention of lipofuscin development in neurons by anti-oxidants. *Virch. Arch. Path. Anat.*, **409**, 583–93

71. Gedigk, P. and Fischer, R. (1959). On the origin of lipo-pigments in muscle fibers. Studies in experimental Vitamin E deficiency on rats and organs of man. *Virch. Arch. Path. Anat.*, **332**, 431–68

72. Sokol, R.J. (1988). Vitamin E deficiency and neurologic disease. *Annu. Rev. Nutr.*, **8**, 351–73

73. Fahn, S. (1989). The endogenous toxin hypothesis of the etiology of Parkinson's disease and a pilot trial of high dosage antioxidant in an attempt to slow the progression of the illness. *Ann. N.Y. Acad. Sci.*, **570**, 186–9

74. Frei, B., England, L. and Ames, B.N. (1989). Ascorbate is an out-standing antioxidant in human blood plasma. *Proc. Natl. Acad. Sci. USA*, **86**, 6377–81

75. Sadrzadeh, S.M. and Eaton, J.W. (1988). Hemoglobin-mediated oxidant damage to the central nervous system requires endogenous ascorbate. *J. Clin. Invest.*, **82**, 1510–15

76. Halliwell, B. (1989). Oxidants in the central nervous system: some fundamental questions. *Acta Neurol. Scand.*, **126**, 23–33

77. Burton, G.W. and Ingold, K.U. (1984). B-carotene: an unusual type of lipid antioxidant. *Science*, **224**, 569–73

78. Peto, R., Doll, R., Buckley, J.D. and Sporn, M. (1980). Can dietary beta-carotene materially reduce human cancer rates? *Nature (London)*, **290**, 201–8

79. Janzen, E.G. (1980). A critical review of spin trapping in biological systems. In Pryor, W.A. (ed.) *Free Radicals in Biology*, pp. 115–54. (New York: Academic Press)

80. Floyd, R.A. (1990). Role of oxygen free radicals in carcinogenesis and brain ischemia. *FASEB*, **4**, 2587–97

81. Halliwell, B. and Gutteridge, J.M.C. (1986). Oxygen free radicals and iron in relation to biology and medicine: some problems and concepts. *Arch. Biochem. Biophys.*, **246**, 501–14

82. Halliwell, B. (1989). Protection against tissue damage *in vivo* by deferrioxamine. What is its mechanism of action? *Free Radic. Biol. Med.,* **7,** 645-51

83. Aust, F.D. and White, B.C. (1985). Iron chelation prevents tissue injury following ischemia. *Adv. Free Rad. Biol. Med.,* **1,** 1-17

84. Ben-Shachar, D., Eshel, G., Finberg, J.P.M. and Youdim, M. (1991). The iron chelator desferrioxamine (desferal) retards 6-hydroxy dopamine-induced degeneration of nigral striatal dopamine neurons. *J. Neurochem.,* **56,** 1441-4

85. Sengstock, G.J., Olanow, C.W., Dunn, A.J. *et al.* (1992). Iron induces degeneration of substantia nigra neurons. *Brain Res. Bull.,* in press

86. Crapper-McLachlan, D.R., Dalton, A.J., Kruck, T.P.A. *et al.* (1991). Intramuscular desferrioxamine in patients with Alzheimer's disease. *Lancet,* **337,** 1304-8

87. Blake, D.R., Winyard, P., Lonec, J. *et al.* (1985). Cerebral and ocular toxicity induced by desferrioxamine. *Q. J. Med.,* **219,** 345-55

88. Braughler, J.M., Pregenzer, J.F., Chase, R.L., Duncan, L.A., Jacobsen, E.J. and McCall, J.M. (1987). Novel 21-aminosteroids as potent inhibitors of iron-dependent lipid peroxidation. *J. Biol. Chem.,* **262,** 10438-40

89. Hall, E.D. and Younkers, P.A. (1988). Attenuation of post-ischemic cerebral hypoperfusion by the 21-aminosteroid U74006F. *Stroke,* **19,** 340-4

90. Hall, E.D., Younkers, P.A. and McCall, J.M. (1988). Attenuation of hemorrhagic shock by the non-glucocorticoid 21-aminosteroid U74006F. *Eur. J. Pharmacol.,* **147,** 299-303

91. Hall, E.D. (1988). Effects of the 21-aminosteroid U74006F on post traumatic spinal cord ischemia in cats. *J. Neurosurg.,* **68,** 462-5

92. Hall, E.D., Younkers, P.A., McCall, J.M. and Braughler, J.M. (1988). Effects of the 21-aminosteroid U74006F on experimental head injury in mice. *J. Neurosurg.,* **68,** 456-61

93. Lim, K.H., Connolly, M., Rose, D., Segman, F. *et al.* (1986). Prevention of reperfusion injury of the ischemic spinal cord: use of recombinant superoxide dismutase. *Ann. Thorac. Surg.,* **42,** 282-6

94. Chan, P.H., Longar, S. and Fishman, R.A. (1987). Protective effects of liposome in trapped superoxide dismutase on post traumatic brain edema. *Ann. Neurol.,* **21,** 540-7

95. McCord, J.M. (1985). Oxygen derived free radicals in post-ischemic tissue injury. *N. Engl. J. Med.,* **312,** 159-63

96. Hayaish, M. and Slater, T.F. (1986). Inhibitory effects of Ebselen on lipid peroxidation in rat liver microsomes. *Free Rad. Res. Commun.,* **2,** 179-85

97. Olanow, C.W. (1992). A rationale for dopamine agonist as primary therapy for Parkinson's disease. *Can. J. Sci.,* in press

98. Hefti, F., Melamed, E. and Bhawan, J. *et al.* (1981). Administration of L-dopa does not damage dopaminergic neurons in the mouse. *Neurology,* **31**, 1194–5

99. Perry, T.L., Young, V.W., Ito, M. *et al.* (1984). Nigrostriatal dopaminergic neurons remain undamaged in rats given high doses of L-dopa and carbidopa chronically. *J. Neurochem.,* **43**, 990–3

100. Quinn, N., Parkes, J.D., Janota, I. *et al.* (1986). Reservation of substantia nigra neurons and locus coeruleus in patients receiving levodopa (2 mg) plus decarboxylase inhibitor over a four year period. *Movement Dis.,* **1**, 65–8

101. Rinne, U.K. (1985). Combined bromocriptine-levodopa therapy early in Parkinson's disease. *Neurology,* **35**, 1196–8

102. Mouradian, M.M. and Chase, T.N. (1988). Hypothesis: central mechanism and levodopa response fluctuations in Parkinson's disease. *Clin. Neuropharmacol.,* **11**, 378–85

103. Felten, D.L., Felten, S.Y., Fuller, R.W. *et al.* (1992). Chronic dietary pergolide preserves nigrostriatal neuronal integrity in aged Fischer 344 rats. *Neurobiol. Aging,* in press

104. Michel, P.P. and Hefti, F. (1990). Toxicity of 6-hydroxydopamine and dopamine for dopaminergic neurons in culture. *J. Neurosci. Res.,* **26**, 428–35

105. Clemens, J.A. and Phebus, L.A. (1988). Dopamine depletion protects striatal neurons from ischemia-induced cell death. *Life Sci.,* **42**, 707–13

106. Curnutte, J.T. and Babior, B.M. (1987). Chronic granulomatous disease. *Adv. Hum. Genet.,* **16**, 229–97

107. Dormandy, T.L. (1988). In praise of peroxidation. *Lancet,* **2**, 1126–8

108. Bodis-Wollner, I., Chung, E., Ghilrdi, M.F., Glover, A., Onofrj, M., Pasik, P. and Samson, Y. (1991). Acetyl-levo-carotene protects against MPTP-induced parkinsonism in primates. *J. Neural Transm.,* **3**, 63–72

109. Siliprandi, N., Siliprandi, D. and Siman, M. (1965). Stimulation of oxidation of mitochondrial fatty acids and of acetate by acetyl-carnitine. *Biochem. J.,* **96**, 777–80

110. Olney, J.W. (1989). Excitotoxicity and N-methyl-D-aspartate receptors. *Drug Dev. Res.,* **17**, 299–319

111. Meldrum, B. (1985). Excitatory aminoacids and anoxic/ischaemic brain damage. *Trends Neurosci.,* **18**, 47–8

112. Alberts, G.W., Goldberg, M.P. and Choi, D.W. (1989). N-methyl-D-aspartate antagonists: ready for clinical trial in brain ischemia? *Ann. Neurol.,* **25**, 398–403

113. Graybiel, A.M. (1990). Neurotransmitters and neuromodulations in the basal ganglia. *Trends Neurosci.*, **7**, 244–54
114. Bergman, H., Wichmann, T. and DeLong, M.R. (1990). Reversal of experimental parkinsonism by lesions of the subthalamic nucleus. *Science*, **249**, 1436–8
115. Klockgether, T. and Turski, L. (1990). NMDA antagonists potentiate antiparkinsonian actions of L-dopa in monoamine-depleted rats. *Ann. Neurol.*, **28**, 539–46
116. Turksi, L., Bressler, K., Rettig, K.J., Lo'Schmann, P.A. and Wachtel, N. (1991). Protection of substantia nigra from MPP$^+$ neurotoxicity by N-methyl-D-aspartate antagonists. *Nature (London)*, **349**, 414–18
117. Sonsalla, P.K., Nicklas, W.J. and Heikkila, E. (1988). Role for excitatory amino-acids in metamphetamine-induced nigrostriatal dopaminergic toxicity. *Science*, **243**, 398–400
118. Pellegrini-Giampietro, D.E., Cherichi, G., Alesiani, M., Carla, V. and Moroni, F. (1988). Excitatory amino acid release from rat hippocampal slices as a consequence of free-radical formation. *J. Neurochem.*, **51**, 1961–3
119. Komulainen, H. and Bondy, S.C. (1988). Increased free intracellular calcium^{2+} by toxic agents; an index of potential neurotoxicity? *Trends Pharm. Sci.*, **9**, 154–6
120. Gelmers, H.J., Gorter, K., DeWeerdt, C.J. and Wiezer, H.J.A. (1988). A controlled trial of nimodopine in acute ischemic stroke. *N. Engl. J. Med.*, **318**, 203–7
121. Yamada, T., McGeer, P.L., Baimbridge, K.G. and McGeer, E.G. (1990). Relative sparing in Parkinson's disease of substantia nigra dopamine neurons containing calbindin-D$_{28k}$. *Brain Res.* **526**, 303–7
122. Hyman, C., Hofer, M., Barde, Y.A. *et al.* (1991). BDNF is a neurotrophic factor for dopaminergic neurons of the substantia nigra. *Nature (London)*, **350**, 230–2

12

Current roles and future applications of trophic factors

C. W. Shults

INTRODUCTION

A possible role for trophic factors in the treatment of Parkinson's disease has emerged from studies of transplantation of fetal dopaminergic cells and adrenal medulla into the striatum in animal models of Parkinson's disease. These investigations have indicated that trophic factors may be useful because of two mechanisms. First, trophic factors have been demonstrated to promote survival of adrenal medullary cells transplanted to the striatum, and to induce chromaffin cells to assume a more neuronal morphology. In the future, trophic factors may be used to enhance survival and promote dopamine production by fetal mesencephalic, adrenal medullary or other catecholaminergic cells transplanted into animal models of Parkinson's disease, and ultimately in parkinsonian patients. Second, more recent studies have suggested that trophic factors may induce residual dopaminergic neurons in the mesencephalon and their axons to the striatum to sprout collateral axons, reinnervate the denervated regions of the striatum, and induce a behavioral recovery.

Other studies, which were carried out in animal models of Parkinson's disease and in cultures of mesencephalic dopaminergic neurons, have indicated that trophic factors can promote survival of acutely injured dopaminergic neurons. These studies and those of the effects of trophic factors on transplanted catecholaminergic cells suggest that trophic factors could potentially be used to slow the progressive loss of dopaminergic neurons in the mesencephalon, which remains the fundamental problem in Parkinson's disease.

TROPHIC FACTORS ENHANCE SURVIVAL OF ADRENAL MEDULLARY GRAFTS

Shortly after the initial reports that transplantation of fetal mesencephalic cells to the striatum could reverse behavioral deficits in animal models of Parkinson's disease, investigators began to search for alternate sources of catecholaminergic cells. Two groups noted that transplantation of adrenal medulla into the ventricle adjacent to the denervated striatum or into the striatum itself caused reduction in rotational asymmetry[1,2]. However, the number of surviving chromaffin cells was low, and investigators began to search for ways to increase the survival of the transplanted chromaffin cells. Studies *in vitro* had demonstrated that nerve growth factor (NGF) supported survival of neonatal rat adrenal medullary cells and promoted extension of neurites from the cells[3]. In a rat model of Parkinson's disease, Stromberg and colleagues[2] found that administration of NGF with the grafts of adrenal medulla increased the number of surviving chromaffin cells and induced transformation of the chromaffin cells to a more neuronal phenotype. The NGF-treated adrenal grafts also had greater adrenergic fiber outgrowth than grafts not treated with NGF. Animals that received grafts treated with NGF had significant and sustained reduction in rotational asymmetry after administration of apomorphine. Pezzoli and colleagues[4] confirmed this observation but also noted that intraventricular infusion of NGF in conjunction with ventricular implantation of adipose tissue or sciatic nerve, caused a marked reduction in apomorphine-induced rotational behavior in rats whose substantia nigra pars compacta (SNpc) had been unilaterally lesioned with 6-hydroxydopamine (6-OHDA). Pezzoli did not observe an increase in survival of chromaffin cells in animals treated with NGF. This difference may be explained by a number of difference in technique between the two studies.

Gash and colleagues[5] extended these observations by co-grafting C glioma cells with adrenal medullary cells as well as grafting adrena medullary cells alone and C6 glioma cells alone. C6 glioma cells have been shown to produce NGF and other trophic factors[6]. Interestingly all three treatment groups demonstrated a reduction in rotation after administration of amphetamine, but there was greater reduction in animals that received the co-grafts. Co-grafting of C6 glioma cells with adrenal medullary cells promoted survival of the chromaffin cells and transition of the chromaffin cells to a more neuronal appearance.

There have been surprisingly few reports of attempts to use trophic factors to increase the survival and extension of axons of fetal mesencephalic dopaminergic cells transplanted to the striatum in animal models of Parkinson's disease[7,8]. However, investigators have shown that NGF can enhance the effects of transplants of hippocampus in animal models of Alzheimer's disease[9].

TROPHIC FACTORS MAY PROMOTE SPROUTING OF DOPAMINERGIC AXONS

In the course of studies of transplantation in animal models of Parkinson's disease, a number of investigators noted that certain manipulations in the striatum caused residual mesencephalic dopaminergic cells and their axons to the striatum to sprout collateral axons and reinnervate the striatum. The manipulations also caused improvement in behavioral deficits. Bankiewicz, Plunkett, and co-workers[10-12] noted that in MPTP-treated monkeys a wound or transplantation of various tissues to the striatum caused varying degrees of sprouting of residual dopaminergic axons into the striatum. The dopaminergic fibers appeared to arise largely from the nucleus accumbens and ventral striatum, projection areas of the ventral tegmental area (VTA) and medial SNpc. The various operations also resulted in varying degrees of improvement of parkinsonian symptoms. Transplanted fetal mesencephalon caused the greatest behavioral recovery, but transplantation of adult adrenal medulla and cavitation alone also caused improvement. Transplants of fetal mesencephalon survived, and the dopaminergic cells extended axons which did not extend beyond the graft. However, dopaminergic axons, which appeared to emanate from the intact ventral striatum, were noted in the caudate ventral to the graft site. Bankiewicz and Plunkett also noted sprouting of dopaminergic fibers from the ventral striatum toward a simple cavity in the caudate, which had not received an implant. Although the various operations caused both sprouting of dopaminergic fibers and improvement in parkinsonian symptoms, a causal relationship between sprouting and behavioral improvement is not yet established. It is likely, however, that among the changes induced in the striatum by wound or transplantation, reinnervation of the striatum by sprouting dopaminergic fibers plays a crucial role in reversal of parkinsonian symptoms. Gash and colleagues found similar results in MPTP-treated monkeys[13,14] and 6-OHDA treated rats[15] after transplantation of adrenal medulla to the striatum. Similarly, Bohn[16] found that implantation of adrenal medulla into the striatum of MPTP-treated mice quickened the regeneration of dopaminergic fibers. Felten and colleagues[17] replicated Bohn's finding but found that aged mice had less recovery of dopaminergic axons than young mice. One must critically evaluate studies carried out in MPTP-treated mice. In young, mature mice treated with MPTP, the mesencephalic dopaminergic neurons may not degenerate despite loss of tyrosine hydroxylase immunoreactive (TH-IR) axons and reduction in levels of dopamine in the striatum. With time the mesostriatal dopaminergic fibers may spontaneously regenerate[16,18-20]. Two features common to the various manipulations that induced sprouting of collateral dopaminergic axons were the presence of inflammatory cells and reactive astrocytes at the site of manipulation. Weber and colleagues[21] made the interesting observation that in rats with selective unilateral lesions of the SNpc, transplantation of activated leukocytes to the denervated striatum induced reinnervation of the striatum and reduction in rotational asymmetry after administration of amphetamine.

A number of laboratories undertook studies to identify specific molecules that promote collateral sprouting of mesostriatal dopaminergic axons. These studies have been carried out both *in vitro* and *in vivo*. One must interpret carefully the results of *in vitro* studies because a trophic factor could act either directly on the dopaminergic neurons to support neurite outgrowth or indirectly through other cells in the culture, for example glia, to stimulate production of trophic factors, extracellular matrix molecules, or cell surface molecules, which are the actual stimuli for neurite outgrowth from the dopaminergic neurons. Also, although certain neuronal populations may respond to a trophic factor during development, these same populations may no longer be responsive to the trophic factor in the adult central nervous system. As mentioned above, one must also critically interpret studies carried out in MPTP-treated mice because of spontaneous recovery.

The specific molecules that induce and support sprouting of mesen-cephalic dopaminergic axons remain to be elucidated. In the past decade, a number of polypeptides have been identified which support the survival and neurite extension of neurons. Three trophic factors, basic fibroblast growth factor (bFGF), acidic fibroblast growth factor (aFGF) and brain-derived neurotrophic factor (BDNF) have been demonstrated to have a trophic effect on mesencephalic dopaminergic cells.

FIBROBLAST GROWTH FACTORS

During the past 5 years, data have accumulated to indicate that bFGF and aFGF have trophic effects on mesencephalic dopaminergic cells. In 1986, Walicke and colleagues[22] demonstrated that bFGF and aFGF increased survival and promoted neurite outgrowth of fetal hippocampal cells grown in chemically defined media. Ferrari and co-workers[23] subsequently showed that bFGF increased survival and neurite outgrowth of fetal mesencephalic dopaminergic cells cultured in a chemically defined media. Knüsel[24] recently demonstrated that bFGF was one of a number of trophic factors that increased uptake of tritiated dopamine in cultures of fetal mesencephalic cells which had been plated at high density and supplemented with fetal calf serum.

As studies of the effects of bFGF and aFGF on neural cells *in vitro* were being carried out, studies of adrenal to striatal transplantation in animal models of Parkinson's disease were beginning to indicate that bFGF and aFGF could have an effect on mesencephalic dopaminergic cells *in vivo*. Bohn and colleagues[16] demonstrated that adrenal medullary tissue implanted into the striatum of mice that had been treated with MPTP enhanced recovery of dopaminergic innervation of the striatum. Baird had previously shown that bFGF is contained in the adrenal gland[25], and Westermann[26] demonstrated that bFGF is contained in the chromaffin cells. Otto and Unsicker[27] recently reported that implantation of gel foam, which had been soaked in bFGF, into one striatum in mice treated with MPTP increased the levels of dopamine and tyrosine hydroxylase activity in the striatum bilaterally. Implantation of the gel foam also increased the density of tyrosine hydroxylase immunoreactive axons in the striatum but only in the side in which the gel foam had been implanted. This effect was noted if the bFGF was administered at the time of MPTP administration or 8 days later. Felten's group[28] noted a similar phenomenon in young mice which received intrastriatal injections of aFGF at 2, 7 and 12 days after administration of MPTP. However, administration of aFGF in aged mice treated with MPTP had no effect.

Basic FGF and aFGF were the first members of the FGF family of growth factors to be isolated and are the most thoroughly characterized[29]. So far, five other members of the FGF family have been identified: INT 2, HST, FGF 5, FGF 6, and KGF[30]. The high degree of homology between members of the FGF family suggests that they are derived from a common ancestral gene. Basic FGF and aFGF are each encoded by a single gene which contains three exons and two introns. The primary translation product for either bFGF or aFGF is composed of 155 amino acids. Proteolytic cleavage of the first nine amino acids of bFGF or the first 15 residues of aFGF results in generation of shorter forms. The 155 amino acid forms of both bFGF and aFGF do not contain a signal peptide. The apparent lack of a signal peptide is consistent with the observation that cultured cells that produce bFGF release little of it into the media. There is considerable evidence that bFGF is not released in a soluble form but rather is bound to a component of the extracellular matrix and cell surface, heparan sulfate[31]. Heparan sulfate protects bFGF from degradation and may act as a reservoir for bFGF. Degradation of heparan sulfate, which is insoluble in the extracellular matrix, could serve as a mechanism for releasing bFGF.

A cDNA clone for the bFGF receptor in the chick was recently isolated and sequenced[32]. The bFGF receptor is a tyrosine kinase. It appears to be a member of the immunoglobulin supergene family because of the presence of three characteristic immunoglobulin-like domains, each containing two cysteine residues. The sequence for the chick bFGF receptor has considerable homology with the human flg gene, suggesting that flg encodes for the human bFGF receptor. Work from Reid's laboratory[33] indicates that there appear to be multiple FGF receptors in the mouse brain which are tyrosine kinases. Wanaka and colleagues[34] isolated a cDNA clone from rat which had 91% and 97% homology with the human and mouse sequences for the bFGF receptor within the 300 nucleotides that they sequenced. Wanaka carried out *in situ* hybridization studies and found a wide distribution of the message for the bFGF receptor in the rat brain. The neurons of the SNpc and VTA showed moderate binding. Little signal for the bFGF receptor could be detected in the striatum. Ferguson[35] demonstrated that iodinated bFGF injected into the lateral ventricle or striatum was retrogradely transported to the SNpc.

NEUROTROPHINS: NGF, BDNF, NT-3

Recent studies have indicated that a member of the neurotrophin family, BDNF, can have a trophic effect on mesencephalic dopaminergic cells *in vitro*. Hyman and colleagues[36] noted in cultures of embryonic mesencephalic cells that a single application of BDNF increased the survival of dopaminergic cells 1.9-fold 8 days later and repeated treatments with BDNF increased survival 2.7-fold 11 days after the initial plating. The response to BDNF appeared to be dose-dependent and NGF was without effect. Knüsel and colleagues[37] observed in cultures of fetal rat mesencephalon that after 6 days *in vitro* and 4 days of treatment with BDNF, uptake of tritiated dopamine was approximately 100% greater than in untreated cultures. No effect was noted with neurotrophin-3 (NT-3). Previous studies from this and other groups had shown that NGF had no effect on the dopaminergic cells[38,39].

NGF, BDNF, and NT-3 are homologous and appear to have evolved from a common gene. The primary structure of mouse NGF was determined by Angeletti and Bradshaw[40], and the mouse and human cDNA clones were first isolated in 1983[41,42]. In 1989, Barde and colleagues[43] determined the partial amino acid sequences of BDNF, which had been purified from pig brain, and constructed oligonucleotides that were used to prime the amplification of a pig genomic template using polymerase chain reaction. This group was able to determine the nucleotide sequence of the mRNA coding for BDNF of the pig and mouse. BDNF was noted to share approximately 50% amino acid homology with NGF. One of the most conspicuous similarities between the two trophic factors was absolute conservation of six cysteine residues that in NGF have been shown to form three disulfide bridges. The amino acids flanking these cysteine residues are the most highly conserved regions of the molecules. These regions of homology stimulated and enabled molecular biologists to search for additional members of the

NGF/BDNF family. Again utilizing oligonucleotides based on these regions of homology coupled with polymerase chain reaction or other techniques, four groups[44-47] identified from mouse, rat, and human genomic libraries clones similar to those of NGF and BDNF. This third member of the NGF/BDNF family was designated NT-3. The predicted structures of the three molecules share a number of features. The precursor form of each begins with a putative signal sequence, which contains significant homology between the three molecules. The signal sequence is followed by a prosequence which is presumably involved in folding and proper formation of the disulfide bridges of the three molecules. A single potential glycosylation site is located just upstream to the putative cleavage site for generation of the mature forms of NGF, BDNF, and NT-3. The mature proteins are similar in size: mouse NGF contains 118 amino acids, pig BDNF contains 119 amino acids, and mouse and rat NT-3 contain 119 amino acids. There is approximately 50% homology in the mature forms of the three proteins. In the mature form of the polypeptide, in each of the three neutrophins there appears to be four variable regions which presumably confer specificity on each of these proteins. Maisonpierre and colleagues[46] have evidence to suggest that there are long as well as short precursor forms of BDNF and NT-3 as there is for NGF.

The distributions of mRNA for NGF, BDNF, and NT-3 in the brain have been described using techniques of both Northern blot analysis and *in situ* hybridization[48-51]. The highest concentration of mRNA for each member of the neurotrophin family is in the hippocampus, and the distributions are partially but not entirely overlapping. The distribution of mRNA for BDNF is more widespread than that of NT-3 in the cortex. Using *in situ* hybridization, the signal for mRNA of BDNF and NT-3 in the striatum has not been noted to be above background[49,50]. However, Hofer[49] specifically mentioned detection of a weak signal for BDNF in the striatum by Northern blot. Studies to date have not commented on the presence of mRNA for BDNF or NT-3 in the SNpc. The apparent very low levels of mRNA for BDNF in the adult striatum and SNpc stands in contrast to the trophic effect that BDNF has been reported to have on fetal mesencephalic dopaminergic neurons. Potential explanations for this discrepancy include the possibility that BDNF produced in the striatum may exert a trophic effect on mesencephalic dopaminergic cells at very low concentrations in the adult. Alternatively, BDNF may be present in the striatum and have an effect on mesencephalic dopaminergic cells only during the period of development of the mesostriatal dopaminergic system. A third explanation is that there is a fourth member of the neurotrophin family which is structurally similar to BDNF and present in the striatum.

INSULIN AND INSULIN-LIKE GROWTH FACTORS I AND II

Knüsel and colleagues[24] reported that insulin and insulin-like growth factors (IGF) I and II stimulated the uptake of tritiated dopamine by cultures of fetal mesencephalic cells which had been plated at high density and in media supplemented with fetal calf serum. Insulin, IGF I, and IGF II are structurally similar polypeptides that appear to have derived from a common ancestral gene[52]. Studies utilizing *in situ* hybridization indicate that insulin appears not to be produced in the brain except perhaps in a few periventricular cells of the hypothalamus[53]. A sensitive solution hybridization assay has demonstrated the expression of mRNA for both IGF I and II in the brain of the adult rat[54]. The levels of message for both were higher in the fetal than adult brain, and the levels of the message for IGF II were considerably higher than for IGF I. The levels of mRNA for IGF I were substantially lower in the brain than in the liver, the major source of IGF I. The levels of message for both IGF I and IGF II in the striatum were rather modest. It should be noted that studies utilizing *in situ* hybridization techniques have failed to demonstrate message for IGF II in neuronal or glial cells but have noted expression in the choroid plexus and leptomeninges[55,56]. The receptors for insulin and IGF I are structurally similar[57]. The receptor for IGF II, which is composed of a single polypeptide chain and may be closely related, or identical to, the mannose-6-phosphate receptor, is structurally different from the insulin and IGF I receptors. Autoradiographic studies utilizing radiolabelled insulin, IGF I, and IGF II have been carried out to localize the receptors for insulin, IGF I, and IGF II in the brain. In the rat, receptors for IGF I were noted to be present in low concentrations in the caudate/putamen, and the density of binding of IGF II was noted to be present at moderate levels in the SNpc and caudate/putamen[58]. Adem[59] likewise demonstrated only low levels of the IGF I receptor in the caudate and SN in the human brain. These studies must be interpreted carefully because of the presence of insulin-like growth factor binding proteins in neural tissue[60]. The roles of insulin, IGF I, and IGF II in development and function of the mesostriatal dopaminergic system require further studies.

EPIDERMAL GROWTH FACTOR

Epidermal growth factor (EGF) is a single chain polypeptide, which in humans has 53 amino acids[61]. EGF has been shown to support the survival of cortical neurons *in vitro*[62]. Studies of the effects of EGF on fetal mesencephalic cells in culture have produced conflicting results. Casper and associates[63,64] noted that EGF caused an increase in uptake of dopamine in fetal mesencephalic cells cultured in a chemically defined media. However, Knüsel[24] noted little effect of EGF. As mentioned above, one must interpret carefully studies of the effects of trophic factors on fetal dopaminergic cells in culture. A growth factor may not directly interact with the dopaminergic neurons but indirectly have a trophic effect on these neurons by stimulating other cells, such as glia, to produce trophic factors, extracellular matrix molecules, or cell surface molecules, which exert a trophic action on the dopaminergic cells. EGF has been demonstrated to be a mitogen for astrocytes[65].

GANGLIOSIDES

Gangliosides are normal constituents of plasma membranes of cells. They consist of a hydrophobic ceramide portion, which is located in the outer leaflet of the plasma membrane and hydrophilic oligosaccharide chain, which extends into the extracellular space. The hydrophilic portion may be involved in intercellular recognition or adhesion, and the hydrophobic portion may be involved in signal transduction[66]. Unlike the trophic factors discussed earlier, gangliosides are not polypeptides and would not be considered to be growth factors under a narrow definition of such. However, a number of experiments have demonstrated that administration of gangliosides can ameliorate an injury to the brain and enhance recovery. Agnati and colleagues[67] reported that administration of the ganglioside GM1 to rats that had received unilateral partial transection of the mesostriatal tract resulted in maintenance of the number of dopaminergic cell bodies in the SNpc and terminals on the lesioned side. Lesion-induced dopaminergic receptor supersensitivity did not occur in rats that received GM1, and apomorphine-induced rotations were decreased by the treatment. A number of groups have studied the effects of administration of gangliosides in mice treated with MPTP. Hadjiconstantinou and colleagues[68] noted that administration of GM1 for 23 days after 7 days of treatment with MPTP resulted in recovery of striatal dopamine levels to approximately 83% of control levels. They also noted that treamtent with GM1 did not affect the number of remaining dopaminergic neurons in the SNpc but increased the cell body size above controls in mice treated with GM1 alone or MPTP and GM1. Schneider and Yuwiler[20] noted that GM1 administered shortly after MPTP, and continuing for 2–4 weeks after MPTP treatment, caused significant increases in the levels of striatal dopamine. The duration of GM1 therapy appeared to influence the level of dopamine. They also noted that treatment with GM1 that was delayed for 3 days after completion of MPTP treatment still increased the striatal levels of dopamine. However, the levels were not as great as in animals which received GM1 at the time of administration of MPTP. These studies indicate that gangliosides can ameliorate injury to mesencephalic dopaminergic neurons and may promote collateral sprouting from remaining dopaminergic axons.

OTHER TROPHIC FACTORS

A number of other trophic factors have been isolated and shown to influence neural cells *in vitro*. These include platelet derived growth factor and ciliary neurotrophic factor. In addition, cytokines, e.g. interleukin-1, have been postulated to have a trophic effect on neurons either through a direct mechanism or by stimulation of astrocytes[69]. The effects of these trophic factors on mesencephalic dopaminergic neurons have not been reported.

METHODS OF ADMINISTRATION

For a trophic factor that has been demonstrated to enhance graft survival or promote sprouting of collateral dopaminergic axons in an animal model of Parkinson's disease, the optimal method for delivery of the trophic factor will need to be determined. Some simple methods of administration, such as direct injection into the striatum[28] or infusion into the ventricle[4] have been shown to have an effect. Novel methods for delivery of trophic factors to the brain are being developed. Gage[70] has pioneered the technique of genetically engineering cells to produce trophic factors and then implanting the cells into the brain. Langer[71] and Aebischer[72] have developed controlled release polymer systems which gradually release molecules loaded on to the polymer.

CONCLUSION

Increased understanding of the pathology of Parkinson's disease and neurochemistry and physiology of the basal ganglia has led to a remarkable succession of new therapies for the disease. These treatments, some of which seem ordinary today, include levodopa, dopaminergic agonists, antioxidative agents, which may slow the progression of the disease, and transplantation of dopaminergic cells to the brain. Trophic factors may someday be used to slow the progressive loss of dopamine neurons in the SNpc. Trophic factors also hold the promise of improving the survival and efficacy of catecholaminergic cells transplanted to the brain, or of inducing sprouting of collateral axons from residual dopaminergic neurons in the mesencephalon and their axons to the striatum. By these mechanisms, trophic factors may slow or even reverse the loss of dopaminergic innervation to the striatum and cause a functional improvement in patients.

ACKNOWLEDGEMENTS

The author appreciates the thoughtful comments of Drs Andrew Baird, Denis Baskin, and Mike Rosenberg. The author was supported in preparation of this chapter by the United Parkinson Foundation and the Parkinson's Disease Foundation.

REFERENCES

1. Freed, W.J., Morihisa, J.M., Spoor, E., Hoffer, B.J., Olson, L., Seiger, A. and Wyatt, R.J. (1981). Transplanted adrenal chromaffin cells in rat brain

reduce lesion-induced rotational behaviour. *Nature (London)*, **292**, 351–2

2. Stromberg, I., Herrera-Marschitz, M., Ungerstedt, U., Ebendal, T. and Olson, L. (1985). Chronic implants of chromaffin tissue into the dopamine-denervated striatum. Effects of NGF on graft survival, fiber growth and rotational behavior. *Exp. Brain Res.*, **60**, 335–49

3. Unsicker, K., Miller, T.J. and Hoffmann, H.D. (1982). Nerve growth factor requirements of postnatal rat adrenal medullary cells *in vitro* for survival aggregate formation and maintenance of extended neurites. *Dev. Neurosci.*, **5**, 412–7

4. Pezzoli, G., Fahn, S., Dwork, A., Truong, D.D., de Yebenes, J.G., Jackson-Lewis, V., Herbert, J. and Cadet, J.L. (1988). Non-chromaffin tissue plus nerve growth factor reduces experimental parkinsonism in aged rats. *Brain Res.*, **459**, 398–403

5. Bing, G., Notter, M.F.D., Hansen, J.T., Kellogg, C., Kordower, J.H. and Gash, D.M. (1990). Cografts of adrenal medulla with C6 glioma cells in rats with 6-hydroxydopamine-induced lesions. *Neuroscience*, **34**, 687–97

6. Westermann, R., Hardung, M., Meyer, D.K., Ekhrhard, P., Otten, U. and Unsicker, K. (1988). Neurotrophic factors released by C6 glioma cells. *J. Neurochem.*, **50**, 1747–58

7. Steinbusch, H.W.M., Vermeulen, R.J. and Tonnaer, J.A.D.M. (1990). Basic fibroblast growth factor enhances survival and sprouting of fetal dopaminergic cells in the denervated rat caudate-putamen: preliminary observations. *Prog. Brain Res.*, **82**, 87–94

8. Steinbusch, H.W.M., Dolleman-Van der Weel, M.J., Nijssen, A. and Fuller, F. (1990). Effects of basic fibroblast growth factor and heparin on transplanted fetal dopaminergic neurons and astrocytes in the denervated rat caudate-putamen. *Soc. Neurosci. Abstr.*, **16**, 341.17

9. Tuszynski, M.H., Buzsaki, G. and Gage, F.H. (1990). Nerve growth factor infusions combined with fetal hippocampal grafts enhance reconstruction of the lesioned septohippocampal projection. *Neuroscience*, **36**, 33–44

10. Bankiewicz, K.S., Plunkett, R.J., Kopin, I.J., Jacobowitz, D.M., London, W.T. and Oldfield, E.H. (1988). Transient behavioral recovery in hemiparkinsonian primates after adrenal medullary allografts. In Gash, D.M. and Sladek, J.R. Jr. (eds.) *Prog. Brain Res.*, **78**, pp. 543–9. (Amsterdam: Elsevier Science)

11. Bankiewicz, K.S., Plunkett, R.J., Jacobowitz, D.M., Porrino, L., di Porzio, U., London, W.T., Kopin, I.J. and Oldfield, E.H. (1990). The effect of fetal mesencephalon implants on primate MPTP-induced parkinsonism. *J. Neurosurg.*, **72**, 231–44

12. Plunkett, R.J., Bankiewicz, K.S., Cummins, A.C., Miletich, R.S., Schwartz, J.P. and Oldfield, E.H. (1990). Long-term evaluation of hemiparkin-

sonian monkeys after adrenal autografting or cavitation alone. *J. Neurosurg.*, **73**, 918–26

13. Fiandaca, M.S., Kordower, J.H., Hansen, J.T., Jiao, S.S. and Gash, D.M. (1988). Adrenal medullary autografts into the basal ganglia of Cebus monkeys: injury-induced regeneration. *Exp. Neurol.*, **102**, 76–91

14. Hansen, J.T., Kordower, J.H., Fiandaca, M.S., Jiao, S.S., Notter, M.F.D. and Gash, D.M. (1988). Adrenal medullary autografts into the basal ganglia of Cebus monkeys: graft viability and fine structure. *Exp. Neurol.*, **102**, 65–75

15. Bing, G.Y., Notter, M.F., Hansen, J.T. and Gash, D.M. (1988). Comparison of adrenal medullary, carotid body and PC12 cell grafts in 6-OHDA lesioned rats. *Brain Res. Bull.*, **20**, 399–406

16. Bohn, M.C., Cupit, L., Marcianoa, F. and Gash, D.M. (1987). Adrenal medulla grafts enhance recovery of striatal dopaminergic fibers. *Science*, **237**, 913–16

17. Date, I., Felten, S.Y., Olschowka, J.A. and Felten, D.L. (1990). Limited recovery of striatal dopaminergic fibers by adrenal medullary grafts in MPTP-treated aging mice. *Exp. Neurol.*, **107**, 197–207

18. Ricaurte, G.A., Irwin, I., Forno, L.S., DeLanney, L.E., Langston, E. and Langston, J.W. (1987). Aging and 1-methyl-4-phenyl-1,2,3,6-tetrahydro-pyridine-induced degeneration of dopaminergic neurons in the substantia nigra. *Brain Res.*, **403**, 43–51

19. Zuddas, A., Corsini, G.U., Schinelli, S., Johannessen, J.N., di Porzio, U. and Kopin, I.J. (1989). MPTP treatment combined with ethanol or acetaldehyde selectively destroys dopaminergic neurons in mouse substantia nigra. *Brain Res.*, **501**, 1–10

20. Schneider, J.S. and Yuwiler, A. (1989). GM_1 ganglioside treatment promotes recovery of striatal dopamine concentrations in the mouse model of MPTP-induced Parkinsonism. *Exp. Neurol.*, **105**, 177–83

21. Weber, R.J., Ewing, S.E., Zauner, A. and Plunkett, R.J. (1989). Recovery in hemiparkinsonian rats following intrastriatal implantation of activated leukocytes. *Soc. Neurosci. Abstr.*, , 54.1

22. Walicke, P., Cowan, W.M., Ueno, N., Baird, A. and Guillemin, R. (1986). Fibroblast growth factor promotes survival of dissociated hippocampal neurons and enhances neurite extension. *Proc. Natl. Acad. Sci. USA*, **83**, 3012–16

23. Ferrari, G., Minozzi, M.-C., Toffano, G., Leon, A. and Skaper, S.D. (1989). Basic fibroblast growth factor promotes the survival and development of mesencephalic neurons in culture. *Dev. Biol.*, **133**, 140–7

24. Knüsel, B., Michel, P.P., Schwaber, J.S. and Hefti, F. (1990). Selective and nonselective stimulation of central cholinergic and dopaminergic

development *in vitro* by nerve growth factor, basic fibroblast growth factor, epidermal growth factor, insulin and the insulin-like growth factors I and II. *J. Neurosci.*, **10**, 558–70

25. Baird, A., Esch, F., Mormède, P., Ueno, N., Ling, N., Böhlen, P., Ying, S.-Y., Wehrenberg, W.B. and Guillemin, R. (1986). Molecular characterization of fibroblast growth factor: Distribution and biological activities in various tissues. *Rec. Prog. Horm. Res.*, **42**, 143–205

26. Westermann, R., Johannsen, M., Unsicker, K. and Grothe, C. (1990). Basic fibroblast growth factor (bFGF) immunoreactivity is present in chromaffin granules. *J. Neurochem.*, **55**, 285–92

27. Otto, D. and Unsicker, K. (1990). Basic FGF reverses chemical and morphological deficits in the nigrostriatal system of MPTP-treated mice. *J. Neurosci.*, **10**, 1912–21

28. Date, I., Notter, M.F.D., Felten, S.Y. and Felten, D.L. (1990). MPTP-treated young mice but not aging mice show partial recovery of the nigrostriatal dopaminergic system by stereotaxic injection of acidic fibroblast growth factor (aFGF). *Brain Res.*, **526**, 156–60

29. Baird, A. and Böhlen, P. (1990). Fibroblast growth factors. In Sporn, M.B. and Roberts, A.B. (eds.) *Handbook of Experimental Pharmacology*, Vol. **95/1**, *Peptide Growth Factors and Their Receptors I*, pp. 369–418. (Berlin, Heidelberg: Springer-Verlag)

30. Benharroch, D. and Birnbaum, D. (1990). Biology of the fibroblast growth factor gene family. *Isr. J. Med. Sci.*, **26**, 212–19

31. Saksela, O., Moscatelli, D., Sommer, A. and Rifkin, D.B. (1988). Endothelial cell-derived heparan sulfate binds basic fibroblast growth factor and protects it from proteolytic degradation. *J. Cell. Biol.*, **107**, 743–51

32. Lee, P.L., Johnson, D.E., Cousens, L.S., Fried, V.A. and Williams, L.T. (1989). Purification and complementary DNA cloning of a receptor for basic fibroblast growth factor. *Science*, **245**, 57–60

33. Reid, H.H., Wilks, A.F. and Bernard, O. (1990). Two forms of the basic fibroblast growth factor receptor-like mRNA are expressed in the developing mouse brain. *Proc. Natl. Acad. Sci. USA*, **87**, 1596–1600

34. Wanaka, A., Johnson Jr., E.M. and Milbrandt, J. (1990). Localization of FGF receptor mRNA in the adult rat central nervous system by *in situ* hybridization. *Neuron*, **5**, 267–81

35. Ferguson, I.A., Wanaka, A. and Johnson Jr., E.M. (1990). bFGF undergoes receptor-mediated retrograde transport in CNS neurons. *Soc. Neurosci. Abstr.*, **16**, 343.5

36. Hyman, C., Hofer, M., Barde, Y.-A. and Lindsay, R.M. (1990). Brain derived neurotrophic factor promotes survival of dopaminergic neurons of the embryonic rat mesencephalon. *Soc. Neurosci. Abstr.*, **411**, 10

37. Knüsel, B., Winslow, J.W., Rosenthal, A., Burton, L.E., Seid, D.P., Nikolics, K. and Hefti, F. (1991). Promotion of central cholinergic and dopaminergic neuron differentiation by brain-derived neurotrophic factor but not neurotrophin-3. *Proc. Natl. Acad. Sci. USA*, **88**, 961–5

38. Korsching, S. (1986). The role of nerve growth factor in the CNS. *Trends Neurosci.*, Nov/Dec., 570–3

39. Knüsel, B. and Hefti, F. (1988). Nerve growth factor promotes development of rat forebrain but not pedunculopontine cholinergic neurons *in vitro*; lack of effect of ciliary neuronotrophic factor and retinoic acid. *J. Neurosci. Res.*, **21**, 365–72

40. Angeletti, R.A. and Bradshaw, R.A. (1971). Nerve growth factor from the mouse submaxillary gland: amino acid sequence. *Proc. Natl. Acad. Sci. USA*, **68**, 2417–20

41. Scott, J., Selby, M., Urdea, M., Quiroga, M., Bell, G.I. and Rutter, W.J. (1983). Isolation and nucleotide coding sequence of a cDNA encoding the precursor of mouse nerve growth factor (NGF). *Nature (London)*, **302**, 538–40

42. Ullrich, A., Gray, A., Berman, C. and Dull, J.J. (1983). Human β-nerve growth factor gene sequence highly homologous to that of mouse. *Nature (London)*, **303**, 821–5

43. Leibrock, J., Lottspeich, F., Hohn, A., Hofer, M., Hengerer, B., Masiakowski, P., Thoenen, H. and Barde, Y.-A. (1989). Molecular cloning and expression of brain-derived neurotrophic factor. *Nature (London)*, **341**, 149–52

44. Hohn, A., Leibrock, J., Bailey, K. and Barde, Y.-A. (1990). Identification and characterization of a novel member of the nerve growth factor/brain-derived neurotrophic factor family. *Nature (London)*, **344**, 339–41

45. Kaisho, Y., Yoshimura, K. and Nakahama, K. (1990). Cloning and expression of a cDNA encoding a novel human neurotrophic factor. *FEBS Lett.*, **266**, 187–91

46. Maisonpierre, P.C., Belluscio, L., Squinto, S., Ip, N.Y., Furth, M.E., Lindsay, R.M. and Yancopoulos, G.D. (1990). Neurotrophin-3: A neurotrophic factor related to NGF and BDNF. *Science*, **247**, 1446–51

47. Rosenthal, A., Goeddel, D.V., Nguyen, T., Lewis, M., Shih, A., Laramee, G.R., Nikolics, K. and Winslow, J.W. (1990). Primary structure and biological activity of a novel human neurotrophic factor. *Neuron*, **4**, 767–73

48. Ernfors, P., Wetmore, C., Olson, L. and Persson, H. (1990). Identification of cells in rat brain and peripheral tissues expressing mRNA for members of the nerve growth factor family. *Neuron*, **5**, 511–26

49. Hofer, M., Pagliusi, S.R., Hohn, A., Leibrock, J. and Barde, Y.-A. (1990).

Regional distribution of brain-derived neurotrophic factor mRNA in the adult mouse brain. *EMBO J.*, **9**, 2459–64

50. Maisonpierre, P.C., Belluscio, L., Friedman, B., Aldeerson, R.F., Wiegand, S.J., Furth, M.E., Lindsay, R.M. and Yancopoulos, G.D. (1990). NT-3, BDNF, and NGF in the developing rat nervous system: Parallel as well as reciprocal patterns of expression. *Neuron*, **5**, 501–9

51. Phillips, H.S., Hains, J.M., Laramee, G.R., Rosenthal, A. and Winslow, J.W. (1990). Widespread expression of BDNF but not NT3 by target areas of basal forebrain cholinergic neurons. *Science*, **250**, 290–4

52. Recio-Pinto, E. and Ishii, D.N. (1988). Insulin and related growth factors: effects on the nervous system and mechanism for neurite growth and regeneration. *Neurochem. Int.*, **12**, 397–414

53. Baskin, D.G., Wilcox, B.J., Figlewicz, D.P. and Dorse, D.M. (1988). Insulin and insulin-like growth factors in the CNS. *Trends Neurosci.*, **11**, 107–11

54. Rotwein, P., Burgess, S.K., Milbrandt, J.D. and Krause, J.E. (1988). Differential expression of insulin-like growth factor genes in rat central nervous system. *Proc. Natl. Acad. Sci. USA*, **85**, 265–9

55. Beck, F., Samani, N.J., Byrne, S., Morgan, K., Gebhard, R. and Brammar, W.J. (1988). Histochemical localization of IGF-I and IGF-II mRNA in the rat between birth and adulthood. *Development*, **104**, 29–39

56. Stylianopoulou, F., Herbert, J., Soares, M.B. and Efstratiadis, A. (1988). Expression of the insulin-like growth factor II gene in the choroid plexus and the leptomeninges of the adult rat central nervous system. *Proc. Natl. Acad. Sci. USA*, **85**, 141–5

57. Werner, H., Woloschak, M., Adamo, M., Shen-Orr, Z., Roberts Jr., C.T. and LeRoith, D. (1989). Developmental regulation of the rat insulin-like growth factor I receptor gene. *Proc. Natl. Acad. Sci. USA*, **86**, 7451–5

58. Lesniak, M.A., Hill, J.M., Kiess, W., Rojeski, M., Pert, C.B. and Roth, J. (1988). Receptors for insulin-like growth factors I and II: autoradiographic localization in rat brain and comparison to receptors for insulin. *Endocrinology*, **123**, 2089–99

59. Adem, A., Jossan, S.S., d'Argy, R., Gillberg, P.G., Nordberg, A., Winblad, B. and Sara, V. (1989). Insulin-like growth factor I (IGF-1) receptors in the human brain: quantitative autoradiographic localization. *Brain Res.*, **503**, 299–303

60. Ocrant, I., Fay, C.T. and Parmelee, J.T. (1990). Characterization of insulin-like growth factor binding proteins produced in the rat central nervous system. *Endocrinology*, **127**, 1260–7

61. Laurence, D.J.R. and Gusterson, B.A. (1990). The epidermal growth factor. A review of structural and functional relationships in the normal

organism and in cancer cells. *Tumor Biol.*, 11, 229–61

62. Morrison, R.S., Kornblum, H.I., Leslie, F.M. and Bradshaw, R.A. (1987). Trophic stimulation of cultured neurons from neonatal rat brain by epidermal growth factor. *Science*, 238, 72–5

63. Casper, D., Blum, M. and Mytilineou, C. (1989). Epidermal growth factor is neurotrophic in rat embryo mesencephalic primary culture. *Soc. Neurosci. Abstr.*, 15, 287.6

64. Casper, D., Mytilineou, C. and Blum, M. (1990). Epidermal growth factor is a mitogen and increases dopamine uptake in rat embryo mesencephalic primary culture. *Soc. Neurosci. Abstr.*, 16, 413.18

65. Wang, S.-L., Shiverick, K.T., Ogilvie, S., Dunn, W.A. and Raizada, M.K. (1989). Characterization of epidermal growth factor receptor in astrocytic glial and neuronal cells in primary culture. *Endocrinology*, 124, 240–7

66. Baker, R.E. (1988). Gangliosides as cell adhesion factors in the formation of selective connections within the nervous system. In Boer, G.J., Feenstra, M.G.P., Swaab, D.F. and Van Haaren, F. (eds.) *Prog. Brain Res.*, 73, pp. 491–508. (Amsterdam: Elsevier Science)

67. Agnati, L., Fuxe, K., Calza, L., Benfenati, F., Cavicchioli, L., Toffano, G. and Goldstein, M. (1983). Gangliosides increase the survival of lesioned nigral dopamine neurons and favour the recovery of dopaminergic synaptic function in striatum of rats by collateral sprouting. *Acta Physiol. Scand.*, 119, 347–63

68. Hadjiconstantinou, M., Mariani, A.P. and Neff, N.H. (1989). GM$_1$ ganglioside-induced recovery of nigrostriatal dopaminergic neurons after MPTP: an immunohistochemical study. *Brain Res.*, 484, 297–303

69. Gage, F.H., Olejniczak, P. and Armstrong, D.M. (1988). Astrocytes are important for sprouting in the septohippocampal circuit. *Exp. Neurol.*, 102, 2–13

70. Gage, F.H. (1990). Intracerebral grafting of genetically modified cells acting as biological pumps. *Trends Pharmacol. Sci.*, 11, 437–9

71. Langer, R. (1990). New methods of drug delivery. *Science*, 249, 1527–33

72. Aebischer, P., Salessiotis, A.N. and Winn, S.R. (1989). Basic fibroblast growth factor released from synthetic guidance channels facilitates peripheral nerve regeneration across long nerve gaps. *J. Neurosci. Res.*, 23, 282–9

13

Designing clinical trials in Parkinson's disease

R.A. Hauser and C.W. Olanow

INTRODUCTION

Clinical trials in Parkinson's disease examine the relationship between an intervention and one or more outcome variables in a group of Parkinson's disease patients followed over time. Study designs vary in their ability to minimize unwanted influences such as the placebo effect, bias and random chance that can obscure the nature or extent of this relationship. Challenges specifically posed by Parkinson's disease trials include difficulty with accuracy of diagnosis, progression of disease during the trial, and confounding drug-induced adverse effects such as fluctuations in motor response. An understanding of these influences is vital to the optimal design and interpretation of clinical trials in Parkinson's disease.

UNWANTED INFLUENCES

The *placebo effect* refers to any improvement (or worsening) due to the psychological effects of participating in a trial. Patients may feel more important, receive more attention, or attempt to please the examiner. An informal 'support group' may form among study participants[1]. The placebo effect may also have an organic component, as psychological influences can induce both pharmacological and physiological changes which can mitigate a patient's disease or clinical status[2].

Bias is a systematic error leading to a discrepancy between what one attempts to do and what is actually done. Bias can be introduced during any stage of a clinical trial, including the selection, randomization, treatment and assessment processes. It can be the result of intentional or unintentional acts, and can profoundly affect the observed outcome.

A *differential bias*, or differences in the way groups to be compared are selected or handled, can influence the outcomes observed between treatment groups. A differential selection bias can result in treatment groups that are not comparable with respect to sex, age, disease severity, or to prior or concurrent treatment. A differential bias can also occur during treatment. Patients may differentially receive drugs or treatments other than the intended intervention. The greater use of minor anti-parkinsonian drugs such as trihexyphenidyl (Artane) or amantadine (Symmetrel) in one treatment group compared to the other can affect the observed outcome. Similarly, a physician might influence outcome unintentionally by behaving either more or less enthusiastically with one treatment group. An ascertainment bias is introduced through systematic errors in patient evaluations and can result from an intentional or unintentional desire to demonstrate an improved outcome in a particular treatment group.

Random chance variations in outcome cannot be avoided and are handled statistically through the use of significance level testing. A probability value of $p < 0.05$ indicates that there is less than a 5% probability that an observed outcome is due to random chance alone. By tradition, this is deemed to represent a real rather than a chance relationship, and is considered 'statistically significant'.

MINIMIZING UNWANTED INFLUENCES

The unwanted influence of the placebo effect and bias can be minimized through the use of control groups, randomization and blinding. The effect of random chance can be reduced by increasing the sample size and can be defined through the appropriate use of statistics.

A *control group* serves as a basis for comparison with a study group and consists of patients who are comparable to those receiving the desired intervention. They are treated in exactly the same manner as the study group except with regard to the active treatment. The two groups can then be compared in order to determine the specific effects of that treatment. In *single-group designs*, patients serve as their own controls and are compared before and after the application of an intervention. This study design is vulnerable to the placebo effect and time-dependent confounding variables such as the natural history of the disease. Without an independent control group, changes that are due to the natural course of the disease cannot be clearly delineated. This is an important consideration in a progressive disorder such as Parkinson's disease. *Between-group designs* compare outcomes observed in two or more groups that receive different interventions. If the investigator intends to compare the efficacy and side-effects of two different drugs, the study cohort is divided into two groups and each receives one of the study medications. In a placebo-controlled trial, the study group receives the acting drug and the control group receives placebo. Similar designs can be used to evaluate drugs as adjuncts to a standard treatment. For example, the symptomatic benefits of a new monoamine oxidase inhibitor or dopamine agonist can be compared to placebo as an adjunct to Sinemet.

Randomization of the study cohort into control and study groups minimizes the risk of bias due to baseline differences. If the sample size is sufficiently large, there should be no meaningful differences between randomized study and control groups. Ideally, randomization should be performed in a pre-determined fashion according to a random number list or computer-generated program and carried out at a site which is remote from the study center. After baseline data have been collected and the patient determined to be eligible for the study, randomization should be requested and treatment group assigned.

Blinding both the investigator and the patient to the intervention minimizes the risk of bias following randomization. If the investigator is unaware of patient assignments, one group cannot be treated differently from the other. Blinding the patient minimizes the risk of a differential placebo effect between the study groups. Because each patient is treated identically and receives an unknown drug, psychological effects should be comparable for each group.

Increasing the *sample size* reduces the effect of random chance on outcome. The larger the sample size, the smaller the probability that an outcome of a given magnitude is due to random chance alone. This is reflected in the statistical analysis.

PLANNING THE TRIAL

Prospective clinical trial designs exist on a continuum from open-label to randomized triple-blind. Generally, the more rigorous the trial the greater the expenditure of time, effort and money. The stringency of the study design should be appropriate for the question being asked. Open-label clinical studies are often employed initially when animal studies or a theoretical hypothesis suggest the possible efficacy of a drug or treatment. These trials suggest the appropriate dosage range, common side-effects and possible efficacy of the drug.

Randomized blinded trials are then performed to provide stronger evidence of a causal relationship between the drug intervention and the clinical improvement and any side-effects observed. The prospective randomized placebo-controlled blinded trial is the gold standard of clinical designs and is generally reserved for relatively mature research questions.

In planning a clinical trial, the investigator states the hypothesis to be examined and estimates the sample size likely to yield a meaningful result. The hypothesis is stated in advance, and delineates the primary outcome variable or endpoint that will serve as the basis for statistical analysis.

A *null hypothesis* is defined which states that there is no association between the intervention and the outcome variable. If the results of the study demonstrate that the null hypothesis is sufficiently unlikely ($p < 0.05$), the investigator rejects the null hypothesis and accepts the alternative hypothesis that the intervention and the outcome variable are related. For example, if the investigator plans to assess the efficacy of a drug, the null hypothesis would state that the drug has no clinical effect. If statistical analysis demonstrates that the outcome of the trial has less than a 5% probability of being due to chance alone, the investigator rejects the null hypothesis and accepts the alternative hypothesis that the drug does have a clinical effect. The *alternative hypothesis* may be one-tailed or two-tailed. The 'tails' refer to the two ends of a random distribution curve (Figure 1(a)). This bell-shaped curve represents the frequency distribution of outcomes due to random chance alone if increasing magnitude of improvement is plotted in one direction and increasing magnitude of deterioration in the other. Outcomes at either end of the curve are those least likely to occur on the basis of

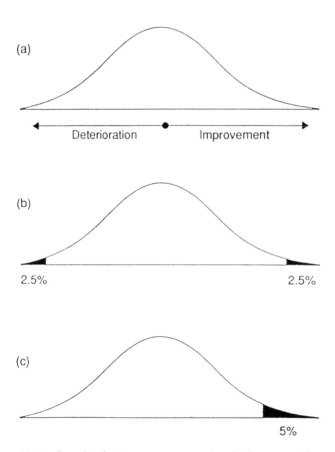

Figure 1 (a) Random distribution curve representing the frequency of outcomes of increasing magnitude of improvement or deterioration expected on the basis of chance alone. (b) The two shaded areas at the ends of the curve, or 'tails', represent the least likely 5% ($p \leq 0.05$) of outcomes due to chance alone using a two-tailed alternative hypothesis. If the outcome of a trial using a two-tailed alternative hypothesis falls within one of these two areas, the probability that the outcome is due to random chance alone is deemed sufficiently unlikely ($\alpha = 0.05$) to reject the null hypothesis. (c) The shaded area at one end of the curve represents the least likely 5% ($p \leq 0.05$) of outcomes due to chance alone using a one-tailed alternative hypothesis. If the outcome of a trial using a one-tailed alternative hypothesis falls within this area, the probability that the outcome is due to random chance alone is deemed sufficiently unlikely ($\alpha = 0.05$) to reject the null hypothesis

chance alone. A two-tailed alternative hypothesis states that an association exists but does not specify the direction of association. This is necessary if two drugs are being compared. One might be more efficacious (positive association) or less efficacious (negative association) than the other. Both of these possibilities, represented by the two tails of the distribution curve, need to be examined in order to define the relationship between the two drugs. The 2.5% of unlikely outcomes at each end of the curve comprise the 5% of outcomes that are least likely on the basis of chance alone ($p \leq 0.05$) when a two-tailed alternative hypothesis is used (Figure 1(b)). To compare the efficacy of a new drug to placebo, a two-tailed alternative hypothesis is required. The active drug might cause improvement *or* worsening.

A one-tailed alternative hypothesis states that there is an association between the intervention and the outcome *and* designates the direction of that association. A one-tailed hypothesis can only be used if only one direction of association is meaningful or makes sense. For example, when the side-effects of a drug are compared to placebo, it would not be meaningful to examine the hypothesis that the placebo has a greater frequency of side-effects than the active drug. In this case, it is appropriate to use a one-tailed alternative hypothesis, examining only the possibility that side-effects are more common with the active drug. If a higher frequency of side-effects occurs in the placebo group, this is assumed to be due to random chance. A one-tailed alternative hypothesis examines outcomes only at one end of the distribution curve and implies that outcomes in the opposite direction of association must be due to chance. The 5% of unlikely outcomes in the single designated direction of association define $p \leq 0.05$ when a one-tailed alternative hypothesis is used (Figure 1(c)). The advantage of a one-tailed alternative hypothesis is that it permits a smaller sample size. However, if the investigator incorrectly chooses a one-tailed alternative hypothesis when a two-tailed hypothesis is called for, an outcome in the opposite direction of association will erroneously be attributed to chance, and statistical analysis of an outcome in the designated direction of association will yield a p value that is one-half its true value. For example, if statistical analysis of a data set using a two-tailed alternative hypothesis yields a p value equal to 0.10, a one-tailed alternative hypothesis examining the same set of data will generate a p value equal to 0.05 and potentially change the conclusion of the study.

The *sample size estimate* depends on the type of statistical analysis to be used, the size and variability of the effect that the investigator wishes to detect, and the predetermined probability of reaching an erroneous conclusion that the investigator is willing to accept. The choice of the appropriate statistical tests should be made prior to the initiation of the study, generally in consultation with a biostatistician. The choice of statistical test is dictated by the type and number of predictor and outcome variables. Predictor variables are the treatment regimens that define each study group. Outcome variables are the parameters that will be evaluated to judge the effect of the intervention.

Predictor and outcome variables are nominal, ordinal, interval or ratio. A nominal (or classificatory) scale employs variables which consist of mutually exclusive, unordered, named categories, such as diagnosis (e.g. Parkinson's disease, progressive supranuclear palsy and olivoponto-cerebellar atrophy) or blood type (A, B, AB and O). An ordinal, or ranking, scale employs variables that are descriptive and ordered. Examples of ordinal scales include descriptions of disease severity – mild, moderate or severe, or stages of a disease, such as the Hoehn-Yahr scale. An interval scale employs variables that have units of measurement, such as centimeters, seconds or degrees centigrade. The distance between any two consecutive integers on an interval scale is constant and the distance between any two points is a known quantity. Because of this, interval variables can be added or multiplied – e.g. 1 centimeter plus 2 centimeters equals 3 centimeters. A ratio scale consists of ratios of interval numbers and is zero at its origin. The proportion of time awake with dyskinesia and hemoglobin concentration are examples of ratio scales. Nominal and ordinal scales are qualitative, or descriptive, whereas interval and ratio scales are quantitative, or numeric.

The choice of statistical test depends, in part, on whether the variables used in a clinical trial are parametric or nonparametric. Parametric variables are quantitative, offer a large number of choices, and fit a distinct distribution (e.g. a bell-shaped curve). If the variable is qualitative, or the data do not fit a distinct distribution, it is nonparametric.

Rating systems used in assessing Parkinson's disease typically employ ordinal numbers whose assignment is based on descriptive terms such as mild, moderate or severe, and reflect an order or ranking of severity. Here, therefore, there are no units of measurement. A score of 3 is worse than a score of 2 by definition, but there is no way of discerning by how much. Ordinal numbers are not additive. A score of 3 is not equal to the sum of a score of 2 plus a score of 1. Because of this, nonparametric tests such as the χ^2 test or the Mann-Whitney U (Wilcoxon rank-sum) test should be employed. Means and standard deviations, as well as all the statistical tests that use them, are parametric and are inappropriate for use with ordinal scales. The use of parametric statistics for the analysis of ordinal data is a common error which should be avoided[3-5]. Parametric statistics are appropriate for ratio scales such as hours 'off' per day, or percentage of time awake with dyskinesia. In most clinical trials the predictor variable is dichotomous (allowing one of two possible choices) i.e. the presence or absence of an intervention. Outcome variables may also be dichotomous (e.g. improved or not improved). If both the predictor and outcome variable are dichotomous, a z statistic should be used. The χ^2 test is a two-tailed z statistic. If the predictor variable is dichotomous and the outcome variable is parametric, a t-test (comparison of means) can be employed. If three or more groups are being compared and the outcome variable is parametric, an analysis of variance (ANOVA) can be used. In most clinical trials in Parkinson's disease, the predictor variable is dichotomous and the outcome variable is ordinal. In this case, a nonparametric statistical test such as the Mann-Whitney U (Wilcoxon rank-sum) test, which compares medians, should be employed.

Another important statistical method is *survival analysis*[6], which describes the probability of a designated event occurring over a period of time. The endpoint can be any defined event that occurs over a variable length of time, such as death, the development of dyskinesia or the development of disability necessitating symptomatic therapy. For example, the recently published DATATOP study evaluated the ability of Deprenyl (Eldepryl) to reduce a patient's risk over time of developing disability warranting treatment with Sinemet[7]. The Kaplan-Meier statistic[8] and the actuarial life table method[9] are the two most commonly used methods to calculate survival. These analyses calculate hazard ratios, or the risk of reaching endpoint over intervals of time, by taking all available data into account, including those from patients who do not reach endpoint, drop out of the study or are lost to follow-up. If, in a 1-year study, a patient does not reach endpoint in 6 months and then drops out, survival analysis will reflect the fact that he 'survived' through the first 6 months. For the next 6 months it is assumed that his risk of reaching endpoint would have been the same as the other patients who did not reach endpoint in the first 6 months and who remain in the study.

After the type of statistical analysis to be used is determined, the standardized effect size is estimated. The *effect size* is the magnitude of change in the primary endpoint which the investigator would like to be able to detect, based on a clinically relevant estimate of the expected magnitude of change from baseline. For example, in a symptomatic trial the investigator may wish to be able to detect a defined quantity of improvement in the Unified Parkinson's Disease Rating Scale (UPDRS) as evidence of a drug's efficacy. In a trial to evaluate protective therapy (the ability of a drug to slow the progression of disability), he may wish to be able to detect a defined reduction in the rate of deterioration of UPDRS score as evidence of a drug's efficacy. The smaller the magnitude of change to be detected, the greater the sample size required. In addition, the greater the *variability in outcome* or endpoint the more difficult it is to detect a given effect size, and the larger the sample size required. For example, if all patients deteriorated at exactly the same rate, then, a small change in the rate of deterioration would be easy to detect. If patients vary widely in their rate of deterioration, then a small change in the rate of deterioration is more difficult to detect. Effect size and variability are often combined into the standardized effect size (E/S, where E is the effect size and S is the standard deviation).

Sample size is also determined by the degree of certainty the investigator wishes to have regarding the accuracy of the conclusion. A *type I error* (false-positive) occurs when the investigator rejects a null hypothesis that is actually true. In this case, he will conclude that a treatment is efficacious when in reality it is not. The probability of making a type I error is termed 'α' and is set prior to the initiation of the study to represent the level of statistical significance which will be required to reject the null hypothesis. On completion of the study, statistical analysis will yield a p value which represents the probability that the study results have occurred by chance alone, assuming the null hypothesis is true. If p is less than α, the null hypothesis is rejected in favor of the alternative hypothesis.

A *type II error* (false-negative) occurs when the investigator fails to reject a null hypothesis that is actually false. In this case, he will conclude that a drug is not efficacious when in reality it is. The probability of making a type II error is termed 'β'. The quantity $1 - \beta$ describes the power of the study. This is the likelihood of observing an effect in the study population if an effect of the specified size or greater actually exists.

Ideally, the investigator would wish to eliminate the possibility of false-positive and false-negative conclusions, but this would require an infinitely large sample. Sample-size determination seeks a compromise between certainty in drawing a conclusion and feasibility of performing the study. In many trials, α is set at 0.05 and 'β' at 0.20 (power = 0.80). Using these values, the investigator will reject the null hypothesis if there is less than a 5% probability that the study results could be due to random chance alone ($p < 0.05$), and there is an 80% probability (power = 0.80) of observing an effect of the designated size in the study population if it actually exists. After the appropriate statistical test is selected, α and β are set, and the effect size estimated, charts or formulas can be used to determine the sample size required[10]. Allowances must be made for anticipated dropouts, non-compliant subjects and inaccurately diagnosed patients.

PERFORMING A RANDOMIZED BLINDED TRIAL

Several basic steps are carried out during a randomized blinded trial. Inclusion and exclusion criteria are defined and a study cohort is selected. Baseline data are gathered and subjects are blindly randomized into two or more study groups. Predetermined outcomes and adverse effects are then ascertained in a blinded fashion at preset points in time. When the trial is completed, statistical analysis is performed to compare findings between treatment groups.

The study cohort for a clinical trial is selected to be representative of a larger group of patients (target population) for whom the results of the trial will be generalized. A set of inclusion criteria to define the primary characteristics of the target population is established. Exclusion criteria are then developed to exclude those individuals who will not be considered for participation in the study because of excessive risk, the likelihood of diminishing the quality of data, or ethical considerations. Inclusion and exclusion criteria should be tailored to permit the investigator to study the desired population. Failure to define the target population clearly, or the use of excessive exclusion criteria, may jeopardize the generality of the study.

The method of *patient selection* may be influenced by the patient population available for study. If the investigator has access to a large number of patients who meet the eligibility criteria, he may choose simply to select those individuals who appear well-suited to participate in the trial. However, this type of judgemental sampling is vulnerable to selection bias, as patients selected in this fashion may be more highly motivated, have milder disease or appear more in need of treatment. More stringent sampling techniques help avoid sampling bias and maintain the generality of the study. Consecutive sampling is the preferred technique and involves offering entry to each patient who meets eligibility criteria until a predetermined number of study subjects is reached or a defined time period has elapsed. Systematic sampling consists of selecting every second or third individual who meets eligibility criteria, and random sampling consists of selecting participants according to a set of random numbers applied to eligible individuals.

If only a small number of patients meet the eligibility criteria, the investigator might feel pressured to offer entry to patients who do not strictly fit these criteria and who would otherwise be excluded. This can create a study cohort that is not representative of the target population. Selection bias may also occur if the accessible target population is not representative of the defined target population. Patients who present to subspeciality Parkinson's disease clinics may be more highly motivated or have disease that is more difficult to diagnose or manage.

Entry bias can occur if patients who accept entry into the study differ from those who do not. For example, patients with more advanced disease may not be able to visit the clinic as frequently as is required to participate in a trial. The best way to minimize entry bias is to use practical eligibility criteria and promote as high an acceptance rate as possible.

Errors in diagnosis reduce the power of the study. As there are currently no reliable laboratory or radiographic markers for Parkinson's disease, the diagnosis relies on clinical criteria. Patients with atypical parkinsonisms (e.g. progressive supranuclear palsy, striatonigral degeneration, olivopontocerebellar atrophy, etc.) may be difficult to distinguish from those with Parkinson's disease and may comprise as many as 20% of the patients who present with clinical features of parkinsonism[11,12]. Clues to the diagnosis of atypical parkinsonism include: early and prominent speech and balance involvement, lack of resting tremor, greater axial than appendicular rigidity, relatively rapid progression, and a poor response to levodopa therapy[11,12]. High field-strength (1.5 Tesla) T_2-weighted magnetic resonance imaging may be of help in identifying patients with some forms of atypical parkinsonism, as the majority demonstrate signal attenuation in the putamen which equals or exceeds that in the globus pallidus[13]. Despite this, errors in diagnosis may be unavoidable and sample-size calculations should be adjusted accordingly. Difficulty with accuracy of diagnosis is greatest in the early stages of the disease when the clinical picture may not yet have fully evolved, and patients may not have received an adequate trial of levodopa. Diagnosis is more reliable later in the disease when the clinical picture and response to levodopa therapy are better defined.

The *randomization* procedure should be designed so that members of the research team cannot influence the allocation of patients into study groups. Assignments are best made according to a computer-generated randomization schedule managed by individuals who are not in contact with study subjects. Prior to randomization, the potential participant is evaluated to determine eligibility for inclusion into the study and informed consent is obtained. The name and study number of the subject are then forwarded to the randomization site or responsible person and the predetermined randomization code used to make the group assignment. Less rigorous randomization procedures can create intentional or unintentional differences between groups. For example, if an investigator were able to influence group assignment, he might subconsciously direct patients with more severe disease toward the therapy believed to have the greatest likelihood of benefit. If the investigator has prior knowledge of the assignment code, a patient in need of treatment, but scheduled for randomization to the placebo group, might not be offered entry into the trial.

Randomization minimizes the risk of confounding variables at baseline, but does not protect the study from unintended interventions that can occur during treatment. These are best prevented by *blinding*. There are three 'participants' to consider in any study – the patient, the investigator applying the intervention and the investigator judging the outcome and adverse effects. In many clinical trials the same investigator applies the intervention and judges the outcome. If both the investigator and patient are blind to the intervention, the study is designated 'double-blind'. If separate blinded investigators apply the intervention and judge the outcome, the study is designated 'triple-blind'. Partially blinded designs are also possible. A double observer, single-blind study is one in which the treating investigator-therapist and the patient are aware of the intervention, but the investigator-evaluator is blinded.

In blinded drug trials, study and placebo capsules which are identical in appearance, taste and smell are employed. Labelling and dispensing systems must be developed which maintain the blindness of the study and provisions must be made to allow the code to be broken on an emergency basis if a patient becomes acutely ill.

Complete blinding is often difficult to achieve. Even when 'look-alike/taste-alike' capsules are used in a drug trial, the subjective effects may not be the same. This is particularly true in Parkinson's disease, as dopaminergic drugs often induce a recognizable sensation or energy surge. Side-effects such as nausea, dyskinesia or hypotension may also unblind the subject or investigator. If the active treatment does lead to improvement, this too may cause unblinding, and can lead to an amplification effect that overestimates the drug's true benefit[14].

Laboratory tests are another potential source of unblinding and, ideally, should be reviewed by an outside investigator. All participants cannot be blinded to certain interventions, such as surgery, physical therapy and psychotherapy.

One way to assess potential unblinding is to have subjects and investigators provide their best guess and level of confidence as to each patient's group assignment at the completion of the trial. Statistical analysis can then be performed to determine if the patients or investigators correctly identify a greater proportion of treatment assignments than would be expected by chance. In addition, unblinding should be suspected whenever differences in outcome appear only in subjects whose treatment assignment is correctly identified.

Dosing and *compliance* must also be considered. If an inadequate dose of the active drug is used, no effect will occur. On the other hand, doses that are too high may cause a high incidence of side-effects. Most dopaminergic drugs must be administered to begin with at relatively low dosages and then slowly increased. If the dose is increased too quickly, a high proportion of patients may experience otherwise avoidable side-effects. Compliance is important because the power of a study is reduced in relation to the degree that subjects fail to comply with the protocol.

Compliance can be increased by discussing the study thoroughly with each patient before entry. If possible, simple instructions and a convenient dosing schedule should be employed. Attempts should be made to monitor compliance using pill counts, diaries and measurements of drug levels or other informative laboratory markers.

The *clinical evaluation* of patients should be performed using a standard and widely used rating scale. Currently, the Unified Parkinson's Disease Rating Scale (UPDRS)[15] is the most commonly used scale to assess parkinsonian signs and symptoms. Others used include the Columbia University Rating Scale[16], the North-Western University Disability Scale[17], the Webster Rating Scale[18] and the Schwab-England Disability Scale[19]. Disability scores describing improvement from base-line (expressed as percentages) vary considerably between these scales, as they measure or emphasize different aspects of parkinsonism[20]. Therefore, comparisons between results of studies using different scales may not be valid and the universal use of a single rating scale is to be encouraged. It should also be noted that these scales are ordinal and therefore non-linear. A given numerical change or percentage change from baseline may not represent the same degree of functional change in patients with varying disease severity. A further limitation of the currently available rating scales is their relative insensitivity to subtle changes. Scoring systems may occasionally be modified or abbreviated to fit the purpose and limitations of a particular study, but if too few functions are assessed, the sensitivity of the scale will be further diminished. In order to avoid inter-observer error, patients should be assessed by the same observer before and after the application of the intervention.

Motor fluctuations complicate the assessment process. If patients fluctuate in response to medication, assessments of motor function and disability should be obtained for both the 'on' and 'off' states. Ideally, patients should be examined while 'on' and 'off' at each visit, although this is often not possible. However, attempts should be made to examine the patient at approximately the same time relative to drug administration at each visit, and the patient's response state should be recorded. This helps to minimize the effect of motor fluctuations on assessment. An historical assessment of disability in both the 'on' and 'off' states should be obtained from the patient and family, reflecting the patient's function at his best and worst. The proportion of time spent in the 'on' and 'off' states can be determined by asking the patient to complete a diary which reflects his status at hourly intervals throughout the day.

Videotape recordings of study subjects can be made at baseline and at present points during the course of a clinical trial. On completion of the study, the recordings of each patient can be placed in a random sequence and scored by a blinded observer. Because recordings from all of a patient's visits can be reviewed at one time, this technique may make improvement or deterioration easier to judge. Video analysis could potentially serve as the primary method of evaluation, but some parkinsonian features, such as rigidity, are not satisfactorily evaluated in this way.

The evaluation of '*wash-in*' and '*wash-out*' periods may be helpful in discriminating between protective effects (which slow the underlying disease process) and symptomatic effects. 'Wash-in' refers to the introduction of treatment and 'wash-out' refers to the discontinuation of treatment. Symptomatic effects can be evaluated on either the initiation or discontinuation of treatment. Protective effects can be evaluated by comparing patients' baseline untreated status to their untreated status following an interim period of treatment and wash-out.

The *statistical analysis* to be performed at the conclusion of the trial should be determined in advance in consultation with a statistician. Methods to deal with drop-outs, early terminations, and outlying statistical values should be included.

In order to preserve the full value of randomization, it is best to use an *intention-to-treat analysis*. For this, all available outcome data is analyzed according to group assignment, regardless of whether the patient actually received the intended intervention. Because compliant patients may respond differently than non-compliant patients to treatment[21], analysis which is limited to compliant patients can create a post-randomization selection bias and affect the observed outcome. The disadvantage of the intention-to-treat method is that noncompliant patients reduce the power of the study. This makes a high compliance rate extremely important.

Subgroup analyses can provide useful additional information but they are easy to misuse and can lead to erroneous conclusions. Subgroup analyses based on post-randomization factors are of particular concern. When one makes multiple subgroup comparisons based on the data generated during the study, significance level testing becomes more likely to detect differences which are due to chance variation alone. If, for example, one evaluates outcomes in 100 subgroups, five can be expected to be 'significant at the $p \leq 0.05$ level' by chance alone. The same is true when one performs multiple outcome variable testing, such as looking for differences in tremor, rigidity and bradykinesia separately. Simulation studies have shown that even when subset analyses are based on only three patient characteristics, 20% of trials will yield at least one false-positive comparison at the $p \leq 0.05$ level. These analyses can provide useful clues for further research, but should not be interpreted as providing evidence of a causal relationship.

Early stopping rules are often incorporated into the design of long-term studies so that the trial can be terminated prematurely if benefit or harm become evident. To accomplish this, outcomes are evaluated at preset points during the course of the study. This is best performed by an independent advisory group which is given responsibility to stop the study if predetermined p value levels are exceeded. The investigator is not made aware of the result of these interim analyses unless the study is to be terminated. The problem with performing repeated analyses during the course of the trial is that it increases the likelihood of obtaining a false-positive outcome. Simulation studies have shown that if four periodic evaluations are performed (three during the trial and one at the completion of the trial) at '$p \leq 0.05$', 17% of studies will yield a false-positive conclusion compared to the expected 5%[22]. This means that if four analyses of outcome are performed over the course of a study at '$p \leq 0.05$', the probability of obtaining a false-positive outcome due to random chance alone is actually 17%. One way to minimize the effect of taking multiple 'peeks' at the data is to require that very small p values (e.g. $p < 0.001$) must be exceeded to stop the study. The method of O'Brien and Fleming[23] requires p values of less than 0.001, 0.004, 0.018 and 0.042 for four sequential analyses and maintains the overall experimental error rate (α) at 5%. In this way, only strikingly significant differences between groups will be detected during the course of the study. Sample size requirements will not be affected and the probability of terminating the study prematurely will be minimized.

VARIATIONS OF THE RANDOMIZED BLINDED DESIGN

The *run-in design* is a useful technique to increase the proportion of the study cohort that is compliant. After selecting the cohort and obtaining consent, all subjects initially receive placebo treatment. Following a specified period of time, those who have complied with this intervention are blindly randomized to placebo and active drug groups. Non-compliant patients are excluded from the study, thereby increasing its power. A variation of this design uses the active drug for the run-in period. The investigator can then choose an intermediary variable (one that occurs between the intervention and the outcome) as a criterion for randomization. A particular subset of patients is thereby selectively removed for inclusion in the experimental phase of the trial. One could assess, for example, the efficacy of a drug amongst only those who were able to tolerate it, or the side-effects of a drug amongst only those who were improved by it.

The *2 × 2 factorial design* allows the investigator to compare two active treatments against placebo and with each other. Patients are randomized into four groups. One group receives treatment A, the second receives treatment B, the third receives both treatments and the fourth receives placebo only. The study cohort can then be compared with regard to the two drug treatments. In addition, the investigator can assess additive and inhibitory effects of the two drugs combined, making this design extremely efficient. It requires fewer patients and less expenditure of time and money to generate the same amount of information than separate studies. This design also reduces (to 25%) a given patient's chances of receiving placebo alone.

In a *crossover design*, patients first receive one treatment and then 'crossover' to the other. Most commonly, one-half of the group of patients is randomly assigned to receive placebo first, then the active treatment, while the other half receives active treatment first and then placebo. The major advantage of this design is that each patient serves as his own control, thereby eliminating baseline confounding variables. In addition, the effect of time-dependent confounding variables, such as the natural progression of the underlying disease, is minimized since half of the study cohort receives active treatment early and half receives active treatment late. The major concern in a crossover study is that of possible carryover effects, due to the continued effect of a drug after patients are crossed over to the other treatment. To minimize this risk, the investigator can introduce an untreated wash-out period, but it is often difficult to know with certainty how long such a period should be.

REFERENCES

1. Diamond, S.G., Markham, C.H. and Treciokas, I.J. (1985). Double-blind trial of Pergolide for Parkinson's disease. *Neurology, 35,* 291–5
2. Kojo, I. (1988). The mechanism of the psychophysiological effects of placebo. *Med. Hypotheses, 27,* 261–4
3. Kurtzke, J.F. (1986). Neuroepidemiology. Part II: Assessment of therapeutic trials. *Ann. Neurol., 19,* 311–19
4. Forrest, M. and Anderson, B. (1986). Ordinal scales and statistics in medical research. *Br. Med. J., 292,* 537–8
5. Watson, J.P. (1986). Use of ordinal scales in clinical trials. *Br. Med. J., 292,* 413
6. Reznick, R.K. and Guest, C.B. (1989). Survival analysis: a practical approach. *Dis. Colon Rectum, 32,* 898–902
7. The Parkinson Study Group. (1989). Effect of deprenyl on the progression of disability in early Parkinson's disease. *N. Engl. J. Med., 321,* 1364–71
8. Kaplan, E.L., Meier, P. (1958). Nonparametric estimation from incomplete observations. *J. Am. Stat. Assoc., 53,* 457–81
9. Berkson, J., Garge, R.P. (1950). Calculation of survival rates for cancer. *Mayo Clin. Proc., 25,* 250
10. Hulley, S.B. and Cummings, S.R. (1988). *Designing Clinical Research: An Epidemiological Approach.* (Baltimore: Williams and Wilkins)
11. Jankovic, J. (1989). Parkinsonism-plus syndromes. *Movement Disorders, 4,* S95–119
12. Quinn, N. (1989). Multiple system atrophy – the nature of the beast. *J. Neurol. Neurosurg. Psych.,* (Suppl.) 78–89
13. Olanow, C.W., Alberts, M., Djang, W. and Stajich, J. (1991). MR imaging of putamenal iron predicts response to dopaminergic therapy in parkinsonian patients. In Calne, D. (ed.) *Early Markers of Parkinson's Disease,* in press
14. Kramer, M.S. and Shapiro, S.H. (1984). Scientific challenges in the application of randomized trials, *J. Am. Med. Assoc., 252,* 2739–45
15. Fahn, S., Elton, R.L. and members of the UPDRS Development Committee. (1987). Unified Parkinson's Disease Rating Scale. In Fahn, S., Marsden, C.D., Calne, D.B. and Goldstein, M. (eds.) *Recent Developments*

in Parkinson's Disease, Vol. 2, pp. 153–64, (Florahm Park, NJ: Macmillan Health Care Information)

16. Yahr, M.D., Duvoisin, R.C., Schear, M.J., Barrett, R.E. and Hoehn, M.M. (1969). Treatment of parkinsonism with levodopa. *Arch. Neurol.,* **21**, 343–54

17. Canter, C.J., de la Torre, R., Mier, M. (1961). A method of evaluating disability in patients with Parkinson's disease. *J. Nerv. Mental Dis.,* **133**, 143–7

18. Webster, D.D. (1968). Critical analysis of the disability in Parkinson's disease. *Mod. Treat.,* **5**, 257–82

19. Schwab, R.S. and England, A.C. (1969). Projection technique for evaluating surgery in Parkinson's disease. In Gillingham, F.J. and Donaldson, M.C. (eds.) *Third Symposium on Parkinson's disease.* (Edinburgh: E. & S. Livingstone)

20. Diamond, S.G. and Markham, C.H. (1983). Evaluating the evaluations: or how to weigh the scales of parkinsonian disability. *Neurology,* **33**, 1098–9

21. The CDP Research Group. (1980). Influence of adherence to treatment and response of cholesterol on mortality in the CDP. *N. Engl. J. Med.,* **303**, 1038–41

22. Fleming, T.R. and Watelet, L.F. (1989). Approaches to monitoring clinical trials. *J. Natl. Cancer Inst.,* **81**, 188–93

23. O'Brien, P.C. and Fleming, T.R. (1979). A multiple testing procedure for clinical trials. *Biometrics,* **35**, 549–56

14

Thoughts on Parkinson's disease

C.D. Marsden

Parkinson's disease was the first, and so far the only, neurodegenerative disease to respond to the principle of neurotransmitter replacement therapy. The discovery that levodopa treatment could reverse all the major motor disabilities of parkinsonism in the late 1960s has been a stimulus to neuroscience in many fields. In this respect, Parkinson's disease has been a pathfinder for other chronic progressive neurological conditions. The paths explored in this volume include all the major challenges faced by those in the field today.

How can we improve on present symptomatic treatment for Parkinson's disease? Levodopa works remarkably well initially, but with the passage of time problems often emerge, the commonest of which are troublesome fluctuations in clinical response and dyskinesias. Considerable experience is required to disentangle the many various types of fluctuations and dyskinesias that can plague the patient with advanced Parkinson's disease. No one pathophysiological mechanism explains all these complications. Pharmacokinetic and pharmacodynamic factors interact in complex ways in different situations. The peripheral pharmacokinetics of levodopa are now reasonably well understood, but changes in central pharmacodynamics remain uncertain. The parkinsonian brain exhibits a plasticity to chronic levodopa therapy which has proved difficult to fathom. Changes in dopamine receptor sensitivity must contribute, but the understanding of dopamine receptors has been thrown into turmoil by the realization that the classical subdivision into cyclase-linked D_1 and cyclase-independent D_2 receptors is an over-simplification. First, D_2 receptor activity modulates D_1 cyclase behavior.

Second, such D_1-D_2 linkage depends upon the species studied and the impact of denervation. Third, molecular biological techniques have led to cloning of further categories of dopamine receptors, whose anatomical siting and agonist–antagonist affinities differ. Understanding the new biology of multiple dopamine receptors will have a profound impact on the design of new antiparkinsonian drugs.

The present range of directly-acting dopamine agonists in clinical use (bromocriptine, lisuride, pergolide and apomorphine) have a proven place in the management of Parkinson's disease. But they have not solved the problems of troublesome fluctuations and dyskinesias. One may look forward to a new generation of directly-acting dopamine agonists, based upon the new biology of dopamine receptors. Meanwhile, one continues to struggle with the problems of the severely fluctuating parkinsonian. Again, longer-acting formulations of levodopa have helped, but have not resolved the problem. Nor have alternative delivery systems (intravenous, subcutaneous, intraduodenal, transdermal and even intraventricular) proved of general value because of their complexity. The dream of some simple implantable remotely-controlled continuous delivery system has not yet been realized.

Against this background, a number of chapters in this volume have dealt with the present state-of-the-art of understanding and treatment of patients with advanced Parkinson's disease with the tools we have available today. What is needed are new tools. In this context the potential of brain grafting is of considerable interest. It seems clear that simple implantation of the patient's adrenal medulla into the striatum is not the answer. However, co-implantation with a source of natural growth factors or synthetic growth factors may prove more effective. Indeed, the role of nerve growth factors in brain repair and therapy of neurodegenerative disease is an exciting area of future research. The place of fetal nigral implantation also is gradually being established, but remains a research endeavor.

Another major focus now is to unravel the many new clues to the cause of Parkinson's disease, and to devise new treatment strategies aimed to halt or reverse progression of the underlying pathology of the illness. The hereditary/environmental, soil/seed debate is alive and kicking again! Early suggestions that inheritance played a significant part in the illness appeared to be dismissed by the findings and interpretation of twin studies. But such a conclusion may have been premature. Re-analysis of such data has led to the conclusion that an inherited contribution has not been excluded. The problem is that clinically unaffected siblings may have the disease pathologically, but have not yet expressed symptoms, and may not do so for many years. In addition, the significance of isolated tremor as a marker of the disease is controversial. Identification of presymptomatic Parkinson's disease in life is an urgent priority to solve this riddle, and in the future to select those who would benefit most from neuroprotective therapy at the earliest opportunity. Positron emission tomography with [^{18}F]dopa has the capacity to detect minor degrees of striatal dopamine depletion and may prove to be the gold standard against which other methods will need to be judged. However, the sensitivity and specificity of this technique, especially its repeatability, need to be critically assessed. Maybe other tracers identifying, for example, gliosis or neuronal loss in substantia nigra will prove more sensitive and reliable. Whatever the best positron emission tomography technique, the cost of the method at present is such that it cannot be used as a simple screening test. Other studies, which might be biochemical, physiological or immunological, must be explored.

Returning to the soil and seed debate, if inheritance does play a role, what could this be? An attractive hypothesis is that one inherits an inability to deal safely with one or more environmental toxins, which lead to selective nigral destruction along the lines of MPTP. Such a notion introduces a degree of complexity in any search for a genetic abnormality or an environmental agent. At the extremes, one can envisage a genetic defect producing a major susceptibility to a minor exposure to a toxin, or a normal genetic background that can be overwhelmed by a massive exposure to the toxin, or any intermediate position. Given this scenario, it may be time to rethink epidemiological approaches. For instance, if a genetic predisposition is identified, for example a difference in P-450 detoxification mechanisms, one might have to take those with the disease exhibiting this genetic marker and compare them in case–control studies to those in the normal population with a similar abnormality, in order to search for an environmental agent.

Another issue is whether the genetic predisposition is common, and the environmental agent is rare, or vice versa. Again, at the extremes, it could be that there is a common genetic defect, but only those exposed to an uncommon toxin develop the illness, or there could be an uncommon genetic defect rendering a minority susceptible to a common toxin. Of course, there may be many different genetic predispositions and many different environmental agents. Parkinson's disease as we know it may have many causes, and Lewy body degeneration of pigmented brainstem nuclei may be the single end-product of a variety of insults.

Another major area of interest is the mechanism of cell death of the substantia nigra in Parkinson's disease. Study of postmortem tissue has led to two novel concepts, both based upon study of the mechanisms whereby MPTP/MPP$^+$ causes nigral destruction. First, there is oxidative stress. There is now some evidence to implicate free radical attack on nigral neurons in Parkinson's disease, and changes in some antioxidant defence mechanisms have been identified in the parkinsonian nigra. Perhaps the most significant finding in this context is the replication of depleted levels of reduced glutathione in nigral tissue, for this is found in pathological presymptomatic Parkinson's disease. Linked to this evidence implicating oxidative stress is the finding of increased levels of iron in parkinsonian nigra, for iron in reactive form can drive free-radical attack. Why there is this change in nigral iron in Parkinson's disease, and whether it is present in a reactive form are uncertain at this time.

Second, there is the exciting demonstration of alteration in the activity of mitochondrial Complex I in the parkinsonian nigra. This seems a robust and disease-specific abnormality. It is not evident in other brain areas, but whether a similar change is apparent in peripheral tissues such as platelets and muscle is controversial at this time. If a Complex I deficit is expressed in platelets, then here may be the simple method of presymptomatic diagnosis.

Two crucial questions surround these findings concerning oxidative stress and mitochondrial abnormalities in Parkinson's disease. First, which is the primary abnormality? Oxidative stress can damage mitochondria, and Complex I deficit can drive oxidative stress. Second, are these changes, or one of them, related to the cause of Parkinson's disease, or are they secondary consequences of some other insult?

Even if oxidative stress and/or Complex I deficit are secondary phenomena, their presence provides novel targets for neuroprotective therapy. An attractive hypothesis is that an unknown insult triggers the beginning of nigral destruction, which then leads to an escalating cascade of secondary changes involving oxidative stress, iron and mitochondrial damage, resulting in exponential nigral cell loss. Hitherto, it has been suggested that the presymptomatic phase of nigral pathology may exist for decades before the clinical illness appears. But this may not be the case. Recent quantitative studies of nigral neuronal loss in presymptomatic cases of Lewy body disease, and at various stages of the illness, suggest a much more rapid process, perhaps over 5 years or less. Sequential positron emission tomography studies of dopamine function are also beginning to hint at a speedier loss than hitherto envisaged. Given this scenario, treatment aimed at preventing this secondary cascade of events at the earliest opportunity may have a profound beneficial effect on the disease process.

An extension of this concept is the notion that Parkinson's disease is not fundamentally a selective system degeneration of certain brain regions, but a much more widespread disease. Recent neuropathological studies have indicated that Lewy bodies, when looked for carefully and with the help of ubiquitin immunostaining, are present far more widely than hitherto realized. For example, they are found in cerebral cortex in virtually every case. Does this mean that the agent(s) causing Parkinson's disease attacks the whole brain, but to begin with it produces a motor disorder because the substantia nigra, for other reasons, is selectively vulnerable?

A working hypothesis as to the cause(s) of Parkinson's disease might run as follows. An inherited trait renders some individuals susceptible to an environmental toxin(s), with which they cannot deal safely. This toxin(s) causes minimal damage to most brain regions (and to extracerebral tissues), at least initially. For two possible reasons, however, the substantia nigra is selectively vulnerable. First, the toxin may be concentrated into nigra via uptake mechanisms and binding to neuromelanin, like MPP^+. Second, the nigra is particularly susceptible to its actions because of the high oxidative stress imposed by dopamine metabolism. This sets in train an escalating cascade of secondary changes, culminating in selective nigral cell death and a profound motor disorder.

Now the scene is set to think about novel neuroprotective therapy in Parkinson's disease. A number of approaches are being considered, for example aggressive antioxidant therapy, iron chelation and mitochondrial repletion. Maybe a combination treatment will be required.

Whatever is chosen as practical at this stage can be put to the test, thanks to the demonstration of the effects of deprenyl in the DATATOP study. The latter has shown that it is possible, using the enthusiasm and expertise of 'Parkinsonologists', to set up and run the large multicenter trials required to assess the impact of novel neuroprotective treatments. These are, yet again, exciting times for Parkinson's disease. The authors in this volume, and the editors, are to be congratulated for capturing this excitement in their chapters, which provide a contemporary overview of the many practical and research avenues being explored at this time.

Index